THE
HEART
HEALERS

The Misfits, Mavericks, and Rebels
Who Created the Greatest Medical
Breakthrough of Our Lives

JAMES S. FORRESTER, M.D.

St. Martin's Griffin ✿ New York

www.stmartins.com

Designed by Patrice Sheridan

The Library of Congress has cataloged the hardcover edition as follows:

Forrester, James, 1937–
    The heart healers : the misfits, mavericks, and rebels who created the greatest medical breakthrough of our lives / by James Forrester, M.D. — First edition.
        p. cm.
    ISBN 978-1-250-05839-3 (hardcover)
    ISBN 978-1-4668-6255-5 (e-book)
    1. Cardiology—History.   I. Title.
    RC666.5.F67 2015
    616.1'2—dc23

                                                                    2015017977

ISBN 978-1-250-10540-0 (trade paperback)

Our books may be purchased in bulk for promotional, educational, or business use. Please contact your local bookseller or the Macmillan Corporate and Premium Sales Department at 1-800-221-7945, extension 5442, or by e-mail at MacmillanSpecialMarkets@macmillan.com.

First St. Martin's Griffin Edition: August 2016

10 9 8 7 6 5 4 3 2

Praise for *The Heart Healers*

"A stunning survey of cardiology's 'Golden Age' and the 'misfits' who made it so. . . . It's a book of marvels."

—*Publishers Weekly* (starred review)

"Forrester brings history to life and explains complex procedures for lay readers in this excellent book for readers interested in medical history and those who want to understand modern medical procedures."

—*Library Journal* (starred review)

"Dr. James Forrester's *The Heart Healers* is a fast-moving tale told by someone who has lived through many of the developments he describes. Forrester is a gifted writer whose prose flows effortlessly and is, by turns, both inspired and irreverent. He always keeps the narrative moving quickly, letting readers in on the fact that that success was not inevitable, describing false starts and blind alleys along the way. *The Heart Healers* is deepened by the fact of James Forrester's career, his contact with patients and colleagues, and the personal stories of patients he has treated and woven into the narrative."   —W. Bruce Fye, M.D., author of *Caring for the Heart: Mayo Clinic and the Rise of Specialization*

"James Forrester is one of the great medical storytellers of our era. In *The Heart Healers*, he applies his exceptional talent to illuminate—and tell the backstories of—the momentous milestones in cardiovascular medicine and surgery."   —Eric Topol, cardiologist, author of *The Patient Will See You Now* and *The Creative Destruction of Medicine*

"This book is a great read! Even if one is familiar with some of the players who contributed to breakthroughs in cardiovascular medicine, to learn the backstories from an expert who lived through the events is a very enriching experience. Dr. Forrester makes a very compelling case that the misfits, mavericks, and rebels who persevered with their ideas truly impacted our society in ways that we cannot fully appreciate since we now take those things for granted. This is a story of disruptive innovation before that term was even invented!"

—Elliott Antman, M.D., professor of medicine,
Brigham and Women's Hospital, Harvard Medical School;
and president, American Heart Association, 2014–15

This book is filled with stories of courage in the face of adversity.
One I do not tell is that of my oldest son, Jeffrey,
who personified this quality as he edited this book,
and my family who support him.

CONTENTS

PART IV: HOW TO CONQUER CORONARY ARTERY DISEASE 251

ACKNOWLEDGMENTS

THANKS FROM ALL four chambers of my heart to Stuart Horowitz, Jeffrey Forrester, and Michael Flamini, each of whom made superb crucial editing contributions at different stages of the book. Treasured friends who read the draft and provided invaluable medical and nonmedical critiques and insights include Dr. France Doyle, Dr. Alex Dubelman, David Bancroft, and Richard Cain. Elizabeth Wilson and Margaret Knill saved me endless aggravation by skillfully tracking down copyrights for many of the illustrations. Although I never typed until after medical school, I can now text and email, and I surprised myself by typing the entire manuscript.

AUTHOR'S NOTE

AS AN AUTHOR I have many debts. My narrative stands squarely on the shoulders of the many authors who researched, compiled, interviewed, and wrote in the years before me. In particular I am indebted to the biographers of several of the characters in this chronicle. I have sought to acknowledge this debt in the Notes section. My narrative also rests heavily on my own direct personal interaction with the physicians and scientists who populate these pages. The essence of a remembered experience is often clear, but the details of old memories are not. No doubt some who shared these experiences will feel my views about people unfair or inaccurate, or they may recall events quite differently. Some individuals who have made huge scientific contributions to cardiovascular medicine will be disappointed that I have not recognized them explicitly, given the attention I have accorded others of lesser scientific stature. My primary motive, however, is to recount a compelling adventure as I experienced it rather than to identify each giant in his field.

I use patient experiences to give a human dimension to the breakthroughs I describe. So I have a heavy debt to the many patients and families who have taught me so much about humanity, dignity, and courage over these years. Many of the patients that appear in these pages are well known locally. Some are internationally known. In compliance with recently enacted extremely strict federal Health Insurance Portability and Accountability (HIPAA) privacy legislation with associated penalties, except where specifically noted, I have used pseudonyms and significantly altered personal details like occupations and locations to conceal every patient's identity, both living and dead. To help your understanding of the vast complexity of doctor-patient interactions from the first symptom through the conundrums of cardiac diagnosis to its culmination in the heroic life-saving treatments, in one case I have merged two patient stories into one. The sum of these disclaimers is that every patient story is inspired by real events, but my hope is that no one will imagine they recognize the patients in this narrative. If they think they do, however, I would ask them to respect the privacy of these patients and their families.

In preparing this manuscript, I identified five international thought leaders in cardiology, each of whom is known for his expertise in a different area. On behalf of the American College of Cardiology (ACC), I conducted lengthy recorded interviews, which are now part of the ACC's Digital Historical Archives. I want to express my deep appreciation to Drs. Lawrence Cohn (cardiac surgery), Douglas Zipes (electrophysiology), Eugene Braunwald (acute coronary care), Spencer King (interventional cardiology), and Bruce Fye (cardiology historian), each of whom recalled wonderful stories and insights about the characters who appear in this book.

Finally, as I tell the story of how patients and doctors have won their individual battles with heart disease, I seek to show you how to prevent and to overcome heart disease in your own life, so throughout the book I offer both advice and opinions on management of heart disease. While it is fair to assume that my views and advice are in line with most of my fellow "thought leaders" in cardiology, they cannot be taken as a guide to treatment in any specific case. The reason, as we will see, is that decision-making about heart disease in an individual patient depends upon clusters of details. To sift and give the proper weight to each detail, you need a face-to-face discussion with an up-to-date cardiologist.

PROLOGUE

ABOUT A THIRD of the world's deaths, 15 to 20 million people annually, are due to cardiovascular disease. In just one year, heart disease claims more lives in the United States than all Americans lost in the wars of the past century. Perhaps worse, an astonishing eighty million U.S. citizens currently suffer from cardiovascular disease. Do not imagine yourself immune. No one gets a free pass because they have no symptoms of heart disease: among the nation's 400,000 annual sudden deaths, about half of the men and two-thirds of the women have no preceding symptoms. It spares no age, sex, or era. It strikes newborns and children, young athletes in their prime, and adults in apparent perfect health.

But medical statistics are patients with the tears wiped away. So let's enter this story when I did, as the first rays of dawning sun filter through the grimy windows of a medical ward in a mid-1960s hospital in Philadelphia. A thirty-eight-year-old man has been admitted in the middle of the night with chest pain. His first name is Willie; I no longer recall his real last name. As I walk onto the ward in my white pants and the starched short white coat that marks me as a doctor in training, I instantly recognize Willie from our prior meetings in the outpatient clinic.

I think back to the first time I met Willie. With only our wits and a stethoscope as our primary diagnostic tools, I was taught to be a medical Sherlock Holmes, focusing on tiny details from the moment I saw a new patient. This is what I saw: Willie was just under six feet tall, with thinning, neatly trimmed black hair speckled with gray. His rheumy brown corneas had rims of white, as he peered cautiously out from beneath bushy graying eyebrows. His prominent well-shaven jowls reminded me of a chipmunk. Tiny blood vessels spread over his small upturned nose. Perched on an exam table with his legs dangling over the side, Willie reminded me of photos of the legendary Yankee slugger Babe Ruth. He had a barrel chest, a gut that protruded prominently over his belt, and mismatched sticklike legs that peeked from beneath a faded threadbare county-issue smock. As we shook hands, I noticed Willie's palms were flushed pink. His nails were trimmed and clean but had a dusky tinge. On his bare arms and legs I saw that he had a few raised, waxy yellow bumps. Before we spoke, I silently made my initial diagnosis: Willie was an alcoholic who was a reformed heavy smoker. He had emphysema in his lungs, cirrhosis in his liver, and atheroma in his coronary arteries.

How did I arrive at these conclusions? Willie's barrel chest and dusky fingernails suggested emphysema, almost always caused by smoking. But his fingers had no nicotine stains, so he probably had given it up. The dilated blood vessels on his nose, flushed palms, large abdomen with skinny legs, and chipmunk face were all signs of alcoholic liver disease. Most of these signs reflected failure of the liver to metabolize circulating steroids, particularly the female hormone estrogen. The white arc in the cornea in early middle age and the yellow bumps on the arms and legs (called xanthoma) were telltale signs of an inherited high level of blood cholesterol.

In an understaffed overworked hospital the lowest-ranked person in the training program often is the first to see patients and typically spends the most time with them. Willie was one of my favorite patients. He had a huge welcoming smile. He remembered the name of each doctor, nurse, and patient. Willie told hilarious stories, but he was as willing to listen as to talk. We had much in common. We had grown up in neighboring small towns in the Central Pennsylvania Dutch country. Willie loved the Phillies. I knew every player's batting average. "You call me Willie the Phillie," he'd urge. He was a reformed alcoholic, sober for three years. Willie was a traveling auto parts salesman. To me he was the incarnation of Willy Loman in Arthur Miller's classic play *Death of a Salesman*, played that year by the legendary Lee J. Cobb and two decades later in 1985 by Dustin Hoffman. Willie was the "low-man" on society's ladder, trampled by his boss, his former wife, his teen-age son, even his customers. Yet he retained Willy Loman's faith in the American Dream. He had an abiding faith in me as his doctor, too, since the day in the outpatient clinic when I prescribed nitroglycerin pills for his newly developed chest pain with exercise, and it worked. "When you hang out your shingle, Doc, I'll be your first patient," he'd tell me on each subsequent visit.

On the ward I greeted Willie. The night before, he had been jolted awake in the middle of the night by severe chest pain. "It felt like a vise being tightened around my chest," he said. "It squeezed the air out of me. I took a nitroglycerin. But this time nothing happened. I took another, but instead the pain just kept getting worse. I took another nitro, and felt so light-headed I couldn't even sit up. For a half hour I lay there, unable to move. Then the vise started to relax. As soon as I could, I got out of bed and drove here to the emergency room. By the time I got on the ward, the pain was gone." I knew Willie's diagnosis from the textbooks. He had what we then called preinfarction angina and now call unstable angina. Although the patient feels fine between episodes, it is often the harbinger of a full-blown, potentially lethal heart attack.

The treatment for preinfarction angina in those years was strict bed rest. Over the next two days Willie continued to have episodes of prolonged chest pain at rest, but between the episodes he felt fine. Toward the end of the third day, as I stood at his bedside chatting about the Phillies, Willie grimaced. His right hand flew to the center of his chest, and contracted into a tight fist. "The pain is coming back, Doc," he said. Small beads of sweat appeared just below his hairline. His breathing became labored. His eyes widened with fear. He looked beseechingly into my eyes. "Doc, this one is worse, I feel like I'm gonna die. Help me," he pleaded. I put a nitroglycerin under his tongue. No response. Willie was right . . . this one was worse.

I called the ward nurse to summon my medical resident, and anticipating his arrival, I told her to draw up a syringe of morphine right away. Everything now began to whirl past me at triple speed. Willie's systolic blood pressure, which was usually 140, fell to 115. I gave him another nitroglycerin. No relief. The morphine arrived, but no resident. So I gave Willie the morphine by intravenous injection. Almost immediately he began to experience relief of pain. But over the next few minutes his blood pressure continued to slip lower . . . 110, 105, 100. I told the nurse to wheel the ward's cardiograph (ECG) machine—we had no TV monitors in those days—to his bedside. Willie's tracing showed all the ECG hallmarks of a heart attack. I felt like David facing Goliath with an empty slingshot. I was responsible for Willie's care and I had no effective therapy to offer.

We were now three or four minutes into his pain, and the resident had still not appeared. When Willie's blood pressure fell further to 90, I ordered a medication to support his blood pressure, fearing it would be of little value. As it was being infused into his intravenous line, I kept my eyes on his panicked face and my fingers on his pulse. My own heart began to pound furiously when I felt Willie's pulse rate suddenly triple and weaken further. I recorded another strip of the ECG. Willie's normal heart rhythm was gone. In its place was ventricular tachycardia—a very fast, life-threatening rhythm that often comes just before ventricular fibrillation, the rhythm of sudden death. Now in near panic I shouted Code Blue, medicine's universal message of disaster, its urgent plea for help from any nearby doctor. A few seconds later, Willie's eyes rolled to the ceiling and he lost consciousness.

In the preceding months, we had learned of a new approach called cardiac resuscitation. I had not yet seen a resuscitation; my first experience would be performing one. Behind me I heard a sudden explosion of running doctors, nurses frantically pushing carts. Someone yanked the curtain around Willie's bed, concealing all but white pant legs and white stockings. Willie's heartbeat disappeared completely. I recorded another strip of ECG. There it was: the rhythm of death, ventricular fibrillation.

A staff doctor in a long white coat charged in to assume the role of foreman. "Who's his doctor?" he asked. When no one answered, the nurse pointed to me. He swiveled toward me and shouted, "Pump!" I began rhythmically pressing on Willie's chest. A defibrillator was rolled to the bedside. Long Coat showed me where to press the two paddles on Willie, one on his upper right chest, the other on the lower left, and handed them to me. "Hands off the bed!" he shouted and nodded to me. Like Ben Franklin's key, you did not want to be touching metal when the lightning struck. I fired the defibrillator by depressing the thumb switch on the right paddle. I jumped back reflexively as Willie's whole body flexed in a violent convulsion, like he had the sudden impulse to sit up. Then just as quickly he flopped back. To my horror I saw my intervention had left his body crumpled, head angled crazily, hair disheveled, mouth agape. My entire body recoiled as I felt—I saw—the terrible indignity of death. I dropped the paddles, and resumed pumping on Willie's chest. Someone ran another strip of the ECG. Still ventricular fibrillation.

A minute later an anesthesiologist, panting from running the hallways, shoved aside the surrounding curtains, grasping a breathing tube. I stepped aside as she flexed Willie's neck back. It took her about a minute to insert a metal flange into his mouth, pass a breathing tube into his trachea, and connect a breathing bag. I resumed pumping. After a few minutes of furious pumping on his chest I was drenched in sweat and near exhaustion. Another trainee replaced me.

Long Coat handed me a large syringe filled with a heart stimulant that we hoped might restore the heartbeat. The syringe was connected to a menacing six inch long needle. "Stick it in the fourth intercostal space," he said. "Keep going until you are inside the heart." I shoved the needle deep between Willie's ribs, almost to the hub, then pulled back on the barrel of the syringe. Blood poured into the syringe. I was inside the heart. I injected the concoction.

Over the next twenty minutes, with the rest of the ward in morbid silence, the slurp of suction tube, loud thumps, and heavy breathing rose above the turmoil from behind Willie's curtain. Above the cacophony, two terse words repeatedly declared our abject failure. "Still v fib." We could not resuscitate Willie.

By thirty minutes, the others were wordlessly looking at Long Coat for a decision. He turned to the anesthesiologist.

"What do you think?"

"I think he's gone," she said. Her words fell like a guillotine..

He turned to me. "He's your patient, Doctor. What's your call?"

His question was like a punch to my solar plexus, unexpected, stunning, painful, taking my breath away. Why me? I was still just a twenty-something kid. An apprentice. This was my friend Willie the Phillie. Was Long Coat being cruel beyond imagination? He knew I wasn't remotely qualified or prepared, and he yet he seemed to be taunting me by putting this final responsibility for Willie's death on my shoulders.

Wasn't this final responsibility clearly his, not mine? Or was he treating me with profound respect, calling me "doctor" before my time, admitting me to the fraternity of shared exhilaration and grief between doctor and patient, letting me know that although we had failed, I had done enough to earn his respect? I will always wonder and never know.

I had never come face-to-face with such a profound, wrenching decision. I felt submerged, unable to breathe. In that moment of total silence, I could only look at my shoes, engulfed in impotent failure. We had done everything to save my thirty-eight-year-old patient, yet in that moment I realized that for people with heart disease, we had almost nothing to offer. Nitroglycerin under the tongue was a mismatch worse than Crimea against the Russians. I raised my eyes to rest them on Willie's ashen face for a long moment of resignation. In that moment I accepted my responsibility. I was Willie's friend, but as he said, I was his doctor.

"We should terminate Mr. Loman's resuscitation. I will record that the patient was pronounced dead at 11:58 a.m.," I choked out, staring at the wall well above the tattered white curtains.

Long Coat delivered a final insight. "He had coronary disease. It was his time." His subtext was clear. Willie's misfortune was that he had coronary disease. With coronary disease, there was nothing a doctor could do.

Routine returned. The anesthesiologist extracted her tube, then sidled around the still closed curtain. The nurses silently, respectfully smoothed and folded Willie's sheets around him, and over his face. I slipped out from behind the curtain and, avoiding eye contact with my other patients on the ward, trudged to the nurses' station to make my final entry in Willie's chart. Trained in medicine's language of facts devoid of feelings, I wrote, "Cardiorespiratory arrest at 11:27 a.m. Unresponsive to intracardiac medications, intubation, and defibrillation. Pronounced dead at 11:58 a.m." I called Willie's next of kin, knowing that on this charity ward, typically no one would come. Watching Willie's tiny cubicle surrender his lingering identifiers and a gurney wheel his shapeless mass past unshaven men with averted eyes, I felt like a prison warden overseeing the last walk of an innocent man. As I closed his chart, I reread my note: it seemed like I was ushering Willie into eternity with neither a name nor a tear.

My impotent witness to Willie's sudden death left me staring into an emotional chasm, a doctor's version of post-traumatic stress syndrome. I felt that although our treatment was bankrupt, we accepted the satisfied conventional wisdom that this was the best cardiology could do. Had he survived his heart attack, my mentors would prescribe a minimum of three weeks of strict bed rest for Willie's injured heart to heal from injury, after which they would conduct an erudite discussion of when it would be safe for him to dangle his legs over the side of the bed. We needed to discover a better way. Impossibly self-delusional as I may have been, I decided to enter cardiology. And that is why I write today.

When I entered cardiology, we faced a new virulent illness. Epidemics are nothing new. In the early 1300s a new disease appeared in China, joined travelers along the Silk Road to Crimea, then moved on to Europe, carried by Oriental fleas living on black rats, the ubiquitous denizens of merchant ships that plied the Mediterranean Sea. In the half century that followed, the Black Death killed half of Europe's population, cutting the world population by an estimated seventy-five million people. For seven centuries, the plague stood as mankind's greatest scourge. At the middle of the twentieth century heart disease erupted in exactly that way, as a scourge before which we stood helpless. Heart disease began to kill five to twenty million people worldwide every single year. In my country, the United States, when I entered medicine, more lives were being lost in a single year than in all of World War II.

If you want to understand this enemy, you have to begin with the normal heart. Its principal function is to deliver life-giving oxygen to all the body's organs. To do this, the heart consists of four components. Muscle that pumps blood. An electrical system to control the pump's rate. Valves that control the flow of blood through the heart. And coronary arteries to supply oxygen to the other three components.

A glitch in any one of these four systems gives you heart disease, each with a different constellation of symptoms. Disordered muscle and valve function cause arrhythmias (abnormal heart rhythms), manifest as light-headedness, fainting, and even sudden death. Diseased coronary arteries shows up as angina (chest pain on exertion), heart attack, and sudden death.

I knew all this on that humid Philadelphia morning and still in my own heart I realized that as a doctor, I knew nothing of enduring value to

Willie the Phillie. Our medical establishment was largely bereft of effective treatment to reverse his condition. Yet today my heart sends me a different message, one of considerable hope. If I could have shared with Willie what I now know, he would have lived to see his grandchildren graduate.

FOR MUCH OF my professional career I served as director of one of the National Heart, Lung, and Blood Institute's nine multimillion-dollar Centers for Research in Ischemic Heart Disease, and later as director of the division of cardiology at one of the nation's leading medical centers. So I have been fortunate to have a role in what was and continues to be the most astonishing medical advance of our lifetime. I think I am most proud of my role as a mentor for hundreds of clinician-scientists, challenging them to think differently, to find innovative solutions to all forms of heart disease. A few years ago my efforts were honored when I was selected as the second-ever recipient of the American College of Cardiology's highest honor, the Lifetime Achievement Award. I know full well that my mentees, my mentors, my colleagues, my profession, and our patients are the ones who really deserve this honor. Our shared achievement is that we have humbled what was the scourge of the twentieth century. As I spin out the story of how our nation's number one killer, coronary artery disease (CAD), became a preventable disease, I aim to teach you how to prevent or conquer heart disease in your own and your family's lives.

Since I know personally most of the doctors in this story, I should explain why I dub them "misfits." It's fascinating to me how many of them share some unusual personality traits. They reject the common wisdom. They rely on their own intuition. In their private lives they are risk-takers. They ignore the criticism of their peers. They persist in the face of failure. Unlike most of us, they are nonconformists, iconoclasts who refuse to knuckle under to society's norms, regardless of the potential consequences. Does this tell us something about creativity? I think it does. I concur with Steve Jobs on this:

Here's to the crazy ones. The misfits. The rebels. The troublemakers. The round pegs in the square holes. The ones who see things differently. They're not fond of rules. And they have no respect for the status quo. You can quote them, disagree with them, glorify or vilify them. About the only thing you can't do is ignore them. Because they change things. They push the human race forward. And while some may see them as the crazy ones, we see genius. Because the people who are crazy enough to think they can change the world, are the ones who do.

Let me introduce just a few of the misfits we will meet on our journey: we will begin with a bullheaded battlefield surgeon named Dwight Harken. Along the way we will meet cantankerous heart surgeon Charles Bailey, scandalously outspoken cardiologist Mason Sones, utopian maverick Argentine surgeon René Favaloro, life-of-any-party Andreas Gruentzig, establishment-challenging Japanese biochemist Akira Endo. I suspect most readers will not recognize a single name but, today, if a family member, a friend, or you have experienced relief or been cured of heart disease, these men stand unseen behind the doctor responsible for the cure.

THAT'S THE ESSENCE of our tale: the past, present, and future of heart disease. But it's the tree without the branches. The beauty, the fascination of our chronicle, as with all stories, lies in people: the doctors and the patients who live it. Since I know most of the patients and doctors you will meet, I tell both stories from my own personal perspective. To me this drama casts an illuminating oculus on both the progress of science and on the human soul. In living these experiences, I have seen incredible risk-taking, scintillating intuition, perseverance, hubris, bullheadedness, indomitable courage, commitment, selflessness, love, and hope. And so, the story I set out to tell about my experience in medical science becomes a story about all of us. As Ecclesiastes tells us, "The race is not always to the swift, nor the battle to the strong, nor riches to men of understanding, nor favor to men of skill; but time and chance happen to us all." In the spirit of Ecclesiastes, I offer you a testament to one of the most life-altering, indeed heart-healing, stories of our times.

PART I

ESCAPE FROM THE DARK AGES

1

A DAY LIKE ALL DAYS

A shocking occurrence ceases to be shocking when it occurs daily.

—Alexander Chase, American journalist

EVERY DOCTOR HAS his favorite organ. Hannibal Lecter prefers the liver; I prefer the heart. Surely it is our body's hardest worker. Imagine performing 90,000 very forceful push-ups a day, with no time-out for rest. How is it possible, when few of us could clench and unclench our fist at that rate for even an hour? Try doing that for eighty years with not one second off for good behavior. Complex in structure yet simple in function, yet so perfect in performance, the heart is truly Nature's engineering masterpiece.

Midway in size between a baseball and a softball, its oblong football shape still fits nicely in your hand. Squeeze it. It feels firm and muscular but also hollow. Turn it around in your hands, looking at its surface. Three prominent coronary arteries with lots of branches spread over the heart's surface before diving into the muscle to supply all the heart cells with blood.

Since it feels hollow, let's open the heart to see what is inside. In the heart, as in architecture, form follows function. We see four separate chambers. The two chambers on the right (the "right heart") are responsible for collecting blood from the body and the pumping it to the lungs where oxygen is added. The two chambers on the left (the "left heart") are responsible for collecting oxygenated blood from the lungs and delivering it to all the organs of the body. The heart's structure reflects its dual collecting and pumping function. Both the right and left hearts consist of a thin-walled collecting chamber (ancients coined it the "atrium") and a thicker walled pumping chamber (the "ventricle").

But why does the heart contract about sixty times a minute when we are resting and as much as 180 times a minute when we exercise? What controls the pump? Specialized cells embedded in the right atrium (the blood-collecting chamber of the right heart) spontaneously emit an electrical impulse at about once per second at rest. The impulse causes the atrial muscle to contract. The contraction forces blood across a one-way valve between the atrium and right ventricle. At the same time, the electrical impulse travels also into the ventricle (the pumping chamber). So about two-tenths of a second after the atrium contracts, the ventricle is shocked into vigorous contraction. What a shrewd innovation by the celestial design committee! When it contracts, the atrium "loads" the ventricular pump with blood, and then two tenths of a second later the ventricle fires off, slamming the one-way valve shut and sending blood rocketing to the lungs. It's like the ticktock of a grandfather clock: the valve is opened, closed, opened, closed.

Exactly the same process occurs at the same time in the left heart, sending blood to the body's organs. Repeat that every second, and you have a pumping system that circulates oxygen to body's organs, and returns the deoxygenated blood to the lungs to be reoxygenated.

Because of the valve system, blood flows continuously in only one direction (it "circulates"). It's the same principle as the locks on the Panama Canal. When the inflow valves close, the outflow valves open. Like the needle of a metronome swinging back and forth, the two pairs of valves in the right and left heart open and close in perfect synchrony: the ticktock lasts a lifetime. And of course both the right and left hearts receive and eject blood through large vessels. The most important of these vessels is called the aorta, which delivers blood from the left ventricle to the entire body.

The muscle, valves, and electrical system do the work of the heart. Its fourth component, the coronary arteries, delivers oxygen-giving energy for all this hard work. The two coronary arteries, right and left, are the very first branches to come off the aorta; first dibs for life-sustaining oxygen goes to the body's most important organ. The coronary arteries send branches that cover the entire surface of the heart and also plunge deep into the heart muscle so that no cell is deprived of oxygen.

When the aorta delivers blood into each organ, the red blood cell that transports the energy-giving oxygen changes in color from bright red to dark blue. Now it's time to deliver the blood back to the lungs, add oxygen, and repeat the cycle. The blood from all the organs is collected in larger and larger veins and returned back to the right atrium where the process of reoxygenation begins anew. Arteries deliver blood; veins return it. It takes about sixty heartbeats to complete one cycle at rest.

The heart's oxygen delivery system functions like a perfect machine because its form (anatomy) is so ingeniously integrated with its function. The muscular pump consists of collecting and pumping chambers. Circular flow is created by its system of one-way valves. The muscle meets its own intense need for an energy supply by first delivering oxygen to itself through its coronary arteries. And finally the whole system is exquisitely sensitive to the needs of its client, the body. Need more oxygen because you are in Yosemite, running from a black bear? No problem. Your heart can quintuple the flow of blood in seconds by tripling the heart rate and increasing the vigor of ventricular contraction.

Now that you know how your own heart actually works, let's meet our first patient, who could one day be you.

ALONE WITH HER morning mug of coffee, Greta Adams stood on her patio trying to savor this daily solitary moment she cherished. Thirty-five years old, she loved the moist morning fog that rolled off the Pacific Ocean to be momentarily trapped in the hills above her home in Pacific Palisades, a small community northwest of Los Angeles. Each year nature repainted the canvas behind her, as the torrential rains and mudslides of February led to the explosion of yellow and purple mountain flowers of April, the now-green hills of June, and then finally the dry gray chaparral tumbling before the hot dry Santa Ana winds of September. How could anyone say California has no seasons?

This morning, though, the misty sea and mountain vista did not shake her free from a sense of foreboding. On most days her first thought was how to squeeze in an hour's brisk walk and jog in nearby Will Rogers Park just north of Sunset Boulevard. But jogging, which had been her physical release, was now her bondage. Several weeks earlier she first noticed the discomfort, like a knot in her shoulder. At first, Greta was not so much concerned as she was puzzled. At first she thought it was a muscle cramp from climbing the rope that hung from a tree in her backyard. "I am young and I am healthy," she reasoned. She had had her share of bumps and bruises over the years. Her thought seemed confirmed when she stopped her jog and the cramp rapidly disappeared. When it kept coming back on every morning run, she went to a massage therapist. Massage proved futile. When the knot extended to beneath her breastbone, she began to imagine more fanciful explanations. Could the moist salt air and the morning auto exhaust wafting over from Pacific Coast Highway cause chest pain? Could her discomfort be psychological, precipitated by her worry about a bully at Benjamin's school? No, it wasn't just in her mind, because the knot was now a small insolent fist, more insistent and more menacing with each run. It was time to see a doctor.

Greta and Tyler's drive to my office took her east on Sunset Boulevard past colossal mansions worth tens of millions of dollars. Turning south in a few minutes, a massive eight-story, two-square-block, granite-brown building rose to dominate their view. Its central segment, crowned with a Star of David, stood astride the corner of Gracie Allen Drive and George Burns Road. The unusual street names bespoke a subtle reminder of the prodigious financial support given to Cedars-Sinai Medical Center by the tiny city that surrounds it. Walking the corridors to my fifth floor office, Greta and Tyler would discover that every public corridor is a museum of contemporary art, where huge Rauschenbergs compete with Warhol prints.

Greta made a gallant effort to smile brightly as she stood to greet me in my office, but the smile had already vanished before she spoke. As she sat she brushed a nonexistent hair from her forehead, then clasped her hands tightly in her lap. Greta was shouting fear and anxiety without speaking. So instead of talking about her symptoms, I started with family. I talked about my years coaching Little League, and moved on to ocean sports. Her son, Ben, was starting Little League and her husband Tyler was a surfer, she said, with a big smile. Now we were ready to talk about walks along the ocean and jogs in the hills.

I started with her history. Greta didn't smoke, was still menstruating, and had no history of high blood pressure or diabetes. She had never had her blood lipids checked. Her father had died suddenly at age fifty-seven from a heart attack in the past year. Her mother was in good health; she had no siblings.

In diagnosing the cause of chest pain we begin with uncertainty. At one end of the spectrum Greta's pain could be related to a psychological stress, such as her worry over her son. Or perhaps her father's recent death from heart attack had caused her to obsess over her own risk. At the other end of the spectrum, coronary artery disease (CAD) might be the cause of her symptoms. I knew from large databases like the famous Framingham, Massachusetts, study that a thirtysomething-year-old woman with Greta's demographics has less than 1% probability of having CAD. This woman also had chest pain, which increased the probability of disease, but by how much? In cardiology on most days, I find myself standing at the intersection of science and art, where objective probability meets subjective uncertainty.

I asked Greta about her chest pain. Angina, the pain caused by CAD, has three principal characteristics. Greta had all three. Her pain was located behind the sternum, brought on by exercise, and rapidly relieved by rest. The probability of CAD increases with the number of characteristics, and since she had all three, Greta had "typical angina." If we examine all people with typical angina, 90% have coronary disease. For a young woman who begins with a less than 1% probability of disease, typical angina and a positive family history raises her probability of having coronary disease to about 50%.

I reached toward her and said, "Come, I'll examine your heart."

The hospital is elegant; the examining rooms are not. Greta glanced around the tiny six-by-eight-foot room with its spare undecorated white walls, resting her eyes on the narrow, lumpy three-piece examining table, with a step stool at its base. Her anxiety again filled the room as she sat with her legs dangling uncomfortably from the examining table. I started by resting both hands gently on her arm as I palpated her radial pulse. "Laying on of hands" speaks without words. It says I understand your unspoken anxiety. It recalls a parent's touch that says, "I'm here to take care of you." Greta's pulses were all normal. By finding the tap of her heart on her chest wall, I determined that her heart size was normal. Listening with my stethoscope, I heard her heart valves closing normally, with no heart murmur and normal breathing sounds. With a normal heart size, no murmurs, and no evidence of heart failure, I was confident that congenital and valvular was not the cause of her pain and heart muscle disease was unlikely. That left the coronary arteries. Most people with undiagnosed CAD, like Greta, have a normal physical exam. Greta's history and physical exam brought us face-to-face with the ultimate uncertainty, a 50/50 coin flip about CAD. So we would need a test.

Now I had choices. I could recommend either an exercise stress test, or even the definitive test, a coronary angiogram. Because an angiogram is expensive and invasive, I chose a stress test. There is no "right" choice, but this one cost a lot less, and it was immediately available.

The stress test was distinctly abnormal. In her brief visit, Greta's probability of having CAD had skyrocketed from less than 1% to perhaps 90%. For Greta, a nagging unease over a morning cup of coffee was about to ramp up into a pounding anxiety, like a powerful migraine that obliterated every other thought. The diagnosis of CAD with its sinister implications would be a stunning, life-changing, shattering event.

CAD is due to deposits of fat in blood vessels (called plaques or atheromas). Large ones impede the blood flow particularly when the heart needs more oxygen during exercise or emotional stress. Like all muscles deprived of oxygen, the heart sends a pain signal to the brain. When the need for oxygen diminishes, the pain disappears. So, like Greta's chest pain, typical angina is directly behind the chest, precipitated by stress, and disappears within a minute of termination of the stress. Atheromas create two life-threatening risks. They can cause abnormal heart rhythms, including ventricular fibrillation and sudden death. Rapid complete obstruction of a coronary artery by an atheroma causes heart muscle to die (a heart attack or myocardial infarction).

I was taught in medical school that people under thirty-five seldom contemplate their own mortality. Yet this would be Greta's fate this afternoon. How do I tell a thirty-five-year-old mother that she has life-threatening disease that needs immediate attention, when she has never before been sick? I plodded back to talk with Greta, wondering how my sympathy could possibly match her struggle to absorb this personal tragedy. I stopped by the waiting room to ask Tyler to join me. He jumped to his feet with an expectant smile. We locked eyes; his smile vanished as I said simply, "Please join us." As I ushered Tyler in ahead of me, I took a deep breath, and closed the door. I drew my chair from behind my desk to sit beside Greta and Tyler. "Greta," I began, "let me show you what we found." I showed them the ECG. I knew that neither was trained to interpret what they were looking at, but I felt Greta and Tyler needed assurance that specific, objective information provided a foundation for her diagnosis. Allowing Greta to focus on a piece of paper rather than blurting out the dreadful news directly could give her just a little more emotional space and time; a cushion, however small, for her psychic turmoil.

"What's the next step?" she asked after they had seen the test results. My reply was shaped by uncertainty, cardiology's loyal twenty-first-century companion. We had solved the uncertainty of Greta's diagnosis, only to arrive at a new one. In Edgar Allan Poe's famous 1843 Gothic short story "The Tell-Tale Heart," a murderer is flummoxed by the sound of his dismembered victim's heart that he imagines is still beating beneath the floorboards. Was Greta's heart sending me a message of impending doom requiring immediate action, or did we have time to gradually implement treatment? Should Greta have immediate coronary angiography (X-ray pictures of her coronary arteries), or could she first have a trial of pills, say nitroglycerin, which reduces the pain of angina? I recalled nitroglycerin had relieved Willie's symptoms, but it had not prevented his heart attack.

I gave Greta the argument favoring a trial of pills. Her angina was annoying but not disabling in her daily living. She still drove her car, shopped, cooked, and took care of Benjamin without episodes of angina. Her chest pain bothered her only on walk-jogs. She had not yet tried pills to alleviate the pain, but I felt the probability of pain relief with medication was quite high. Furthermore, I knew from randomized trials comparing medical therapy, angioplasty, and bypass surgery in patients with stable angina that, after five years of follow-up, there was no clear difference in survival among the choices. So one option was to initiate intensive medical therapy and closely monitor her response.

"For you, Greta," I said, "there are two limitations to this choice. First, among those we start on medical therapy, about forty percent are not fully relieved of symptoms and end up going to angiography. More important, however, is that patients with accelerating symptoms of angina are at higher risk of heart attack than those with chronic stable angina. Your chest pain is very recent in onset and has progressed in both frequency and severity. So I cannot tell you that your angina is stable, and that means there is some increased risk for you to go home. There is only one certainty here; it is that there is no absolute best option."

"What do you think I should do?" she whispered.

"This has to be your choice," I replied. From our first days in medical school, we are admonished never to order, only to advise.

"But if I were in your situation, I would choose coronary angiography." I paused to look directly at Tyler before returning to Greta. "Because your symptoms seem to be increasing, I'd have it now, Greta. I wouldn't wait over the weekend." The face of a friend who died suddenly on a Monday morning drive to the cath lab after he'd been sent home over a weekend with recent onset angina flashed in my mind. We sat in silence for a brief moment, then I rose to open my office door.

"Greta, the two of you need to have some time alone," I said. I closed the door of my dimly lit office as I walked into the shimmering sunlight of a Los Angeles summer afternoon, knowing how at that moment how much each soul needed the other.

GRETA'S STORY, AS with all patients suspected of having CAD, spins off in a new direction with the decision for angiography, when the baton of patient responsibility is thrust into the hands of an interventional cardiologist in the catheterization laboratory. Jon Jackson is a superspecialist who spends his waking hours staring at a continuous X-ray image of his catheter and his patient's heart. Like a concert pianist, he must continuously coordinate his foot, which controls the X-ray beam, the visual image from the monitor, and his hands advancing and rotating catheters, wires, and other devices. To be a great interventional cardiologist (one who performs catheterization laboratory procedures) requires the ability to imagine the third dimension of a two-dimensional X-ray image, consummate hand-eye coordination, clearheaded judgment, and the capacity to remain calm under extreme stress.

I spent my cardiology training years in a Boston cardiac catheterization laboratory. Since Greta told me that she cannot recall her catheterization laboratory experience, I will re-create it for her. On her arrival an attendant instructs her to strip off all her clothes, accessories, and undergarments. To cover her otherwise naked body she is offered a flimsy cotton smock, faded and worn from innumerable scalding launderings. The gown, which barely reaches her knees, has ties at the neck and mid-back, leaving a narrow strip of the lower back partially exposed. As Greta would immediately discover, it is impossible to retain any semblance of dignity if she bends over.

When Greta rolls into the cath lab on the gurney, she immediately smells the vague acrid odor of drying disinfectant wafting up from the floor. The lab floor is mopped after every procedure and turnover is rapid. The smell sticks to Greta's nostrils like sunblock. The cath lab recalls for Greta images from the threateningly immaculate surroundings of a futuristic sci-fi horror flick. It is a cool cavernous windowless bunker, bereft of color or decoration. Every object seems to be either gleaming chrome or white, proclaiming its hypermodern sterility to all who enter. Among the unidentifiable nameless devices on rollers that hug the walls, Greta might recognize a particular one if she watches TV programs like *ER* or *House*. It is the one with paddle electrodes used to revive the dead. Otherwise the vast space seems empty, except for a forbidding, centrally placed rectangular block of metal in the shape of a very narrow single bed. About waist-high, the bed's surface has the humorless gleam of hard black plastic.

As a nurse softly introduces herself, nameless souls scurry about behind her in the unisex green pajamas of their trade. All about her, Greta is immersed in controlled urgency: needles forced into vials held aloft, a rolling IV stand, skin patches and wires, monitors snapping alive. With so much distracting sensory input, she can grasp only snippets of conversation about her. Then a voice beside her commands, "Hold still, Greta," and after a 1–2–3 count, four sets of hands grasping the sheet beneath her propel her briefly airborne and quickly deposit her on the hard lonely catheterization table. Suspended above the table are giant circular lights, each with a handle covered by a sterile drape. If Greta squints into the middle of this array, she will see a massive cylinder, heavy enough to eviscerate her, poised high above her chest. The cylinder is the X-ray imager, which will be lowered to almost touch her chest during the procedure. Mounted above the table like appeal court judges, blank-faced monitors stand poised to silently announce their verdict on the rest of Greta's life. CAD or no CAD? That is the question.

At Greta's right side is a metal stand with bulky green packages. The opened packages reveal an array of sterile hemostats, forceps, scissors, and scalpels. Gloved hands replace her blanket with strategically placed sterile blue towels folded just so, creating a large open space over her groin. The bared skin is scrubbed using forceps that held gauze soaked in a cold brown disinfectant. Another set of green-gowned latex-gloved hands extend her arm and tape it to a boardlike extension from the table.

As Greta settles on the cath lab table, Jon and his cardiology fellow assistant enter. With just-scrubbed hands and arms, encased in lead vests that overlap knee-length lead aprons, their mandate is to avoid touching nonsterile objects by walking stiffly with their arms tightly flexed at the elbows like religious supplicants. As a nurse holds up a long gown, Jon forces his arms down into its sleeves. The scrub nurse ties the gown in the back, then holds out sterile gloves into which each doctor in turn plunges his well-scrubbed hands. The solemnity of the gowning ceremony, however, is mocked by the hair bonnets and the foolish-looking bags the doctors wear around their shoes. Frightened, depersonalized, immobilized, and now pinned to this long cold rectangle, the image of masked, gowned doctors incongruously dressed in green burkas completes Greta's vision of the netherworld of the cath lab. A final dislocating incongruity is a faintly audible stanza of Mozart suggesting that her little island was one of peace and tranquility.

Jon's task is to insert a hollow tube, a catheter, into Greta's femoral (leg) artery, then thread it back through the aorta (the body's main artery) until it reaches the origin of the two coronary arteries (which supply the heart with blood). He then injects a dye to create a moving image of each vessel on X-ray film.

All eyes fix on the monitor as Jon injects X-ray dye to outline Greta's left coronary artery. She notices how suddenly the soft background of noise from nurses and technicians ominously falls silent. The TV monitor displays a severe narrowing in Greta's left coronary artery near its origin from the aorta. No wonder she is having chest pain with exercise. An obstruction high in the left coronary artery means that all the heart muscle served by that vessel was in jeopardy. A few minutes later when Jon injects her right coronary artery, another obstruction, high in the vessels appears. Staring at the monitor, Jon's jaw drops. He is looking at the worst of all coronary anatomic conditions: virtually every muscle fiber in the heart of thirty-five-year-old Greta Adams is at risk.

In the room's sepulchral silence, Greta's voice whispered. "What do you see?"

Jon leaned close. It was not into her ears his words were whispered, but into her heart. "Greta, you have blocks in both coronary arteries. These types of obstructions are best treated by a cardiac surgeon."

"When?" was the only word she could croak out.

"This afternoon, Greta. Now."

Those four words shattered whatever was left of Greta's fragile façade. It collapsed as suddenly and totally as an Alaskan glacier. Greta sobbed openly. Tears fell into a pool of words Greta's heart could not express.

Then, the improbable became the impossible. As she lay struggling to close the floodgate of emotion, Greta's heartbeat became irregular. In less than a minute, her systolic blood pressure, initially in the low normal range of 110, faded as fast as a flame without oxygen. Now it was 90, then 80, 70, 60 . . . then suddenly the metronomic beep of the ECG monitor stopped altogether. Her heart was in ventricular fibrillation—the dreaded rhythm of sudden death. Ventricular fibrillation ("v fib" in cath lab parlance) is uncoordinated quivering of the muscle of the ventricle, in which the pumping action of the heart is lost. The quivering is due to chaotic ventricular electrical activity in the ventricle, which is readily apparent on the electrocardiogram as small irregular waves. Untreated ventricular fibrillation becomes a "flat-line" if not treated immediately.

Four hours earlier, thirty-five-year-old Greta Adams strode athletically into the hospital with an unknown malady. Two hours later she was diagnosed with a high probability of CAD. In another two hours she was told she had life-threatening CAD. And three minutes after that stunning diagnosis, she was dead. Greta Adams. Energetic wife. Devoted mother. A happy carefree soul had left her family, had passed to the other side with neither a good-bye, nor a word of protest.

What now? A half a century earlier Greta would have been permanently dead. But today although Greta was dead, she was not gone. Unlike Willie the Phillie whose journey ended abruptly on a 1960s Philadelphia morning, Greta's new life was just beginning. Jon would have to protect her brain from irreversible damage during her cardiac arrest, restore her heartbeat, reopen her closed coronary arteries, keep them open, and prevent further atheroma formation for the rest of her life. How far could Greta tread along this path? As Jon struggles to restore Greta to conscious existence, he will have to use virtually every important cardiovascular advance of the past half century. If she could return to full health Greta Adams's story would, within the life of just a single person, encapsulate the history of what is assuredly the most chaotic, inspiring, and, yes, greatest medical victory of our times. And so we must track back in our medical tale to the days and hours just before cardiac surgery slipped from the womb into the gloved hands of a young battlefield surgeon in World War II.

2

"WHAT MAN MEANT FOR EVIL, GOD MEANT FOR GOOD"

He who wishes to be a surgeon should go to war.

—Hippocrates, Greek physician

OUR STORY BEGINS as the United States mobilizes World War II hospitals throughout Europe and Asia, and surgeon Dwight Harken departs his secure position in the Harvard Department of Surgery to join the U.S. Army Corps group stationed in Luftwaffe-bombed London. Born in Osceola, Iowa, from his early years Dwight Harken had the personality of a man destined to command. With a booming voice, a mane of fiery red hair, and a temper to match, square-jawed Dwight had bulldozed his way to the top of academia, first as a Harvard medical student and later as a young member of the Harvard faculty. As the thirty-five-year-old newly appointed chief of thoracic surgery at the London 160th General Hospital, Harken had never dreamed anything like this as he left Boston: bombs from overhead, fires raging in the streets, and in his operating room, dying soldiers with chests blown wide open, shards of shrapnel scattered throughout their chest cavity, ragged tissue oozing blood. Fresh from university surgical training, Harken now stared down at a patient's operating field in complete chaos. No careful incision exposed the thoracic cavity; rather ragged irregular fragments of white rib framed gaping wounds like the bloody teeth of a great white shark. The lungs were not smoothly retracted to reveal a beating heart. Rather they were shredded, and with each inspiration they oozed blood that welled up into the surgical field faster than one assistant working with gauze or suction could remove it.

Nothing in Harken's training had remotely prepared him for this vision of human ruination. Civilian gunshot wounds create a small round bullet-sized entry wound, and a larger exit wound. Shrapnel was devilishly different. The military offered him no pamphlet of surgical management. No sage professor stood over his shoulder to say, "Let's consider doing it this way." In a battlefield hospital, each young surgeon was on his own. His decisions had to be instantaneous. Like an implacable drill sergeant, the battlefield operating room made three demands: be decisive, be fast, and have good hands. But there was one other requirement. It was psychological. The effective surgeon had to ignore the psychic trauma of his inexperience in the face of such calamities, of his inability to staunch the constant flow of blood, of his failure to save another wounded young soldier's life. Self-criticism and second-guessing became deadly academic relics; this was a new place and time. To do his job, to save a life, the battlefield surgeon needed to be supremely confident and never look back.

I first met Dwight Harken some years later when he was a professor and I was beginning my specialty training as a cardiology fellow learning the newly invented technique of coronary angiography at Peter Bent Brigham (now Brigham and Women's) Hospital in Boston. Years later after I entered academic medicine, we invited Dwight to be a visiting professor at Cedars-Sinai, and on other occasions I felt honored to share the podium with him at national cardiovascular symposia. Dwight Harken was a man you'd never forget. He was the quintessential "can do" American, stepping from the pages of Tom Brokaw's *The Greatest Generation*. When Harken expressed a strongly held opinion, which was pretty much all the time, his face turned bright crimson, leading some of us at Harvard (behind his back of course) to call him the Great Red Man. By the time I met him he dominated every clinical cardiology conference, and at dinner he dominated every conversation. President Teddy Roosevelt's daughter's description of her father seemed to fit Dwight Harken perfectly:

He "always wanted to be the corpse at every funeral, the bride at every wedding, and the baby at every christening."

Like Roosevelt, Dwight Harken was an iconoclast with a font of new ideas, and he expected you to share his enthusiasm. He was unpredictable. He could be deliberately intimidating to young physicians (including me) on hospital rounds. He could shout ferociously at a resident in the operating room, emerge minutes later to be self-deprecating and humble in an interview, and later be hugely entertaining as a cocktail party raconteur. But to me he had one characteristic that overshadowed all others. He had unshakable self-confidence in the operating room. I found myself admiring this man so open with his feelings, an intriguing mix of humility and bombast, sensitivity and arrogance, self-confidence and insecurity.

In his London operating theater Harken confronted dying soldiers with slivers of shrapnel embedded in their beating hearts. Shrapnel is a vicious projectile named after its inventor, eighteenth-century English artillery officer Major General Henry Shrapnel. Placed within the projectile are small balls of lead shot and an explosive charge to scatter the shot and the fragments of the shell casing. Shrapnel's uniquely grisly contribution to the art of human maiming was that he designed his projectiles to burst apart in the air, raining down tiny missiles to penetrate the faces, brains, and chests of soldiers scattered over a wide swath of land below.

As he examined the metal fragments protruding from his soldiers' hearts Harken faced a gruesome choice. If he left a fragment of shrapnel inside a heart chamber, the soldier faced two daunting risks. Blood clots could form on the metal surface, break off and travel to other organs; if one of these biologic bullets lodged in the vessels of his patient's brain it caused a stroke. Equally likely, bacteria could find a home on the metal shards, which served as miniature petri culture dishes, a source to whisk blood-borne infection to every organ throughout the body. This condition, called bacterial endocarditis, was at that time invariably fatal.

Harken's other option was to yank the shrapnel out of the soldier's heart. Now he faced an instant torrent of bleeding from the hole he left behind. In the operating room I have seen sudden unexpected arterial bleeding, like Old Faithful, awesome in its power and bone-chilling in its implication. If the hole is in the main pumping chamber, the left ventricle, each contraction of the heart can unleash a narrow geyser of blood that splatters the operating room ceiling. For me the surge of panic that comes with the unanticipated sudden appearance of arterial bleeding is an indelible memory.

Harken became obsessed by the thought that these young men, still alive with strong, beating hearts, should not be condemned to death by the Hobson's choice of action or inaction. He was looking at hearts too good to die.

Harken knew well the history of surgery on the heart, what there was of it. The most famous case of survival, reported by German surgeon Ludwig Rehn at the turn of the century, bore some resemblance to his problem. Soon after midnight on the morning of September 7, 1896, a drunken twenty-two-year-old gardener's assistant named Wilhelm Justus had lurched along the gravel paths of the scenic park bordering the Main River that bisects Frankfurt, Germany. Fleeing a raucous barroom brawl in the red light district, he stumbled and hit the ground. As he rolled to his feet, a massive form loomed above him in the moonlit sky and metal glinted as a knife hit his chest. Just after 3 a.m., a strolling policeman discovered Wilhelm Justus supine behind a park bench, semiconscious and unresponsive, nostrils flaring as he gasped for breath. His right hand was clenched under his jacket. Kneeling to examine Justus further, the policeman immediately ascertained that the hand covered a small slash that slowly oozed onto a blood-drenched shirt.

At Frankfurt City Hospital the night surgeon found an unconscious young man, with cold and clammy skin and a thready, irregular pulse that briefly disappeared with each inspiration. He carefully inserted a probe into the half-inch wound in the space between the fourth and fifth ribs. Deeper and deeper the probe slid into the body, meeting no resistance. Then it halted and began bobbing in and out of the wound with each heartbeat. As dawn broke the surgeon pronounced his grim prognosis: Justus had a wound to the heart for which there was no treatment. Wilhelm was sent to a private room with the reasonable certainty that, like many thousands of injured warriors over mankind's turbulent history, he would die without regaining consciousness. It was a trivial blessing that unlike so many who preceded him, he would spend his last moments in an environment with a modicum of quiet dignity.

But to Wilhelm Justus was granted the good fortune offered to no one in the prior history of medicine. The chief surgeon at Frankfurt City Hospital was the world-famous Ludwig Rehn. At age forty-seven, Rehn stood as a revolutionary, an innovator who questioned the often tenuous wisdom of his predecessors. When Rehn saw him, Wilhelm was unconscious. Rehn tapped his fingers over the left side of Wilhelm's chest wall to outline the dull resonance of the heart bordered by the air-filled lungs. Whereas the area of cardiac dullness normally extends to the left nipple, he found it now extended to the armpit. Rehn thought about the policeman's account and Wilhelm's symptoms and his physical examination; his fertile imagination visualized what lay unseen within the chest cavity. He knew that in addition to placing the heart behind the bony sternum and ribs, Nature has surrounded and protected it within a tough fibrous sac called the pericardium. Rehn reasoned that when the stiletto slipped between his ribs to enter deep into Justus's chest, it first punctured a small hole in the pericardium and then penetrated further to barely nick the heart muscle. The nick in the heart muscle caused oozing of some blood, but because the hole in the pericardium was small, the blood was all trapped within the firm fibrous sac. As the blood accumulated within it, the blood-filled sac compressed the heart, just as if a hand was gripping it, restricting the inflow of blood into the heart's pumping chambers.

Like Harken a half a century later, when Rehn closed his eyes he visualized a heart too good to die. The heart, with just a nick on its surface, could function normally if he could remove the blood from the sac that was compressing it, and close the nick with a stich or two on the heart's surface to stop further blood accumulation in the sac. Fully aware that many surgeons had failed miserably in similar circumstances he ordered that Justus be taken to the operating room. Opening the chest, Rehn saw the pericardial sac distended with blood to twice its normal size. The heart lay trapped within. He slashed open the sac with his scalpel. Blood gushed from the incision, then within seconds slowed to a tiny trickle. Rehn could now see the heart beating within the sac. Each time the heart filled, blood trickled from a half-inch tear in the wall of the right ventricle. Instinctively, he pressed his left index finger over the cut. The pressure of his finger staunched the bleeding. Justus's heartbeat continued steady but feeble. With his right hand, each time the heart filled Rehn placed a suture to close the wound. The bleeding stopped. And then the surgeon's version of exaltation in Beethoven's Ninth Symphony, the ineffable emotion of snatching a young man's life back from certain death. A century later we can still marvel at the moment's stark contrast to the starched science of Rehn's later description: "bleeding is controlled with finger pressure . . . suture the heart wound tied in diastole . . . bleeding diminished remarkably with the third suture . . . heart rate and respiratory rate decreased and pulse improved." Rehn closed the chest. Two hours later Wilhelm Justus was awake and resting comfortably, with a normal pulse and blood pressure.

Rehn immediately understood the implication of his success. He imagined that his report would galvanize a new surgical era. His lofty aspiration to be a father of cardiac surgery, however, was not to be. Although Rehn's scalpel had laid bare the folly of centuries-old dogma that the heart was off-limits for surgery, his report became an anecdote rather than a breakthrough. In medicine, as we shall see throughout our chronicle, credit goes to the person who convinces the world, not to the one with the first idea. Harken succeeded where Rehn failed because Rehn operated on one man, whereas Harken would operate on another 133-soldiers with shrapnel in their chest cavity, some embedded directly in the heart.

For the half century after Rehn, few dared to operate directly on the human heart, and the few who tried failed. The twin fears of condemnation by colleagues and killing patients outright stayed the hand of even the most adventuresome surgeons. And woe to the surgeon who chose to challenge entrenched authority. The voice of the great Viennese surgeon Theodor Billroth still boomed paternalistically through the decades: "A surgeon who tries to suture a heart wound deserves to lose the esteem of his colleagues." Billroth's eminent English contemporary Stephen Paget pronounced the final, never-to-be challenged, eternal verdict: "Surgery of the heart has probably reached the limits set by Nature to all surgery: no new method, and no new discovery, can overcome the natural difficulties that attend a wound of the heart."

After World War I, Harvard's pioneering surgeon Elliot Cutler attempted to treat severe narrowing of the mitral valve, the valve between the left atrium and the left ventricle, that limits entry of blood into the heart's main pumping chamber. His idea was to make a tiny incision in the heart wall, insert a cutting device through the incision, cut out a piece of the narrowed valve. Cutler's reasoning was only partly correct. Although removing a portion of the valve improved forward flow across the valve, it also allowed torrential backflow when the heart contracted. All but one of seven patients in whom he cut out a portion of the narrowed valve died. Deeply discouraged by so many deaths, Cutler abandoned the procedure. One of the great ironies of research, however, is that we learn more from our failures than from our successes, more from unexpected results than from those we anticipate. Destiny decreed that Elliot Cutler would be Dwight Harken's mentor. Harken learned the details of Cutler's failed technique. Now he would use that knowledge to piece together the shards of Cutler's shattered dream, transforming his failure into an initial baby step on the road to success.

In London's battlefield hospital, Harken devised a plan of action. His idea was simple enough. It was Rehn's finger-in-the-dike strategy. Of course if the hole was bigger than his finger, if his finger slipped off the slick surface of the bleeding heart, if he couldn't completely close the hole with sutures, if the taut silk sutures tore a little further through the heart muscle with each contraction, he would fail. So many ways to fail, so few to succeed. If he failed, his would be the image of a man holding a squirming, writhing, ruptured fire hose gushing five quarts of blood a minute throughout the room for a minute or two, followed by devastating, demoralizing, humiliating, condemning, awesome silence. Death on the table.

When is it ethical to take an action that might kill a patient immediately, particularly if no one had ever done it before? Harken was confronting nothing less than a confrontation with medicine's most hallowed three words: primum non nocere—"First do no harm"—a principle as enduring and as sacrosanct as the Hippocratic Oath. In our story we will encounter this conundrum repeatedly: medical research pits two laudable principles against each other. Medical breakthrough versus benevolence. Progress versus compassion. Harken argued that his conscience was clear: "You have to have a diagnosis that is absolute, a condition that is incurable and, then, if you have any rational concept of how you might attack it, you have the right to try," he said.

Harken argued his case at U.S. Army Corps headquarters. His superiors pointed to the common surgical wisdom of centuries. They buttressed their argument with recent reports that surgeons in the French theater had failed in attempts to extract shrapnel from the heart. Harken countered that since his surgical approach was unique and untested, it deserved to be tried in these dying young men. The balance tipped in his favor when the president of the British Royal College of Surgeons unexpectedly agreed with Harken that at least his proposal was logical, that no one could say with certainty that it wouldn't work. A tepid endorsement, indeed.

In June 1944 Dwight Harken was brought a dying soldier with a gaping injury to his sternum and ribs. The heart's right ventricle lies directly behind the sternum, Nature's impenetrable bony shield. Ancients saw Nature's logic. The word *sternum* descends from the Greek word *sternon*, meaning a soldier's breastplate. As his assistants used retractors to widen Harken's field of view within the chest cavity, he saw shrapnel had penetrated the right ventricle.

For days and weeks leading up to this moment Harken had imagined his every move. First, he placed sutures in a complete circle around the point of shrapnel entry. Harken tried to grasp the end of the protruding fragment of shrapnel, with a clamp (called a hemostat). The ragged sliver of gunmetal bobbed back and forth continuously with each heartbeat, insolently waving at him, a metronome counting down the solder's remaining hours, death by bleeding or by infection. When Harken succeeded in clamping on to the evasive shard, the two men were linked by the soldier's only possible bridge to survival, Harken's hemostat. I can only imagine myself with my own hand on Harken's clamp.

That night Harken described the terrifying sequence of what happened next in a letter to his wife: "For a moment I stood with a clamp on the fragment that was inside the heart, and the heart was not bleeding." Harken steeled himself to commit to the act he had only imagined. He yanked. "Then suddenly with a pop, as if a champagne cork had been drawn, the fragment jumped out of the ventricle, forced by the pressure within the chamber . . . blood poured out in a torrent." He tightened the sutures around the wound. But still the bleeding continued. His patient was bleeding to death on the table. "I told the first and second assistants to cross the sutures and I put my finger over the awful leak. The torrent slowed, stopped, and with my finger in situ [in place over the wound], I took large needles swedged with silk and began passing them through the heart muscle wall, under my finger, and out the other side. With four of these in, I slowly removed my finger as one after the other was tied. . . . Blood pressure did drop, but the only moment of panic was when we discovered that one suture had gone through the glove on the finger that had stemmed the flood. I was sutured to the wall of the heart! We cut the glove and I got loose . . ." Years later, in the macabre humor that characterizes doctors in close encounters with death, we joked (Did I mention, behind his back?) that Harken could have done just as well if he had cut off his finger and left it there.

Emotions surged through Dwight Harken. Exhilaration. He had saved a young man who otherwise would have died. Relief. He had overcome a moment of panic. Vindication. He had proven his skeptics wrong. If he allowed his imagination to roam more broadly, he might even imagine that he had created a brand-new phrase for Webster's dictionary: "cardiac surgeon."

Yet as he stripped off his surgical gloves, even Harken could hardly have imagined how history would revere this day. It was the day of the largest amphibious invasion in world history, when 195,700 Allied personnel in over 5,000 ships landed on a fifty-mile stretch along the beaches of the Normandy coast. It was D-day. Like twins, the turning point of World War II and cardiac surgery would have the same birth date. The world could resist the Nazi army, but not the idea whose time had come. As Walter Cronkite, the great newscaster of the outset of this era, liked to remark: "What sort of a day was it? A day like all days, filled with those events that alter and illuminate our times."

Harken had discovered an unprecedented, lifesaving strategy. In retrospect, I have wondered if he succeeded where others failed because of his instantaneous decision to use two strategies to prevent his sutures from cutting through the muscle with each heartbeat. First, he used "swedges," tiny cloth rolls wedged between the silk sutures and the heart muscle that prevented the sutures from cutting. Second Harken deliberately tied his sutures, as Ludwig Rehn had, during the split second when the heart relaxed and reached its largest volume, so that the heart's alternating expansion and contraction did not place extra stress on the sutures.

Harken, like Rehn half a century before him, understood the implications of his success. Unlike Rehn, however, he took the next step. Over the ensuing months he removed shrapnel from the hearts of sixteen soldiers. Not a single soldier died.

Harken informed the world of his stunning success in the *American Heart Journal* in July 1946. The first sentence of his twenty-page manuscript speaks to the future by recalling the past. Harvard academician to the core, he quotes the Greeks: "Aristotle wrote, 'The heart alone of all viscera cannot withstand serious injury.'" Harken added quotes from Billroth and Paget before proceeding to demolish them with compelling photographs and graphs. On that muggy July day, an idea that stood sacrosanct for two millennia, "Do not touch the heart," vanished from medicine. Of the Nazi shrapnel lodged in the hearts of young soldiers, the trigger of cardiology's first great turning point in the battle with heart disease, it could be said, "although man meant it for evil, God meant it for good."

WHY HAD HARKEN succeeded where other surgeons, including his contemporaries, failed? What was the source of Harken's intuition, his genius, his sixth sense? In his contemporary bestseller *Outliers* Malcolm Gladwell proposes that the person the world sees as an innovative genius is instead often the product of vast experience. Gladwell points to the Beatles' thousands of hours performing in Hamburg, Germany beer halls before they exploded on the world of music, and to Bill Gates's years of writing computer programs in high school at the dawn of the digital era. Could Harken's innovative genius be one more example? Every textbook that relates the history of cardiac surgery describes Dwight Harken's brilliant burst of innovative genius but in none have I found the tale that Harken told his friends.

Prior to the United States's entry into World War II, Harken had been trying to develop a method for removing bacterial infections from the surface of heart valves in the Harvard animal research laboratory. Pathologists, with their penchant for conflating the grisly with the edible, call these infections vegetations. They appear as soft mounds of clotted blood and bacteria attached to the heart valves. Cardiac pathologists have bequeathed us a feast of culinary delights, like the nutmeg liver of heart failure and the bread and butter heart of pericarditis. To develop a surgical approach to vegetations on valves Harken spent countless hours in the animal laboratory trying to develop a model that mimicked the human condition. After many failures he finally hit upon an answer: he speared a dog's mitral valve with a dirty safety pin. A clot and infection quickly formed on the pin. With his model, Harken then spent countless hours trying to surgically extract the pin from the valve without killing the dog in the process. When he was called to the battlefield in World War II, he had just succeeded in extracting a safety pin from within a dog's heart in his Boston laboratory. How difficult was it to make the mental leap from a safety pin to a sliver of shrapnel? And what was the essence of the method for extracting the safety pin? What else but sutures encircling his finger? Dwight Harken's genius in the battlefield operating room, like Bill Gates's genius at the genesis of Microsoft, was real, but the hunch was an educated guess based on years of unheralded prior experience.

And why did Harken tread a path to success whereas Ludwig Rehn with the same result entered a blind alley a half a century earlier in Frankfurt? After all, both had arrived at the same precedent-shattering answer: the heart is a legitimate surgical target.

As we will see, in science the best answers always lead to new questions. The unanswered "yes-but" question that followed Harken's success came from Britain's great thoracic surgeon Lord Brock, who pointedly needled Harken after he demonstrated his technique in the London operating room theater: "Dwight, what useful purpose can this be turned to? After all, no shell fragments presumably are going to appear in people's hearts in a peacetime situation." Brock was of course correct. Harken's achievement seemed little more than a parlor trick. It saved lives, but there were not many men with metal stuck in their hearts back in Boston or London. Ludwig Rehn had not had an answer, but Dwight Harken would.

3

A RIVER OF BLOOD

The tallest trees are most in the power of the winds, and
ambitious men of the blasts of fortune.

—William Penn, founder of Pennsylvania

HISTORIANS HAVE LONG noted that after victory in war, countries often experience an outburst of peacetime creativity. The chaos of war severs the shackles of conventional wisdom, infusing the victor with visions of new vitality. At war's end, the United States was the world's superpower, poised to initiate a phenomenal boom in international innovation and productivity. British Prime Minister Winston Churchill pronounced the verdict, "America at this moment stands at the summit of the world." Optimism infused all walks of life. The economy boomed. The rate of new childbirths escalated to eight every minute. Economist John Galbraith christened "the affluent society" as young couples bought suburban homes, television sets, washing machines, Studebakers or finned Cadillacs, and danced to rock 'n' roll. Belief in the power to create, in both science and medicine, was boundless. After all, the brilliant atomic physicists of the Manhattan Project had brought the war to an abrupt end. In medicine, penicillin, tetracycline, and new antibiotics had suddenly made infections manageable. Life expectancy had increased by twenty-five years in just fifty years. New hospitals were springing up across the country at the rate of two each day, ready to provide cures for every illness.

But the new illnesses were not the old ones. The new diseases were heart disease and cancer, and the old guard of medicine had no remedies for either. Worse, the gray-haired eminences of the medical establishment had no idea where to find them. So just as American's youth was soon to reject the teaching and values of their parents, so did a tiny handful of medical revolutionaries, the young thoracic surgeons returning from World War II, reject the myths and beliefs of their surgical elders. They would be the ones to confront heart disease.

My own early memories of those early postwar years circle around the social life in my house when I was in grade school. Soon after my physician-father returned from the war, we moved into our new postwar home on a street nicknamed Pill Hill because four doctors lived on the same long sloping block. When my father's doctor friends stopped by, I strategically positioned myself beneath a mahogany drop-leaf table my mother had placed against the back of our living room sofa. Unseen but still within earshot I listened as my father, whom I revered, the next-door cardiologist, and the doctors from up the street discussed their patients. When the mystery of a patient's symptoms was solved by my pathologist father's microscope, I beamed with secret delight. But most of all I was moved by the doctors' humanity as they told their patients' stories. Science with compassion. One day I wanted to be like them, beneficence and expert knowledge in a humble white coat.

As I eavesdropped beneath the table I could not imagine that the cardiologist's diagnostic tool kit was limited to a blood pressure cuff, otoscope, stethoscope, an ECG, and a chest X-ray. Worse, his medicine bag had little more than aspirin, digitalis, nitroglycerin, a few topical antimicrobials, and some derivatives of roots. He knew his drugs' safety and efficacy, but virtually nothing about their mechanism of action. The truth was that postwar cardiology could transiently relieve some symptoms of heart disease, but could not alter its course at all. The postwar cardiologist could offer only a modicum more than doctors in Voltaire's time when "the art of medicine consists in amusing the patient while nature cures the disease."

WHEN DWIGHT HARKEN came home, he set out to change that world. It is said that a pile of rocks ceases to be a rock pile when a single man gazes on it bearing within him the image of a cathedral. Dwight

Harken had imagined his cathedral in that battlefield hospital. He would attack mitral valve stenosis, the same disease that had confounded his mentor Elliot Cutler. If he was successful, he would have a permanent place in the history of his profession as the first to operate successfully on the human heart. Harken soon learned that another unknown young battlefield surgeon shared both his vision and his unbounded self-confidence about surgical repair of the mitral valve.

Dr. Charles Bailey of Philadelphia was the polar opposite of Harken. He had been raised by his mother in a dusty small New Jersey town mired in Depression-era poverty. His small-town banker father, destroyed financially in the Depression, died from mitral stenosis at age forty-two, "coughing blood into a basin as my mother tried to soothe him." Bailey was forced to become self-sufficient just as he entered his teenage years when his father died. With only a widowed mother to care for him, both nature and experience stitched combativeness into hardscrabble Charles Bailey's psyche. His mother, a real-life version of Tennessee Williams's Blanche DuBois with ambition, hopes, dreams, and consuming desire to return to better days, focused on Charles becoming a doctor. The devoted son did not disappoint, and did not deviate from the course set for him by his mother. After two years at Rutgers University he entered Hahnemann Medical College, moved to New York to train in surgery, then returned to join the Hahnemann surgical staff at the academic entry level of lecturer, ready to cross scalpels with Harken.

TWENTY-FOUR-YEAR-OLD Housewife Constance Warner had lived a normal childhood until that day she got a fever and a severe sore throat. When she developed joint pain and ring-shaped eruptions on her arms and legs, her mother took her to the doctor. He performed an ECG; it was abnormal. He diagnosed rheumatic fever, the predominant cause of heart valve damage before the discovery of penicillin. In her teens, when Constance seemed to fatigue more easily than others, her doctor said that Constance had a heart murmur. Then soon after the birth of her first child, her health had begun a rapid descent into invalidism. Now she was unable to care for her baby, profoundly weak, and short of breath with the most minimal exertion. Her cardiologist said that rheumatic fever had scarred the valve between her left atrium and left ventricle, leaving it severely narrowed. Her doctors called her condition mitral valve stenosis, and said there was no treatment. Constance rejected her summary verdict: no surgical treatment. Just a condemnation to slow deterioration and a gruesome death drowning in one's own blood.

There *were* two surgeons, one in Boston and the other in Philadelphia, who were willing to tackle the problem, but all they did was make death come quickly . . . in the operating room. Against her family doctor's advice and aware of the risk of almost certain death that she faced, Constance and her husband, Morton, went to Philadelphia to meet Dr. Charles Bailey.

PREMATURELY BALDING WITH closely cropped hair and pursed lips, Bailey could have passed for an easily irritated marine drill sergeant except for the huge professorial wire-rimmed glasses perched on his straight nose. His personality reflected this dichotomy. Bailey was part irascible sergeant and part academic intellectual. Hahnemann lacked the academic cachet of Harken's Harvard. Bailey had none of Harken's panache and people skills. He disdained pretension and seemed intent on making it abundantly clear that he cared not a whit for others' opinions. When he formed a theory he saw each new fact as confirming his ideas. When challenged he was typically aggressive and confrontational. Although he lacked Harken's academic record and Harvard patois, he was Harken's equal in vaulting ambition, self-confidence, and drive to innovate. Bailey's passion, however, was intense and personal, steeped in righteous messianic contempt for the disease that killed his father.

Typically, doctors who become professors earn far less income than those in private practice. The currency of academic medicine, then and now, is recognition. For the academician the sometimes irresistible siren song is acclaim and power, an attraction every bit as seductive and compelling as money. In medicine, there is no greater accomplishment than being the first to successfully implement a treatment that changes the history of medicine. Charles Bailey was tied to no mast. He and Harken both recognized the limitless future of cardiac surgery for congenital heart disease, valve disease, and ultimately the final prize, coronary artery disease.

Both wanted surgery's greatest prize, the mythical title, the public recognition, the worldwide acclaim accorded to the mythical Father of Cardiac Surgery.

Bailey challenged Harken across an academic and cultural gulf that echoed the centuries-old competition between Boston and Philadelphia, The Cradle of Liberty vs. The Birthplace of a Nation, John Adams vs. Ben Franklin, Harvard vs. Hahnemann, Russell vs. Chamberlain. Harken was the charming silk-stocking Bostonian, Bailey the cantankerous Philadelphia proletarian. Although both were iconoclasts, Harken was an academic who reveled in challenging ideas; Bailey reveled in challenging people. He cared little for others' opinions when they conflicted with his own. Convinced of his righteousness Charles Bailey hewed to his own, not society's, behests and standards. Society be damned.

For the two adversaries, the battle was winner take all. If Harken had any thoughts about sharing the pinnacle, Bailey was blunt: "In India, you never find two male tigers on the same hill." By the time a victor was crowned two and a half years later, the psychological endurance of both tigers would be tested almost beyond endurance.

The left atrium collects blood coming from the lungs, and delivers it to the left ventricle, which pumps blood to the body. The mitral valve separates the two chambers. When I look at a normal mitral valve, it reminds me of two white sheets pressed against each other, and each tethered to one side of the inner wall of the ventricle. When the heart is relaxed, its sheets go slack, falling away from each other, allowing blood to flow into the left ventricle. When the ventricle contracts, the force of blood against the sheets causes them to billow backward, just like sails in the wind. The two sheets slam against each other closing the opening between the atrium and the ventricle.

Mitral stenosis is severe narrowing of the opening between the sheets of the mitral valve. A tragic sequel of rheumatic fever, mitral stenosis is like a subway train door at Manhattan rush hour or a closed tunnel exit in a soccer stadium. Blood cells behind the narrowed opening in the valve back up into the lungs "congesting" them. When the blood vessels can swell no more, they burst. If the vessel is large, the patient literally drowns in her own blood.

To relieve the valve narrowing, the purse-string suture Harken had used to encircle shrapnel was the key. Instead of tightening the purse string as he pulled out the shrapnel, he would tighten the sutures as he inserted his index finger into the heart just above the mitral valve. He then blindly would push his finger into the narrowed mitral valve orifice, and by force-fully wiggling his finger back and forth, tear apart the scar tissue that fused sheets (called "leaflets") of the valve. Today I marvel anyone would attempt such an incredibly crude procedure. Even in an era before heart surgery, reasoning that you could treat valve disease by sticking your index finger through a hole in the heart was wildly outside the box. But still, there was also the strange logic that if the surgeon was lucky, the tearing force of his finger could separate the two fused sheets along their original natural lines of separation without shredding them, allowing a marked increase of blood flow across the valve.

In November 1945 Bailey made his move. He operated on a man dying the slow inevitable death of severe mitral stenosis. The details of his surgical strategy were simple in concept. Open the chest to expose the heart. Place a circle of sutures in the left atrium just above the mitral valve. Make a small incision in the atrium within the circle and quickly insert the index finger into the hole. Advance the finger to the mitral valve. Use the finger to blindly tear apart the scar tissue that had fused the leaflets of the valve together. Withdraw the finger while simultaneously tightening the sutures. Voilà, a cure of mitral stenosis. Bailey could visualize it so clearly. No more blood backed up behind the valve, no more bursting vessels in the lung, no more nightmares of his father coughing blood into a basin.

Bailey's first patient was eerily reminiscent of his father. Walter Stockton was thirty-seven years old, with a sixteen-year history of shortness of breath and weakness from mitral stenosis. In the past year he had had severe episodes of coughing up blood. He was quite clearly approaching the catastrophic denouement of his life. On a crisp November 1945 Philadelphia morning in the Hahnemann operating room Bailey made a long incision between the third and fourth ribs. He inserted a rib spreader to create a wider surgical field. As he had practiced in the animal laboratory, he made a small incision in the pericardium, which allowed him to expose the surface of the left atrium. Next, he stitched a circle of sutures (threads) into the surface of the atrium, in the form of a purse string.

His stitches in place, Bailey paused to absorb the full physical and emotional panorama of what was to be a transcendent moment in medical history. Satisfied, he made a small incision in the atrium. He was met instantly by a torrent, a gushing fury of bright red blood, a fierce insistent reply to the audacity of his incision, as if he had released years of the heart's pent-up rage. Bailey immediately inserted his gloved index finger into the incision, as if to stem the sudden surge from a broken dike, while simultaneously tightening his purse-string sutures, just as Harken had described. But the blood kept coming, his patient's life now spilling through his fingers into the open chest cavity, obscuring vision, as sutures meant to close the gap instead shredded the tissue, culminating in chaos as clamps tore even larger rents in the atrium.

Bailey described the carnage: "The purse-string suture was pulled upon and tore out . . . Severe bleeding occurred and a large clamp was hastily applied . . . The clamp cut through the appendage wall . . . It was impossible to get sutures to hold." In the space of a minute or so Bailey witnessed a violent burbling of blood, then gentle spurts, then sporadic pulsations, then nothing but horrifying stillness. In Bailey's terse later description: "Massive uncontrollable hemorrhage resulted in immediate fatality." In a space of a few hundred horrifying seconds, Charles Bailey had utterly failed his thirty-seven-year-old patient. He had failed the memory of his father. He had gained nothing but a new nightmare.

Bailey returned to the animal lab, tinkering with alternate ways to approach the problem. Perhaps the finger was not the best way to reopen the mitral valve orifice. Six months later he was ready to try again. Twenty-nine-year-old Wilma Stevens was a mother of two, already in desperate condition from her disease. She breathed heavily from fluid accumulation in her lungs. Her body was frail but her abdomen was swollen. Her liver was huge and tender. Wilma had the typical signs of end-stage heart failure. This time Bailey fit a tubular metal device over the tip of his finger, then attempted to disrupt the scar that stenosed the mitral valve. When he did so, Wilma turned blue. Bailey withdrew the device and resorted to tearing apart the scar tissue with his finger. Instead of tearing along the lines of fusion of the two leaflets of the valve, however, he shredded them. It was as if he had removed the mitral valve. Each heartbeat now sent torrents of blood flowing backward to the lungs. Wilma was not better, she was much worse. She survived the procedure, but died on the second postoperative day. Whispers depicting horrifying images of operating room chaos found ready ears in the halls of Hahnemann Hospital. Charles Bailey, never an endearing figure, now had acquired a universal new name among the nurses and medical staff. He was Butcher Bailey.

Bailey stood alone, a powerful grizzly surrounded by baying hounds. He pointed to Harken who was up in Boston, matching him patient for patient with similar failures. His colleagues countered that madness in Boston never justified similar behavior in Philadelphia, that his surgeries were unjustifiable, that Hahnemann Hospital had an ethical responsibility to terminate Bailey's human experimentation, that failure to do so betrayed the trust that the city of Philadelphia had invested in the hospital and its physicians. Hahnemann Hospital's headstrong misfit Charles Bailey had to be stopped before it was too late. Cooler heads suggested they reason with Bailey. Dr. George Goekler, Hahnemann's chief of cardiology, asked that Bailey come to his office to discuss the shame he was bringing to his institution, his profession, and to himself.

Bailey recounted the meeting: "First, he allowed me the privilege of the floor, which took up practically the entire interview . . . Then he pulled out a previous typewritten sheet of paper on which he had methodically explained that as a physician it was his Hippocratic duty to do no harm when he could do no good. He ended up telling me it was his Christian duty to keep me from doing any more of these homicidal operations." His response to Goekler's reasoned rebuke was pure Bailey: "I responded with some heat. I told him I believed in this operation, that I was sure I was right . . . and that it was my Christian duty to continue. We shook hands and I departed." No doubt Bailey felt that he had overwhelmed another opponent, that he had quite decisively won his argument with Goekler. If so, his was a Pyrrhic victory. Hours later Charles Bailey's operating privileges at Hahnemann were suspended. He had become Hahnemann's persona non grata.

No problem. Bailey drove down the Delaware River to unsuspecting Wilmington Memorial Hospital. His patient was thirty-eight-year-old William Wilson. Wilson also survived the operative procedure itself. But when Bailey opened Wilson's valve obstruction with his device, he overdid it. His device cut through scar that he was unable to separate with his finger, but it was too crude for finer dissection. The torn valve again lost its capacity to prevent backflow. In medical terms, he had converted mitral stenosis into mitral insufficiency. Wilson died on postoperative day five. When the Wilmington Hospital authorities became cognizant of Bailey's prior history at Hahnemann, Bailey's operating privileges at Wilmington Hospital were suspended. Now with three deaths, at age thirty-eight Charles Bailey had become a pariah among Philadelphia physicians. Discussions began about the possibility of presenting his cases to the Pennsylvania State Board of Medical Licensure in a petition to suspend his license to practice medicine. It seemed clear that one more attempt at "this homicidal operation" would terminate his entire surgical career.

Bailey's response arguably puts him in a class by himself for bullheadedness and hubris. He doubled down. There were two remaining local hospitals where he still retained surgical privileges. He might as well take his best shot: he scheduled two surgeries on the same day, one at each hospital. The 8 a.m. morning surgery was to be at Philadelphia General Hospital, to be followed by his second surgery in the afternoon at Episcopal Hospital on the other side of town. The strategy was as clear as it was cynical. As Bailey explained, "If the operations were done at different hospitals, the probability was great that news of a mortality during the first operation would not reach the second hospital in time to interrupt the performance of the later procedure." He would hope that the car was faster than the telephone.

As day dawned at Philadelphia General Hospital, Bailey opened the chest of thirty-year-old Jerome Randall. Disaster struck immediately. Each time he touched the heart, it responded with a volley of arrhythmia. Despite all available arrhythmia suppressing medications then available, his patient had a cardiac arrest. Bailey managed to revive the heart with manual cardiac massage. Seeing no hope for his patient if Bailey closed the chest and terminated the procedure, Jerome Randall's primary physician, who had accompanied his patient, urged Bailey to continue. Bailey refused, using the feeble reasoning that he would somehow calm his detractors by arguing that this death was not attributable to him, since it had preceded the actual cardiac surgery. Wanting to at least try the surgery yet escape criticism, Bailey then proposed what must be the most bizarre compromise in the history of cardiac surgery. He would agree to operate, but only after Randall's physician declared his patient dead. With the patient declared legally dead, Bailey opened the heart and separated the stenosed mitral valve with his finger. But it was indeed hopeless. Minutes later Jerome Randall's heart stopped forever.

NOW WITH FOUR deaths on his hands, Bailey returned to the dressing room, cleaned up, and headed for Episcopal Hospital to perform the procedure at which he had failed just hours before. Fail this time, and it was all over. At Episcopal Hospital, twenty-four-year-old housewife Constance Warner awaited him. Let's pause for a moment to salute the courage of this young woman, who epitomizes the bravery that we will so often behold in the patients in our narrative. Her chance of survival was remote. But even if she were the first to survive, who could say if she would feel more or less fatigued, more or less short of breath? When Constance Warner underwent anesthesia at age twenty-four, she had to imagine she would never wake up.

Bailey opened her atrium. Perhaps the solution to the dilemma of opening a scarred mitral valve lay in the combination of the device and the finger. He would use the device for crude separation, the finger for finer dissection. He slipped a curved blade over the end of his index finger, and inserted it into her atrium. He moved his finger over the scarred valve. There it was . . . the point at which the two leaflets had fused. The scar was too tough to separate with his finger, but if he could use the blade . . . Bailey used his curved blade to cut through the toughest scar on valve leaflets. Now he had a small groove that separated the fused leaflets. He withdrew his finger and slipped the blade off the tip of his finger. He reinserted his index finger. There was his groove. Now he could use his sense of touch to pry apart the remaining scar. By touch, at least, it seemed like an excellent separation. He withdrew his gloved finger. He closed the hole in her atrium. As he closed the incision in her chest, Bailey looked down at his sleeping patient and allowed himself just a ray of hope. This time, surely his last chance, every part of his surgery had gone well. When he finished, Charles Bailey harbored the hope, however forlorn, that he was discarding far more than his operating gown and mask.

Constance Warner's recovery was different from the very start. She returned to her bed with stable vital signs. By the third post-op day Constance got out of bed. She walked to the bathroom, then the halls. Her breathing, her energy, her sense of well-being already was vastly improved.

As Constance walked the ward, Bailey plotted his vindication. It lay a half continent and a week away, and it was pure Charles Bailey. At the end of the week, he convinced Constance to take a 1,000-mile train trip with him to Chicago. Before a packed auditorium at the annual meeting of the American College of Chest Physicians, the most prestigious professional organization of his peers, Charles Bailey rose to introduce Constance Warner. His presentation electrified the attendees. Sensational world headlines followed. Back in Philadelphia, daggers were sheathed as Bailey's critics fell silent. What had begun two weeks earlier as an outrageous duplicity had become an interesting footnote to a moment in history. Charles Bailey, the dirt-poor kid with the domineering mother, the commoner with unquenchable ambition, the avenging son, the curmudgeon battling pigheaded fools, the Chosen One, had seized the prize. Charles Bailey was cardiac surgery's Neil Armstrong: vaulted forward by the work of others, yet venturing where no person had gone before, he stepped out onto the lunar landscape of cardiac surgery and planted his flag.

AND WHAT ABOUT Constance Warner? When reporters contacted her nine years later in her second-floor walk-up apartment, Constance had a second child and was taking full care of her children. A walk-up apartment had been beyond her imagination a decade earlier. Bailey never failed to stay in touch with Constance as she had two more children, became a grandmother, and lived a full life over the next thirty-eight years. She died at age sixty-two of severe respiratory complications following an episode of herpes simplex.

In the years following his landmark achievement, Bailey continued to be successful. Yet only a man who suffered no fools would end his career as did Charlie Bailey. He had long fumed at what he considered frivolous lawsuits directed against him. At the age of sixty-three he gave up surgery, earned a law degree from Fordham, joined a law firm, and became active in a new battle, medical malpractice law. Bailey left a legacy of trenchant and still relevant insights about medical malpractice and the doctor-patient relationship. At age eighty-one, he confronted another old enemy . . . aortic valve disease. He was successfully treated by Denton Cooley, the world-famous Texas cardiac surgeon of the generation that had learned so much from him and Harken. He died a year later.

As Cooley gently wrote in his obituary, Charles Bailey "could well be considered as the father of direct heart surgery, having demonstrated that the human heart could withstand manipulations which were previously considered impossible" (but his) "professional career was somewhat uneven because of his volatile nature and disregard for his critics" and his "aggressive and often uncompromising convictions" that led to controversy.

But what about Dwight Harken, the race's apparent loser?

4

THE PAIN OF THE
PIONEER

*When you are aspiring to the highest place, it is honorable to
reach the second or even the third rank.*

—Cicero, Roman philosopher

JUST FIVE DAYS after Charles Bailey's waggling finger in the suburbs
of Philadelphia pointed the way to a new era of cardiac surgery, Dwight
Harken announced he had accomplished the same feat in Boston, and a
few weeks later Russell Brock reported a similar success from London.
But as Harken had learned years earlier on his father's Iowa farm, close
only counts in horseshoes.

Dwight Harken, so clearly the father of the idea and the method of
closed heart mitral valve surgery, had lost his place in history. It was not
that he had not tried. Rather it was that Harken's initial results were even
more dismal than Bailey's. He had already operated on six patients when
Bailey first succeeded. All six had died. In clinical research, tragedies precede triumphs. A salvo of ten consecutive deaths preceded the first successful mitral valve surgery. Harken and Bailey had logged a stupefying
twentieth-century proof of the ancient Arab wisdom that "He is not a surgeon who has not killed many patients."

Harken's obstacle to continuing the attempt to successfully operate on
a diseased heart was different from Bailey's, but just as potent. Where Bai-

ley faced fierce external opposition, Harken confronted internal guilt. As Harken recalled, "It was pretty grim. With the sixth death, I was so depressed that I came home in the middle of the morning [the patient had died on the table] and went up to my room and went to bed." For Harken, the torrent of blood in London had transmogrified into a stack of bodies in Boston. Had he crossed a line in the sand that stood for two millennia, drawn by the hand of Hippocrates himself? Primum non nocere. First do no harm. If six deaths were not too many, how many were? Compassion overwhelmed medical progress; Harken had failed, and now he was consumed by guilt. On the day of his sixth consecutive death he vowed to cease his quest, to give up heart surgery.

"No responsible man would continue with the devastation that I have wrought with these people," he said.

The following day his friend cardiologist Lawrence Brewster Ellis came by. Ellis argued the other side of the moral dilemma intrinsic to innovative research, that without surgery his patients were doomed.

"I think that's a terribly selfish attitude you have to waste these people's lives . . . you must have learned something from losing those six people. Don't you think you should put whatever you've learned to good purpose?" In just two sentences, Ellis encapsulated why in medicine tragedies precede triumphs. We humans simply cannot do things perfectly the first time; we must learn from our mistakes.

Wanting to be convinced while retaining his reluctance, Harken demurred. "Well, I do not think any respectable physician would send me a patient."

Brewster Ellis countered, "I'm generally considered respectable. I'm the president of the New England Cardiac Society; I'd certainly send you another patient. I've never sent you a patient who wasn't dying and, if you would be willing to try again, I'd be willing to send you patients." And so Harken agreed to try a seventh time. This time he succeeded, less than a week after Bailey's success. Harken soon proved that he had indeed learned from his failures: after his initial success "only" two of his next fifteen patients died.

After ten successive deaths between them, Bailey and Harken each had a survivor. Like me, some readers may feel queasy at how it came about, when surgeons offered unproven, potentially lethal treatments to vulnerable, desperate patients. Nonetheless that was the accepted ethical norm of the time. But the most critical part of this story is the part that remains true about medical research today: innovators cannot do things perfectly the first time—they learn from their mistakes. The stunning, unspoken consequence is that for great medical advances to occur, patients will be injured and some will die. Later in our story I will confront this wrenching conundrum as a leader of a large research program in a lethal disease, CAD.

With Bailey's success just days earlier, Dwight Harken chafed with the realization that he was destined to be the bridesmaid instead of the bride. "Unless . . . what if . . . ?" Harken pondered. Didn't it really depend on the meaning of "first"? Some might think *first* meant, "first to perform cardiac surgery successfully," but couldn't it just as easily mean, "first to publish a description of successful cardiac surgery"? Fifty years from now, historians would not know the precise date of the original surgery, but they would certainly have the journal in which its first description was published. Harken was in Boston, home of the world's most prestigious medical journal, *The New England Journal of Medicine,* whose editor was his good friend Dr. Joe Garland. As chance would have it, a cynic might say, Harken's manuscript was published that year whereas feisty Charles Bailey's manuscript was not published until the following year. As Harken later lamely suggested, "Whether one gives priority to the first operation or the first publication is a matter of personal opinion."

Time magazine, however, suffered no semantic confusion. On March 25, 1957, Charles Bailey's face appeared alone on its cover. As Harken later admitted to many of us, "He beat me to the punch." Harken's technical knockout defeat in cardiac surgical fisticuffs was to foreshadow an even more sensational and controversial defeat for the world's most talented cardiac transplant surgeon two decades hence.

Harken's shrapnel extraction and Bailey's crude repair of the narrowed mitral valve (mitral stenosis) established the first two signposts in the emergence of cardiac surgery after World War II. It would be nineteen years until the final jewel, coronary artery bypass surgery for CAD, would be inserted in cardiac surgery's crown. In those two decades CAD blossomed and mitral stenosis withered. Today the only mitral stenosis patients I see are immigrants from underdeveloped countries. The reason is penicillin: it effectively prevents acute rheumatic fever in children with streptococcal sore throat. Preventing rheumatic fever has in turn eliminated mitral stenosis among residents of the developed world.

Very early in my career in the 1960s in Philadelphia and much later as a visiting professor in underdeveloped countries, however, I saw my share of mitral stenosis patients. One was a very thin once-athletic twentysomething auburn-haired young woman about the same age as me, now approaching the end of her brief life. She struggled with the routine chores of housewife and mother, as Harken liked to say "preserving her steps like gold pieces." Surgical relief of her mitral stenosis led to one of the most dramatic changes in quality of life that I have seen in my years of cardiology, a life restored by the ten who had lost theirs to Harken and Bailey's learning curve. I believe it was then that I first began to wonder if it would ever be possible for me to reconcile the likely sacrifice of the life of individual patient in high-risk research with its uncertain future benefit to society. I will let you grapple with this question and later give the answer I found for myself.

Within a few weeks of Bailey's and Harken's breakthroughs, Russell Brock succeeded with the same "finger fracture" technique for mitral stenosis in London. With the Philadelphia success confirmed in Boston and London, there could be no doubt, as surgeons now restored vitality to thousands of mitral stenosis victims in the prime of their lives. The era of cardiac surgery had been born, midwifed by shrapnel in the hearts of dying young men, a modern echo of the wisdom of Dominican philosopher Saint Thomas Aquinas that "Good can exist without evil, whereas evil cannot exist without good."

BAILEY'S GROUNDBREAKING REVELATION, that mitral stenosis could be "cured" surgically, led to a new question: can the same technique be used on other valves? The surgeons' new target became the other major valve of the heart, the one between the left ventricle and the aorta, called the aortic valve. When the heart contracts, blood flows into the body's major blood vessel (the aorta) for transport to all the body's organs.

Like all cardiac valves, the aortic valve is prone to both narrowing (called stenosis) and to failure to close completely (called insufficiency or regurgitation).

In the autopsy room, Harken found that he could reach the aortic valve by inserting his index finger through a purse-string suture on the external surface of the ventricle just below the aortic valve. The only difference was that his entry point into the heart was the high-pressure left ventricular pumping chamber rather than the low-pressure left atrial blood-collecting chamber. For his first experiment he chose an older lady from the Massachusetts North Shore whose frequent fainting attacks and heart failure suggested she had a very short life ahead of her. He obtained her consent, even after carefully explaining that he had never performed the procedure in aortic stenosis. In reasoning that he could open the stenosed aortic valve using the same method finger-fracture he had with mitral stenosis, Harken overlooked one critical fact. In severe aortic stenosis the pressure within the ventricular chamber, normally 120 mm Hg, can skyrocket to twice that value because the heart has to generate much greater force to eject blood across the severely narrowed aortic valve. Here is Harken's own description of the horror that ensued: "I exposed the heart; and I put a purse string around the upper portion of the left ventricle; and I made a little stab wound first (and then) insinuated my finger into the ventricle only to discover pressures previously unheard of . . . I tried to stem this hemorrhage by pulling up on the tourniquet around my finger and it only tore and so I put in two fingers and then three fingers and then more bleeding and four fingers and then the dear lady succumbed."

Harken had experienced the uncontrollable fury of the wounded heart that engulfed Charles Bailey in his very first mitral valve surgery. Both men punched a hole in the heart, believing they could control bleeding, desperately applied clamps to control it, lost control within seconds, then stood helpless in the face of exsanguination, facing a task as impossible as stemming the flow from a ruptured fire hydrant. Overwhelmed with his own acute flood of remorse, Harken again retreated to home and went to bed. Harken, always an endearing mix of bombast and uncompromising self-criticism, referred to his decision to enter the high-pressure left ventricular chamber as "my devastating mistake." Doctors who care for terribly ill patients, including me, all know the awful feeling . . . a decision, an action, a path taken, a mistake that cost a patient's life.

During my years in clinical cardiovascular research, I have felt the remorse that Harken felt that day. He called it the Pain of the Pioneer. The pain seems far more intense than that experienced when you have an adverse outcome in the course of patient management. When patients have complications during routine care, the rationalization that I did the best that could be done comes easily enough, since both physicians and patients recognize complications are an inevitable consequence of disease. But when I am testing an unproven new drug or device and experience an adverse outcome, I replace the disease as the cause of the adverse outcome with myself, even though the disease itself may be fatal. The difference is guilt. Whether rational or not, it is a tough emotion to shed. As Harken so poignantly observed, "When we've created the vehicle of death, the bridge to destruction for our patient, that's another kind of pain." He had convinced himself that he would do great good, and now had to confront the reality that instead he had done great harm.

Late that afternoon a woman appeared at the door of Dwight Harken's home, carrying a note she had promised to deliver in the event of her friend's death. Harken opened the note, which read:

> Dear Dr. Harken:
>   Thanks for the chance. A small portion of my estate has been left to see that this doesn't happen again.

The voice of forgiveness had come from the grave.

Remarkably, Harken was not the only surgeon to attempt the closed approach to aortic stenosis. In the South, following Bailey and Harken's lead, young surgeon Dr. Horace Smithy was also gaining success with closed heart surgery on mitral stenosis. He convinced Johns Hopkins Medical Center's renowned thoracic surgeon Dr. Alfred Blalock that they should jointly attempt closed aortic valve surgery. He identified a suitable patient and brought him to Blalock. Smithy had a very personal reason for approaching Blalock. He, too, had aortic stenosis. He knew from experience that once symptoms began he had only a few years to live. If he and Blalock were successful, Smithy wanted to be the famous surgeon's next patient. But when Blalock put a finger-sized hole in the left ventricle, it was like a bullet hole: their patient's heart literally blew up in their faces. Blalock, never enthusiastic about Smithy's idea, now adamantly refused to attempt another case. A few months later, Charleston lost its brilliant young cardiac surgeon when Horace Smithy collapsed and died of aortic and mitral valve stenosis at the age of thirty-four.

Today, aortic valve stenosis and mitral insufficiency are the most common valve deformities in adults. As in Smithy's time, after an aortic valve stenosis patient develops chest pain, heart failure, or fainting, it is particularly deadly. If left surgically untreated, the average survival is only two to four years. Valve surgery, on the other hand, can eliminate symptoms, restore vitality, and add many years of life. A number of American celebrities including Arnold Schwarzenegger, Barbara Walters, Garrison Keillor, and Charles Rose all have suffered from aortic valve disease and publicly discussed their therapy.

HARKEN HAD DISMANTLED the myth that the heart was untouchable. When he and Bailey succeeded in extending his battlefield technique to the treatment of mitral stenosis, an important killer of young adults, they created a scintillating new vision for surgical treatment of heart disease. But in medicine, profound answers always create new questions. While the blind insertion of an index finger into a beating heart provided a crude method for ripping open a scarred valve, operating on a beating heart from its outside surface (called "closed heart" surgery), it was irrelevant to almost all other structural abnormalities within the heart. A child with a hole between the right and left atria (called an atrial septal defect or ASD), or a hole between the right and left ventricles (ventricular septal defect or VSD) could not be helped, since the surgeon had to place stitches inside the heart. Adults with leaky valves were similarly out of luck. And what about CAD, the most pervasive of cardiac disorders? Although the vessels could be touched on a beating heart as they splayed over the surface of the heart, they were only a few millimeters in diameter and were constantly moving with each heartbeat. The coronary arteries of a beating heart were far beyond the reach of even the steadiest surgical hand.

The new question seemed like an insurmountable dilemma. Could they see the inside of the heart, lay it open, perform "open heart" surgery? To progress further they needed to operate on a nonbeating heart. But absence of heartbeat was the definition of death. Now they confronted a hopeless situation, a dead end, an impossible challenge. Or so it seemed.

5

A HILL OF BONES

An essential aspect of creativity is not being afraid to fail.

EDWIN LAND, INVENTOR OF THE POLAROID CAMERA

A SURGEON WHO set out to open up the heart ["open heart surgery"] confronted three new problems that seemed insurmountable. First, the heartbeat had to be arrested to allow surgery, then restarted when the repair was complete. Yet while heart was in arrest, blood still had to be pumped throughout the body. Finally, and most daunting, somehow oxygen had to be added to the blood after it passed through the organs of the body.

At Toronto's renowned Hospital for Sick Children in 1951, surgeon William Mustard had one of his many original ideas. Outrageous notions came easily to Bill Mustard, who on occasion would dive into a fountain in a tuxedo, or swallow a live goldfish, or demonstrate one-armed push-ups at a formal dinner party. If everyone arched an eyebrow, so be it. Bill Mustard relished being unconventional, offbeat, shocking, doing what no else would do.

When Mustard contemplated the challenges of open heart surgery, he figured that if he could solve the problem of oxygenating his patient's blood, he could certainly rig up a pumping system to deliver the blood when he stopped the heartbeat. His hunch was that he knew an efficient, proven oxygenating system: the lungs of a primate. If monkey lungs could be harnessed to oxygenate his patients' blood, then he could backpedal into open heart surgery with some tubes and a pump. Armed with only intuition, indefatigable William Mustard set out to create his own deus ex machina. He anesthetized four monkeys and excised their lungs. To avoid blood mismatch, he thoroughly flushed the lungs clear of blood, "until they were white." He then hung the lungs in sealed jars and ventilated them with oxygen. He connected his patient's venous blood return to a pump, pumped the blood into the monkey lungs, and used an additional set of tubes to return the blood from the lungs to his patient. Voilà! Bill Mustard had created a functioning heart-lung machine. His first patient was a year-and-a-half-old baby with a a hole between the right and left ventricles, called a ventricular septal defect (VSD). Mustard ran into technical difficulties transporting blood from one monkey lung to the next, then into the child's body and back out to the first monkey lung through the maze of tubings. The baby died on the table.

Mustard tinkered with his apparatus, and tried again. This time he completed the procedure but the patient died in the recovery area two hours after surgery. Encouraged by his progress—his patient had survived through the surgical procedure on the machine—Mustard operated on a third patient. And a fourth. Over a period of three years that ended only with others discovering more effective methods of bypassing the heart, Mustard used his system on twelve patients ranging in age from just nineteen days to an adolescent eleven-year-old. The stunning outcome was that every single patient died, mostly on the table or in the recovery room. His longest postoperative survival was two weeks. Whereas Harken's brilliant intuition had triggered a paradigm shift, Bill Mustard's brilliant intuition, equally plausible, was an abject failure. Intuition fails far more often than it succeeds; it is just that failure seldom is recorded for history.

Looking back with current knowledge, we can suggest that Mustard's approach was doomed from the start. He assumed the monkey's lung tissue was inert, whereas the tissue of the monkey lung and his patient's blood probably interacted, courting the same acute reaction that bedevils organ transplantation. In addition his complex apparatus made it almost impossible for him to monitor and control the delicate balance between the volume of blood being pumped in and out of his tiny patients, dooming their organs to periodic flooding and drought.

This tragic record illuminates the essential nature of medical research. As British novelist Arthur Koestler observed, "The progress of science is

strewn, like an ancient desert trail, with the bleached skeletons of discarded theories which once seemed to possess eternal life." William Mustard was indisputably an outstanding surgeon whose many innovations
left the world a far better place. He invented a surgical method for one
form of congenital heart disease that changed 80% mortality in the first
year of life to 80% survival into adulthood. The procedure, which bore his
name, saved thousands of lives. Later in life he was awarded the Officer
of the Order of Canada "in recognition of his many achievements in the
field of medicine," and inducted into the Canadian Medical Hall of
Fame. Yet as we saw with Harken and Bailey, on the way to today's cardiac surgery, our forebears necessarily left many bleached skeletons along
forgotten desert trails. In today's cardiac surgery operating room, the re-
assuring hum of life-preserving blood pulsing through the heart-lung machine belies its source: a river of blood flowing from a tragic path of
premature death of children a half a century earlier.

THE FIRST PROOF that open heart surgery might be feasible emerged
from mankind's particular genius for making implausible associations. Toronto surgeon Dr. Wilfred Bigelow grew up seeing groundhogs scamper
out of the earth in springtime, having slept in the ground during the fierce
winter cold on the Canadian prairie, their bodies the same temperature
as the surrounding earth, a few degrees above freezing.

Gazing at groundhogs and their tunnels on the frozen tundra Bigelow had a flash of intuition. He knew that in the freezing cold, the
groundhog's metabolic rate falls dramatically. With less need for oxygen
supply to the brain and other tissues, the heartbeat also becomes both slow
and sluggish. Bigelow speculated that human brains cooled to these winter temperatures and then subjected to no blood flow might survive longer than four minutes, the limit science set for human brain survival
without a heartbeat. If he could extend that safe period from four minutes to just ten minutes, he speculated that a skilled surgeon might swiftly
repair the simplest and most common of congenital heart defects, like an
atrial septal defect (ASD), a hole between the right and left atrium. Depending on the size of the hole, the lungs can become flooded with blood,
leading to death in early adulthood.

In 1950 Bigelow reported his hypothermia research in 120 dogs, in which he had succeeded in stopping the circulation to the heart and brain, allowing what he called "bloodless heart" surgery at body temperatures of 68 to 70 degrees Fahrenheit. Bigelow proved that hypothermia allowed the duration of absent blood flow to the brain to be doubled or even tripled, without brain damage. He had circumvented the problem of oxygenating blood by ignoring it, by reducing the body's need for oxygen to a bare minimum. Bigelow was ready to try hypothermia in a desperately ill child but his surgical practice was in adults, and despite his years of research he received no patient referrals.

But Bigelow's laboratory report caught the attention of indefatigable Charles Bailey in Philadelphia. Bailey tested Bigelow's idea in his animal lab, where he found that with a body temperature of 81 degrees Fahrenheit animals could survive for twelve minutes without circulation to the brain or heart. By August 1952 Bailey, now restored to good standing at Hahnemann, prepared to toss his second firecracker into cardiac surgery's gas tank. He would perform open heart surgery on a twenty-seven-year-old woman with a hole in the heart, an atrial septal defect (ASD), using hypothermia.

In ASD, since pressure within the left atrium normally exceeds that in the right atrium, blood is shunted from the left atrium to the right atrium. Cells flow in an endless circuit like bumper cars in an amusement park, from left atrium to right atrium to the lungs and then back to the left atrium where they began. The problem created by an ASD is that the flow across the hole is added to the normal blood flow to the lungs. This additional blood distends the veins of the lungs almost to the bursting point. Survival depends upon the size of the shunt. People with small ASDs can survive to adulthood, whereas children with large ASDs are prone to repeated bouts of pneumonia, and over time to either fatal thickening of the blood vessels or to repeated, sometimes catastrophic hemorrhages directly into the lung tissue.

In his OR, Bailey cooled his patient to the target temperature, then clamped off blood flow to and from the heart. His hands flew like a calf roper at a rodeo as he sewed up the defect between the two atria. His surgical expertise was sometimes spectacular: the whole operation was completed in just six minutes, far less than his twelve-minute window.

Delighted with his surgical triumph, he unclamped the vessels to restore blood flow to the heart and brain. Bailey stared in horror as his patient's heart immediately descended into ventricular fibrillation, the rhythm of sudden death that claims so many in our chronicle. With no way to resuscitate her, Bailey had to stand idly by, ignominiously watching as his hopes for a twenty-seven-year-old woman and her own dreams of recovery died on the table. As Bailey looked at the surface of her heart writhing in terminal agony, he was shocked to see that the coronary arteries had become translucent. This was not blood . . . the arteries were frothing with bubbles. Air had entered his patient's circulation as he performed his surgery. The air bubbles had obstructed blood flow to the heart muscle, causing an immediate heart attack. Charles Bailey had succeeded surgically, only to be done in by a simple technical blunder.

Word of Bailey's attempt ricocheted across the heartland. Three days later on September 2, 1952, the University of Minnesota's Dr. John Lewis, fully aware of Bigelow's research and the implication of performing the first successful open heart surgery, rolled the dice for his chance at fame. Lewis operated on tiny Jacqueline Jones, the daughter of traveling carnival workers. Five years old but weighing only twenty-six pounds, Jacqueline had a large ASD. She had suffered recurrent pulmonary infections throughout her short life, and clearly would not survive to adulthood. Lewis anaesthetized Jacqueline, then laid her inert body within a cooling blanket and began lowering her body temperature from the normal 98 degrees Fahrenheit. An excruciating two hours and twenty-six minutes later, her temperature had reached 81 degrees Fahrenheit, well above the temperature used in Bigelow's dog experiments. Putting tourniquets on the veins that returned blood to her still-beating heart to empty it of blood, Lewis went on the clock.

Like Bigelow and Bailey, he estimated that at that temperature her heart and brain could survive for about ten minutes without blood flow. Lewis made his incision. The hole in Jacqueline's heart was laid out in front of him. As his assistant Dr. Walton Lillehei would later say, any seamstress could have sewn it shut. Lewis swiftly closed the hole in Jacqueline's heart with five stitches, a surgical tour de force equal to Bailey's three days earlier. At five and a half minutes, he and Lillehei released the tourniquets, restoring blood flow to her brain. Lewis knew his surgery had progressed well beyond the four-minute limit for brain survival at normal temperature. So either hypothermia worked in humans like it did in dogs or his little patient was brain-dead. Lewis and Lillehei closed little Jacqueline's chest incision, then lifted her inert body to immerse her in a tub of warm water to bring her body temperature back to normal. Nothing fancy there . . . the tub was a farm water trough he had found in a Sears, Roebuck catalog. A few hours later, little Jacqueline awoke, her brain intact. She had not only survived, she now had a heart that would, if she was fortunate, allow her to have a perfectly normal lifespan. On that remarkable morning, a frigid northern Canadian prairie wind had carried hypothermia to a Minneapolis operating room, and with it the world's first successful open heart surgery. The Minneapolis surgeons had proven that in the absence of blood flow, hypothermia slows the death of cells in the heart and brain. As the *Minneapolis Tribune* reported, hypothermia gave surgeons "a method—long sought—of putting the knife into the human heart."

Well, yes and no. Hypothermic heart surgery proved that a surgeon could operate inside the heart. Yet it was a rocket forever locked on its launching pad, a success in theory but not in practice. Hypothermia was hopelessly inadequate for most cardiac problems. Almost all the other cardiac defects simply could not possibly be repaired in less than ten minutes. And so it is an irony of history that it was not Bigelow, who proved the feasibility of hypothermia, nor Lewis, who performed the first open heart surgery, who would ultimately lay claim to being the Father of Open Heart Surgery. It was Lewis's thirty-four-year-old assistant, C. Walton Lillehei, who took the giant step that brought open heart surgery to practical reality.

WITH BLUE EYES and a square face topped with blond hair resembling an early version of Robert Redford, Walt Lillehei was just beginning his cardiac surgery career.

In 1951 he had visited the East Coast to watch the new breed of "closed heart" surgeons in action. About a decade younger than Harken and Bailey,

Lillehei visited Boston, Philadelphia, and Baltimore's Johns Hopkins, returning to Minnesota inspired to make his mark by operating inside the heart.

Walt Lillehei was the eldest boy in his family. His grandfather was an immigrant Norwegian fisherman and his father became a successful dentist in the Minneapolis suburb of Edina. Young Walt emerged as a gifted child early in his life. Walt's particular intelligence lay in his aptitude, fascination, and passion for understanding how things worked. He was a problem solver that loved a challenge. In his superb Lillehei biography, author Warren Miller relates that when, as a teenager, Walt was denied the money to buy a motorcycle, he bought the parts and constructed his own. Walt's creative imagination was clear to his teachers; he skipped two grades, and entered the University of Minnesota at the age of sixteen.

During World War II, Lillehei rose to lieutenant colonel in charge of a Mobile Army Surgical Hospital (MASH) in North Africa where Allied forces battled those of the legendary Nazi Field Marshal Erwin Rommel. At war's end he returned with a Bronze Star to enter surgical training with the University of Minnesota's legendary Dr. Owen Wangensteen.

Inside the hospital Dr. Lillehei was a highly respected surgeon, viewed by his nurses as unusually compassionate, and by surgical colleagues as an innovative genius. But outside the starched hierarchy of the hospital, Walt played by no one's rules but his own. Whereas Charles Bailey scuffled with society's norms, Lillehei simply ignored them. Walt shared a second trait with many of the innovators we will meet later. He was an unmitigated risk-taker. Walt lived life at double speed. Lillehei's days were consumed with thoracic surgery, but his nights were gold chains, a Buick Roadmaster convertible, and late-evening carousing. Early on he discovered that the classic good looks of his Scandinavian heritage, gregarious attitude, personal magnetism, and sensitivity held an irresistible allure for nurses, and throughout his career he was not one to ignore it. "Work hard, play hard," he urged his friends.

If Walt was hedonistic, he had a compelling reason. In his last year of surgical training, Walt noted a small lump in his neck. The biopsy result was chilling. Lillehei had a deadly cancer: lymphosarcoma of the parotid (salivary) gland, with a predicted five-year survival rate of 5 to 10%. After years of college, medical school, internship, and residency training (mine consumed fifteen years, surgeons need even more time), Walt Lillehei had been dealt life's cruelest blow, a sentence of premature death. On the last day of his surgical residency training, instead of celebrating, Lillehei lay down on an operating table. His boss Owen Wangensteen slashed away all the lymph nodes on the affected side of his neck. Wangensteen was operating in the now largely abandoned era of radical cancer surgery, so he plunged into Walt's chest cavity to cut away more tissue. At the end of the surgery the pathologist's microscope shined an oculus on just a tiny sliver of hope: the cancer appeared only on the nodes in his neck. Surgery complete, Lillehei now underwent a course of radiation therapy. His life was dependent on radiation therapy, but his ambition was set free. Told he probably would not survive five years, any stricture on Walt Lillehei's mandate to "work hard, play hard" evaporated. He could hardly have foreseen that his single-minded pursuit of that motto would lead to a career unmatched for its peaks and valleys among all whom I have known in cardiovascular medicine.

IN MEDICINE, WE learn more from our mistakes than from our successes. Error exposes truth. Since we must err, it seems best that our mistakes come first. Bill Mustard's failed monkey lungs taught a critical lesson: it was possible to oxygenate blood outside a patient's body, return it to the recipient circulation, and keep a patient alive while operating on an arrested heart. Knowing that, Lillehei's group made one of those spectacular intuitive leaps of genius that seem obvious in retrospect. Mother Nature offered a better oxygenating system than monkey lungs. When a baby is in a woman's uterus, it cannot breathe, and so it gets its oxygenated blood from the mother. The ingenious method of blood exchange is through the placenta. The placenta is a highly vascular structure that attaches to the inner surface of the mother's uterus. A cord of veins and arteries runs from the placenta to the baby's belly. The placenta collects deoxygenated blood from the baby's organs, sends it to be reoxygenated in the mother's lungs, then returns the oxygenated blood to the fetus. The mother "cross-circulates" her blood with the fetus when it is in her uterus.

Lillehei had an intuition. What worked inside the uterus might work outside the uterus. Instead of inserting just a lung into the circulation as

Mustard had done, why not insert a whole body? Why not connect up the child with a congenital heart defect to his mother or father's arteries and veins? The child's blood could circulate through the parent's lungs, while the surgeon operated on the child's arrested heart. The beauty of this approach was that it eliminated the need for a complex oxygenation strategy, since oxygenated blood would be in constant supply to the child from the parent's normal circulation. If it worked, the procedure would be the essence of simplicity. Only a pump and tubing would be required. Had they come up with the perfect method of oxygenating their patient's blood, by simply mixing it with a compatible living donor?

Lillehei's group bought beer keg tubing and a $500 roller pump that could compress the tubing without being in contact with the blood. This devastatingly simple apparatus also eliminated the cleaning issue that was bedeviling those trying to develop heart-lung machines. Just throw away the tubing at the end of the surgery; use new tubing at the next surgery. In dogs, they discovered that both the recipient dog with an arrested heart and the donor dog awoke quickly and appeared normal after a half hour of cross-circulation. They took another step. They created an artificial ventricular septal defect (VSD) in dogs. A VSD is an abnormal hole between the left and right ventricles, which are normally completely separated by a solid muscular wall. Early anatomists wonderfully dubbed this wall a septum, a derivation of the Latin word *saeptum,* which means a fence. A hole in the fence allows the more powerful left ventricle to pump blood into the right ventricle. As with ASD, the added blood floods the lungs. Most children with VSD do not survive to mature adulthood, unless the VSD is very small.

On his operating table, Lillehei set up cross-circulation between a normal dog and one with his artificial VSD; veins to veins; arteries to arteries. During cardiac arrest on cross-circulation, Lillehei found that he could consistently close the canine VSD with sutures in less than twenty minutes. Walt Lillehei was ready to operate on a child.

The newspapers of March 1954 were dominated by a historic moment in science, the explosion on the Marshall Islands' Bikini Atoll of the fifteen-megaton hydrogen bomb, a thousand times more powerful than the bombs that had leveled Hiroshima and Nagasaki. From my perspective an arguably more important, but less ballyhooed historic event occurred a few weeks later when Walt Lillehei scheduled open heart surgery using cross-circulation at the University of Minnesota Hospital. The donor circulation would be the child's parent, providing their blood type was compatible. It was just a year and a half after Lewis and Lillehei's historic beating heart hypothermic surgery had established the feasibility of open heart surgery.

THE SCHEDULED SURGERY became the University Hospital's own megaton bomb. Walt Lillehei was ready but the University of Minnesota was not. Lillehei possessed Charles Bailey's indifference to criticism, Harken's charm, and both men's supreme self-confidence, but it was not enough. When word leaked out about Lillehei's planned human experiment, as with Bailey at Hahnemann, it precipitated a fierce morality play. The drama pitted the university's two most powerful physicians: Dr. Cecil Watson, chairman of the department of medicine, and Dr. Owen Wangensteen, chief of surgery, against one another. Watson, boiling with righteous moral outrage, felt Lillehei's proposal was an abomination. Given the complete uncertainty about the outcome, Watson imagined that for the first time in the history of medicine Walt Lillehei had come up with an operation with the potential to kill two people at one sitting . . . "a 200% mortality rate!" Operating on a terribly sick child is conceivably justified, he argued, but risking the life of a second healthy person is ethically unacceptable. Once again, Hippocrates made his appearance. Lillehei wanted to stand the oath on its head. Primum non nocere. First do no harm. Lillehei must be stopped.

Lillehei's mentor Owen Wangensteen was Watson's equal in power and prestige, and his argument also was based on uncompromising logic. His department of surgery was world famous for advancing surgery through innovation. His star protégé Lillehei had performed the proposed procedure successfully in animals. If Lillehei was denied, blood would stain Watson's hands . . . a child would die for no other reason than Watson was afraid to try something new. Watson's reaction was his own version of the Bikini Atoll. He felt like the top of his head would blow off with the suggestion that he would be painted as a child killer. He was not the real potential killer of innocents, he raged, pointing a trembling metaphorical finger: it was that man, the one who proposed the research, C. Walton Lillehei.

Here then is the classic, explosive confrontation that has bedeviled groundbreaking research through all my years in cardiology. Just eighteen months earlier Lewis and Lillehei's hypothermic surgery had established the feasibility of open heart surgery. Now where Watson saw risk, Lillehei and Wangensteen saw opportunity. Where Watson saw that both patients might die, Lillehei saw that a child condemned to early death might be given life. The issue as Watson fought Wangensteen on that Minneapolis afternoon was specific to one family, but I see variations on this theme argued in every Institutional Review Board (IRB) meeting, in which we critically review and approve every research project in the medical center prior to its initiation. What criteria are we as a society to use in making such decisions?

My experience provides a bizarre answer. With our human gift of twisted logic, we decide the ethically correct position after we learn the outcome of the research. Charles Bailey was terribly, morally, Hippocratically wrong. Until he was right.

Wangensteen won the argument based on uncertainty: the first-ever human cross-circulation surgery deserved to be tried, because no one could say cross-circulation wouldn't work, and if the Lord was willing and it worked, this form of open heart surgery could save countless numbers of dying children. The gain justified the risk. Wangensteen and Lillehei prevailed, but Watson made it clear that crazy Walt Lillehei was on a very short leash. The winner of the ethical battle would await the result of surgery. Lillehei's first patient, two-year-old Gregory Gittens, seemed to do quite well until the second postoperative week, when he developed pneumonia and died. Rather than resolve the issue, the Gittens experience escalated tension to new levels as both sides saw it proved how right they had been.

AT AGE FOUR Annie Brown was already clearly destined for a very short life. She had a hole in the wall that separated her right and left ventricles, called a ventricular septal defect (VSD). Annie's VSD was large, and her lungs were drowning in her own blood. She could not play with other kids because of progressive fatigue and shortness of breath. She had already undergone repeated hospitalizations for pneumonia. Now she had episodes of coughing up blood as the distended blood vessels in her lungs ruptured. Doctors told her parents Doris and Joseph that she would probably not survive to be a teenager.

Imagine the wrenching decision that now confronted Doris and Joseph. They knew that a young Minneapolis heart surgeon named Walton Lillehei had developed a new way of operating on the heart, called open heart surgery, and that he had tested it successfully—in dogs. But they also knew that his first patient Gregory Gittens, a youngster with the same heart defect as Annie's, had died in the hospital after Lillehei's surgery. Having lived with Annie's progressive deterioration, the Browns had little doubt that Annie had a lethal disease. On the other hand, wasn't the most critical fact that Lillehei's first case lay prematurely in his grave? How does one balance the remote likelihood of cure against the much more real prospect of immediate demise? The Browns, visualizing Annie's future without surgery as recurrent hospitalizations punctuating an accelerating, soul-wrenching, unstoppable march toward death, made a choice. They would gamble Annie's life, and one of theirs, on the young surgeon. Annie would have open heart surgery.

Unaware of this supercharged medical environment, Doris and Joseph Brown gave their consent for Lillehei to operate on little four-year-old Annie. In the university hematology lab, however, they ran into a new wall. Doris's blood type did not match Annie's. The mother could not save her child. But what about Joseph? His blood matched. But he was anemic. The blood bank director decreed that Joseph's hemoglobin level was too low to permit the procedure. Lillehei now flashed the Charles Bailey side of his temperament. He played life by his own rules. He knew more about Annie and Joseph than the hematologist, so the man's opinion was irrelevant. He bulldozed ahead. But now providence intervened. Annie was again hospitalized with pneumonia, requiring postponement of surgery. Was Annie's little body sending headstrong Lillehei a second warning?

When she recovered from pneumonia, Lillehei did not hesitate. The hubris of Lillehei's approach, the intensity of Watson's opposition, and the life-and-death stakes for both little Annie and her father created a crackling electric tension as little Annie and her father, Joseph, were wheeled into the crushingly small white-tiled, green-walled Operating Room II of the University of Minnesota Hospital. Two sets of surgeons awaited, huddled back-to-back over the two operating tables, shoehorned between two anesthesia teams and a bevy of OR nurses. Lillehei was assisted by Dr. Richard Varco, a surgeon many years his senior.

Now captain of the ship, Lillehei recognized he needed more than a perfect surgical procedure. He could lose his patient because of inattention to any number of details. No one knew anything about anesthesia under these conditions. The father, Joseph, had to be asleep, because any movement could lead to catastrophic dislodgement of the complex tubing connections. But little Annie was about a fifth the size of her father. They would be sharing the same blood. Would the anesthetic dose necessary to put Joseph to sleep be fatal for Annie? The father and child had markedly different cardiac output. So the amount of blood entering and leaving Annie's body had to be precisely controlled. If little Annie received either too much or too little blood, her brain might be either starved of oxygen or engorged with blood. The tubing connecting the two patients had to be handled with utmost care. Accidental entry of a small amount of air could obstruct vessels in the brain or heart, causing a stroke or a fatal heart attack.

Two teams of surgeons, packed sardine-close, self-schooled from the same procedure in dogs, connected the maze of tubing. Tubes in Annie's two major veins that return blood to the heart were connected to Joseph's leg vein, which would send Annie's blood on to Joseph's lungs for oxygenation. A second set of tubes delivered the oxygenated blood from Joseph's leg artery back into Annie's aorta.

Lillehei announced he was ready. He turned on the pump and tightened the tourniquets on Annie's two veins. Now Annie's heart and lungs received no blood. Annie was "on bypass." With the pump on and blood from the two souls intermixed, for the first time in biologic history, a child's life-giving blood supply would be dependent on cross-circulation from the father instead of the mother.

Lillehei cut into Annie's right ventricle. He adjusted a headlamp, borrowed from an otolaryngologist (an ear, nose, and throat specialist), to improve his visibility. Its beam was far narrower than those we use in today's cardiac surgery. Magnification, a huge boon to suture placement, would also come later. With the pump on, Lillehei grasped his scalpel, then cut into Annie's heart to expose the ventricular septum. He saw it immediately The gaping hole in the tiny heart appeared to be about the width of two of his gloved fingers. As Varco pulled apart the incision in the right ventricular wall to widen his field of view, Lillehei began placing sutures with consummate hand speed, while observers strained to see from balcony seats.

In training, I found these seats hopeless. Even if you manage to peer through the constantly fluctuating cracks between the surgeons' shoulders, the head surgeon is tying his knots deep within a small hole. As a medical student I spent hours practicing being Lillehei putting thousands of "two hand" and "one hand" surgical knots on bedposts and railings. At the operating table I later learned that although it's easy enough to tie a knot, it is an order of magnitude more difficult to learn to deliver that knot precisely into a deep hole.

Lillehei's hands flashed in constant motion as he deftly placed a knot, then pulled the two ends of the suture material together for Varco's scissors to sever the ends of the thread. Knot, cut. Knot, cut became a silent ballet as they delivered seven sutures in the span of ten minutes. The hole between the ventricles looked like it was completely closed. Lillehei nodded at Varco. They had eliminated the cause of Annie's heart trouble. Vindication, it seemed, would belong to Walt Lillehei.

But as Lillehei began to close his right ventricular incision, disaster struck. Annie's heart rate fell to about thirty beats per minute, half its normal rate. The normally coordinated beating of the atria and ventricles became completely disjointed. The eyes of every surgeon on both teams immediately focused on Annie's ECG, but every doctor already knew. Heart block!

What is heart block? Some tiny blocks in the heart's electrical system are like a grain of sand dropped into a Rolex. In its most severe form, called complete heart block, the electrical impulse activates the atrium but stops there . . . it never reaches the ventricles. When this happens the ventricles have to rely on their own backup generator. But this backup system delivers only about twenty to thirty electrical stimuli per minute, instead of the normal 60 to 100 impulses. The very slow ventricular contraction rate results in insufficient blood flow to the brain, with the likelihood of sudden fainting, seizures, and the ever-present risk of sudden death. In the days before the invention of the pacemaker, complete heart block was a metaphorical Sword of Damocles, a death sentence without a specific execution date.

Lillehei wondered if his last suture had inadvertently compressed her heart's electrical conduits, which pass within millimeters of the VSD. Should he remove that last suture and settle for incomplete closure of the hole, or should he hope that the block would only be fleeting? Uncertainty reared its ugly head. Pacemakers were still in the future. Lillehei had no effective treatment for heart block, as he stood transfixed by the world's first heart block induced by VSD closure. There was no good answer. They had been on cross-circulation for eleven minutes. Lillehei and his surgical teams decided to hope. No doubt some prayed. The room turned deathly still as they stood and watched. With each ticking second, however, hope slipped further through their gloved fingers.

Then at ninety seconds came the miracle. As suddenly as it appeared, the heart block disappeared. Annie's heartbeat more rapidly and coordination returned to the chambers of the heart. At thirteen and a half minutes, Lillehei decreed that the moment of truth had arrived. "Release the tourniquets," he ordered. Lillehei stared down at her heart as the pump was turned off. Annie's heart, now filling with blood, contracted vigorously, a Little Engine That Could. Lillehei placed his hand on the tiny heart. No vibration. His sutures had completely closed the VSD. He and Varco's eyes locked above their white cotton masks and they reached bloody gloves across the table to shake hands. Survival was now up to the rest of Annie's body. If Annie could just recover to grasp more tightly the good fortune that had escaped his first patient Gregory Gittens's tiny fingers, she would have been granted a lifetime in less than fifteen minutes.

As Joseph regained consciousness, he asked about Annie. Lillehei replied that he had found exactly what they expected. He had closed the defect completely. Annie's heart beat vigorously before he closed the chest wall. He was very, very pleased with the result. Joseph's thrilled response to his words proved that Walt Lillehei had finessed Cecil Watson's trump card, the unknown risk to the parent. He had proven that his idea was feasible. But the jury was still out, and he could feel Watson's furious eyes boring into his back.

* * *

ONE WEEK LATER Walt Lillehei held a press conference, a distinctly questionable behavior for a physician in an era of strict rules of professional propriety that prohibited physicians from advertising themselves to the public. The appropriate professional way to announce a scientific advance was to do as Bailey had done with his mitral valve surgery, at a major scientific conference of your peers, who would debate and dissect the strengths and weaknesses of the new method. Walt Lillehei chose the path less traveled. At his press conference, he recounted Annie's and her parents' medical travails prior to surgery. Then came the illustrations. A sensational photograph taken in the operating room on the day of her surgery. Diagrams explaining his method of cross-circulation. Drawings of the heart with a VSD. And then his pitch: "We have long felt that there must be some simple way of working inside the heart. When elaborate machines designed as a substitute for the heart and lungs proved unsatisfactory we tried using the animal's own lungs and substituted the simple mechanical pump for his heart." Next came a four-page handout in case you missed (or failed to grasp) important details for your stories. The slides, photo, and the handout—a masterpiece of medical advertising—were certainly more than enough for any press conference, but not quite enough for Walt Lillehei.

A door to the auditorium was flung open, and there was Annie Brown, preternaturally pretty with dark shoulder-length hair and bangs neatly framing a round face with irresistible big brown eyes. Sitting in a wheelchair pushed by her parents, Annie seemed the picture of health with rosy cheeks and a tiny shy smile. In that profoundly emotional moment, pens and typewriter keys hung in suspended animation. Joseph and Doris then recounted the details of Annie's desperate early years and with glistening eyes spoke of her last days of precarious hold on life prior to surgery. It seemed almost impossible to reconcile her parents' image of that dying child with the one they looked upon now. By the end of the conference, few dry eyes remained in the auditorium. Lillehei had convinced the reporters that they were looking upon a modern miracle, the story of a lifetime, and they intended to report it just that way.

Annie posed for pictures with Lillehei and her parents. In an era when racial tension in the South and confrontation with communism abroad dominated the news, irresistible little Annie's story went viral. *The New York Times* offered the headline: "Impossible Surgery Now Done," while London's *Daily Mirror* gushed that Lillehei's surgery was as "fantastic as any ever written in a shilling science thriller." Walt Lillehei's theatrics had shocked the world, and inevitably torched more bridges with his medical brethren. With some of his conservative surgical colleagues, this time he had crossed the Rubicon. At that moment, however, he hardly needed their support. C. Walton Lillehei ruled the domain of cardiac surgery. As with Caesar, however, he would one day face daggers.

Always photogenic, Annie Brown became Minnesota's most recognizable child. Senator Hubert Humphrey sent her birthday cards. *Cosmopolitan* magazine ran a six-page photo article on Annie and her family. She was chosen Queen of Hearts for the state of Minnesota, and for the American Heart Association.

By the time of his press conference, Lillehei had a second surgical success. Engulfed in the clamor for interviews and a torrent of calls from desperate parents with sick children, reckless Walt Lillehei quietly revealed the other side of his complex personality, the side that endeared him to the friends who would stand by him during future days when the world forsook him. Just four days after the press conference, sensitive and compassionate doctor Walt, so well-known to his patients and nurses, wrote a letter to Gregory Gittens's parents.

> It is still a source of bitter disappointment to me that we were not able to bring Gregory through the postoperative period after the operation had seemingly gone so well. I do wish to tell you again that had it not been for the encouragement gained from Gregory's operation, we would not have had the courage to go ahead with these other children. I feel greatly indebted to both of you.

Frances Gittens's reply captures the heartbreak and hope of an era when heart disease was still untreatable. "Though it is so hard not to feel bitter that little Greg couldn't have lived to rejoice with the other two," Frances wrote, "we just have to accept it as the Lord's will and we know his death wasn't in vain as it has given these two children another chance to live and no doubt many more. May God bless and guide you in the wonderful work you are doing." A half a century later, as both a doctor and father, the grace and nobility of Frances Gittens's Midwestern stoicism captures my own heart. Could anything more poignantly capture that nascent era of cardiac surgery than this mutually bittersweet exchange between doctor and family?

Initially Lillehei's continued success with cross-circulation seemed to make him the unquestioned winner of the ethical debate with Watson. Four months after that first success, however, good fortune completely deserted Walt Lillehei. In a period of nine weeks, he used cross-circulation in seven patients. Six died. Like Bailey and Harken before him, Lillehei was suddenly in danger of becoming an outcast in his own hospital. Blindfolded Lady Justice's scale of ethics and fairness, once so heavily weighted toward Lillehei following the publicity surrounding Annie Brown, now swung toward Watson. Some cardiologists refused to send him patients. When nurses whispered "murderer" it echoed off every wall and down every corridor of the university. And then, just when things could not get worse, they did. In December, now reeling from failure to failure, Lillehei traveled to surgery's most prestigious professional meeting, the annual American College of Surgeons meeting in Atlantic City. Completely suppressing the news of his string of recent failures, he chose to report another spectacular success. He had accomplished the first complete repair of tetralogy of Fallot, the most common of the "blue baby" congenital cardiac abnormalities. We will meet one of my patients with "tet" later, so for now I will just tell you that this surgery is an order of magnitude greater surgical challenge than repair of a septal defect, because the surgeon must also correct stenosis (narrowing) of the pulmonic valve (the valve between the right ventricle and pulmonary artery) and an aorta that is a misconnected to the left ventricle.

His scientific presentation began as a classic Lillehei tour de force. But at least one person who listened that day was not impressed. I have heard both hilarious and embarrassing comments erupt from attendees over years of scientific meetings, but never a single one that comes close to equaling what happened at Lillehei's presentation. An unidentified heckler shouted from the audience: "Admit you have a vegetable in the hospital!"

It was true. In October during his run of bad surgical outcomes, Lillehei's anesthesiologist had allowed air to enter the pump tubing as the equipment was being set up. The curse that had killed Charles Bailey's young lady when air entered her coronary arteries had resurfaced in Lillehei's operating room. Again the simple error was devastating. In Lillehei's case the air had gone to the brain of donor Mildred Jones, the mother of his eight-year-old VSD patient. Lillehei immediately canceled the surgery, but it was too late. Mildred Jones was permanently and severely brain damaged, unable to care for herself or her four small children.

In that sudden reversal of fortune Watson emerged the ethical victor. As world-famous pediatric cardiologist Dr. Helen Taussig sniped at Lillehei's reported success with the tetralogy case, "Too bad, now he'll continue." The Mildred Jones story finalized the decision for most cardiologists and cardiac surgeons. The problem of adding oxygen to blood could not be circumvented by hypothermia or cross-circulation.

Walt Lillehei had proven that the heartbeat could be stopped, that the circulation could be maintained, and that successful surgery could be performed on the arrested heart. In principle no form of heart disease, including CAD, was any longer beyond the surgeon's reach. But as Lillehei and the new breed of cardiac surgeons surmounted these obstacles, they had also proved that cross-circulation carried a terrifying, inescapable, unacceptable ethical risk. To save a life, a healthy volunteer was put at risk of permanent disability or even death. If monkey lungs did not work, hypothermia was inadequate, and cross-circulation was ethically prohibitive, what was left? Was human ingenuity exhausted? Or was there still another way?

6

AN IMPOSSIBLE DREAM

There is no way that the heart-lung machine could have been devised and developed other than through studies on living creatures.

—Professor Sir Norman Browse, President of the
Royal College of Surgeons of England

AT PHILADELPHIA'S JEFFERSON Medical College another war surgeon pursued a quite different dream. Dr. John H. "Jack" Gibbon set out to create a heart-lung machine. Gibbon was the polar opposite of his contemporary fellow Philadelphian Charles Bailey. Son of a prominent Philadelphia doctor, Gibbon was a fifth-generation physician, born to wealth and entitlement. He had an in-town home and a farm home. A Princeton-educated upper-class blue blood, he was both erudite and handsome. To round out his genteel Renaissance Man image, Gibbon also wrote poetry and painted. He and his wife entertained Philadelphia's social elite at large parties with charades, ballet, and music, the privileged life of Gatsby's East Egg. Yet as elegant as he was, John Gibbon was neither aloof nor pretentious. He was down-to-earth, sincerely interested in listening to others and in their ideas. A rather slow and deliberate surgeon, he was an exceptional teacher. His unique breadth of interests, achievements, warm personality, and modesty often led to leadership being thrust upon him.

Jack Gibbon's philosophy of life was quite different from the other surgeons we have met. He enjoyed his surgical career but was not consumed by it. Personally secure, his research was more driven by its pure intellectual challenge than by the competitive desire for peer recognition. I believe this constellation of personal and professional attributes explains what was to be the strangest, most incomprehensible decision I have seen in my years in academic medicine.

In his graduate years, Gibbon was more inclined to creative pursuits than to science. He had to be dissuaded by his physician father from dropping out of medical school in his sophomore year to become a writer. Both smart and connected to the establishment, Gibbon eventually matriculated to surgical training at Massachusetts General Hospital. In those years, every doctor and nurse knew the letters MGH. Those three letters stood for one thing only: the nation's premier hospital. If you worked there you were, by association alone, a superior physician. And if you contemplated leaving the fold, you were reminded to choose your new location well, because you only come from Harvard once.

During his years as an MGH surgical resident, Gibbon was called to assist on the removal of a large blood clot from the pulmonary artery, the vessel that delivers blood from the right ventricle to the lungs, in a desperate effort to save a healthy young woman who had entered the hospital for routine gall bladder surgery. The surgical team extracted the clot, but it was too late. She never regained consciousness. Gibbon was deeply affected by the premature passing of an otherwise healthy young lady of his age: "If only we could remove the blood from her body by bypassing her lungs, and oxygenate it, then return it to her heart, we could almost certainly save her life." Jack Gibbon was describing the genesis of the heart-lung machine. The idea ricocheted within Gibbon's psyche until it became an obsession. Despite universal discouragement from colleagues who bluntly told him that he was wasting a promising career, Gibbon blithely ignored them. Failure was postposed success; persistence was the habit of accomplishment. Like an artist finding joy in a single brushstroke, he was satisfied with the smallest advance. His research would be, as with his surgical technique, tranquil, slow, and deliberate.

Gibbon faced three daunting engineering obstacles that Lillehei had circumvented with cross-circulation. First he needed a method to oxygenate blood. Second, blood outside the body tends to clot, so every surface of his machine, including delivery tubing and the oxygenation device, had to be resistant to blood clot formation. Third, oxygen-carrying red blood cells are extraordinarily fragile. Broken red cells carry no oxygen, and when many cells are disrupted, their fragments obstruct the kidneys causing organ failure. So the entire oxygenation and pumping process had to be exceptionally gentle. In Boston, Jack Gibbon spent ten years tinkering and jiggering one prototype after another without success, but not without reward. One of his coworkers at Harvard, Mary Hopkinson, believed in the unruffled surgeon's dream. As Hitler rampaged through Europe before the war, Mary and John married, then returned to join the staff at Philadelphia's University of Pennsylvania.

As the United States entered World War II, Gibbon was already into his second decade of trying to create a functioning device when he and Mary finally achieved their first modest success. They developed a prototype heart-lung bypass machine, which kept a small laboratory cat alive for twenty-six minutes. But with their first success came terrible disappointment. Japanese bombs terminated their research. John was called to serve four long years as chief of surgical services at the 364th Station Hospital in New Caledonia, a South Pacific island east of Australia. The idea of a heart-lung machine became as remote as the narrow strip of land he now inhabited. Could his lifetime of research survive?

SOME YEARS LATER on a June afternoon in Los Angeles, I sat sorting through a stack of phone messages while watching rush hour traffic from my fifth floor office window. One call had come from Sam Bachner, one of my favorite supporters of our cardiovascular research program. Sam charged enthusiastically though life with the rare and wonderful capacity to be genuinely interested in each person he met, and to draw them into his circle. Sam's perspective on life was captured by his company name, La Mancha, and by his office cluttered with Don Quixote sculptures.

"Jim, I want to get your opinion about a heart problem in a child," Sam said. "My wife and I have a housekeeper from El Salvador who has lived with us for a few years. She sends her money back home to help pay for her kids, who live with her mother in El Salvador. Last week she got a devastating letter about her twelve-year-old daughter, Maria. Here's what

I learned. As a little girl she tired easily, and had episodes where she would start gasping for breath and her lips would turn dark blue. Whenever she had an episode, Maria would squat to relieve her breathlessness. The doctor said Maria was a 'blue baby' and there was nothing he could do for her. Recently her grandmother took her to a doctor because she had begun passing out during these spells. He said that Maria has a heart murmur and that she would probably die in the next year, but that she could live if she had surgery. He said they don't have that kind of surgery yet in El Salvador. So what I am calling to ask is what do you think is wrong with her? And would surgery really save her life?"

I winced, feeling a parent's dismay at knowing her child is dying, a cure exists, but her child is denied. But the doctor in El Salvador was right. Although the heart-lung machine has made reconstructive, curative surgery for all types of congenital heart disease feasible in developed countries, in the developing world congenital heart disease still claims many children.

"I need a lot more information, Sam. If she is a blue baby, the odds are she has a congenital heart condition called tetralogy of Fallot," I said. "But even if we knew her diagnosis we need two more critical pieces of information. Kids with tet often have other cardiac and noncardiac congenital abnormalities. So if you want my opinion, your first step is to get a copy of her doctor's physical examination, and to find out if she has had an echocardiogram back in El Salvador."

A few weeks later, Sam sent over a few crude Polaroid snapshots of echocardiographic images, not the moving video images we typically evaluate. Maria's physical exam apparently had got lost in translation. Even so, I saw she had all four components of the tetralogy. First she had severe stenosis of the pulmonary valve, which separates the right ventricle and the pulmonary artery. Normally, all blood returning from the body is pumped by the right ventricle across this valve on its way to reoxygenation in the lungs. The marked increase in force required to pump blood across a severely narrowed pulmonary valve leads to the second defect of tetralogy, an increase in the mass of the right ventricle (called hypertrophy). I saw that Maria also had the third defect, ventricular septal defect (VSD). Because of this open hole between the two ventricles, some of the deoxygenated blood returning to the right ventricle was being pumped into the left ventricle. The tetralogy was completed by a distorted connection

of the aorta to the left ventricle. Maria turned blue when the deoxygenated blue blood from the right side of her heart was pumped across her
VSD to mix with the left ventricle's oxygenated red blood. When she
squatted, resistance to blood flow into the aorta increased, so that less blue
blood crossed the VSD. Remarkably, before they can talk and even without being told, virtually every child with tetralogy discovers squatting.

I called Sam to deliver the bad news. "Sam, I think it's best that you
are honest with Maria's mother. We haven't seen a child of this age with
untreated tet in years. Here in the United States about half of tets are now
detected before they are born, by fetal echocardiography. The remainder
are detected in the first two years of life, and they all get surgery right
away. So tet in a person of this age nowadays is really confined to children like this little girl, born to poor parents in a poor country."

"So what happens in those countries? What's the treatment?" Sam
asked.

Musing how Lillehei's breakthrough tetralogy case using cross-
circulation forty years earlier was still irrelevant to this little Hispanic
child, I replied, "For these kids the prognosis is dismal. It's the same as it
was here in the United States in the years before cardiac surgery. About a
quarter of infants die in the first year. Most of the rest die before their
teens. I looked up the numbers. About forty percent die by age three, and
seventy percent by age ten. By all odds, Maria should already be dead."

"But she isn't."

"That does not mean she's escaped," I said. "Untreated, only a tiny
fraction, maybe five percent, of tets survive to middle age. Most die during an acute episode of lack of oxygen, gasping for air like a fish out of
water. Or just as bad, their body recognizes that the blood isn't carrying
enough oxygen, and so their bone marrow goes into overdrive, producing
massively more red cells to carry oxygen. But more cells make the blood
more prone to clot. And so they have a stroke. Some even get a brain ab-
scess.

"It is pretty grim," I added unnecessarily, feeling the sterile insensi-
tivity of my statistical recitation.

"So are you telling me it is too late for her, that the doctors in El Salvador are right that she is going to die soon?"

"I'm afraid so," I said. "Fainting is an ominous sign."

"But one doctor also said she has a surgically correctable condition, right? He seemed to be saying that if she did have an operation, she'd have a good chance at a normal life, and yet . . ." Sam said, his voice trailing off.

"That's true too, Sam, it's a personal tragedy played out every day in the third world," I replied. "You are looking at the universal curse of being born poor in a poor country. Life just isn't fair," I said, adding a sop of conventional wisdom to deflect our discussion away from the tragedy of one hopeless little girl.

"So now we know our problem," Sam replied as he said good-bye.

I could hardly miss that. Without any input from me, Sam's maid's daughter's problem had become "our" problem, and in that fleeting instant, I had the sinking feeling that I was about to confront an entirely new problem. I was.

The next day, Sam called again.

"I don't suppose there's any possibility of doing this, but if you don't ask you never know, right? If I pay to fly Maria up here, and put her up in my house before and after surgery, could you get her taken care of?" he asked.

I reflexively tapped my fist against my chin several times before I answered. When you are a chief, this is the kind of request you hate: the impossible problem over which you have no control. I tried diplomacy.

"Sam, I am sorry to tell you that she has no possibility of being done here, or anywhere else in the U.S. that I know of. This is very complex surgery that consumes tens of thousands of dollars in cost just during hospitalization. That's if there are no complications. If the patient needs more prolonged hospitalization, the cost could go into six figures. Our administrators face these kinds of requests all the time. No matter how sad and compelling the story, the medical center just cannot become a charitable institution for needy kids from other countries, when there are a million heartbreaking stories out there."

"OK, then, I'll pay all her hospital fees," Sam replied. "Can you take care of the doctors' fees?"

I sat stunned in my office chair. "Have you ever met this little girl, Sam?"

"I know her mother. That's enough."

"Do you realize that you are talking about an open-ended cost?"

"It's not about money," he said.

"Give me a few minutes to think about this."

I strolled across the hall to the office of Dr. Alfredo Trento, our mul-
tiskilled chief of cardiac surgery. The antithesis of the "surgical personality," Alfredo rose to greet me with his always-welcoming smile, waved at
a sofa next to his desk, and in his charming Northern Italian accent said,
"C'mon in, Jim."

I plunked down in a chair opposite him. Alfredo and I played tennis
together on the weekends when we had time. Our kids played on the same
high school soccer team. Even so this was not going to be an easy conversation.

"I have a once-in-a-lifetime problem, Alfredo," I said. "It involves
three people. There's a poor hard-working mother, a very sick child, and
a remarkable benefactor. And then there's you and me," I added, showing
limited math skills. I told the story of the child we had never seen and a
mother neither of us knew. Then I showed Alfredo the echoes.

"Here's the thing, Alfredo," I said. "If Sam pays the hospital bill, cardiology could do the pre-op evaluation and post-hospital care at no charge.
Is it possible for you to do the surgery at no charge?"

I knew how balanced my question sounded but how unfair it really
was. My part would be easy. I could admit the patient under my name
and handle much of the cardiac evaluation myself. Alfredo's part was far
more complex. He had to convince the physician members of his team and
the anesthesiologist to participate. Then he had to perform the surgery and
commit his team to handling any postoperative problems.

As with Sam, Alfredo's response was stunning. There was not even a
pause for reflection. "I can do it, Jim."

I reached across the desk to shake his hand. "Thanks, Alfredo."

I called Sam to tell him the news.

"I'll do my part, you do yours, Alfredo does his, and providence will
smile on us," he said.

Where Sam thought the problem was solved, I thought it was just beginning. Unlike our usual patients, Maria was coming with a satchel of
unanswered questions. Could the pulmonary stenosis be managed without creating a valve that allowed regurgitation? Would Maria have other

cardiac abnormalities unseen on the Polaroids that could complicate surgery, like a displaced coronary artery? Would she have noncardiac abnormalities like scoliosis? Would she have to be treated for other illnesses before she underwent surgery? Was her body strong enough to sustain her during the time her survival would be totally dependent upon a machine? The heart-lung machine would collect deoxygenated blood returning in the body's veins, add oxygen, and then pump the reoxygenated blood into her arteries, allowing Alfredo to unhurriedly operate on her nonbeating heart. Maria's life would depend on a heart-lung machine.

RETURNING TO PHILADELPHIA after the war, John Gibbon joined the staff of his alma mater, Philadelphia's Jefferson Medical College. Soon after his return, Mayo Clinic surgeon Clarence Dennis, who shared Gibbon's vision of building a heart-lung machine, came to visit. It was to be a critical moment in cardiac surgery. Gibbon cheerfully demonstrated his laboratory prototype and then gave its complete specifications to Dennis. Back in Minnesota, Dennis quickly succeeded in building a functioning device. Dennis leapfrogged Gibbon by testing his device in patients. Both patients died, and with these devastating failures, both Dennis and the heart-lung machine seemed destined to become historical footnotes. But then the heart-lung story took an unforeseeable new direction.

Who could have imagined that the final resolution to Gibbon's apparently insurmountable technical difficulties lay not in his medical domain but in his social life? Gibbon discovered the path that is now the template for all the major technical advances in cardiology. Through his social contacts, Gibbon found a collaborator in industry. Gibbon's angel was the self-made industrialist Thomas Watson, the chief executive officer of International Business Machines (IBM) and one of America's richest men. IBM knew cash registers, high speed sorting of punch cards, and primitive computers, but absolutely nothing about oxygenators and pumps. Watson, captivated by Gibbon's vision, was undeterred. He assigned five IBM engineers to improve Gibbon's device, and funded its development. He added the critical step of sending engineers to Philadelphia to get hands-on experience with the device in Gibbon's laboratory. Working with

Gibbon, the engineers were able to fairly quickly resolve two of three engineering problems: they diminished pump-induced mechanical damage to the oxygen-carrying red blood cells, and they developed a closed system that prevented blood from clotting. Their first device succeeded in bypassing the circulation in dogs, but it was difficult to argue it was ready for human use. About 10% of the dogs died.

Gibbon and the IBM engineers began to attack the most recalcitrant problem, and the one they knew least about: how to add oxygen to the deoxygenated venous (meaning in the veins) blood before returning it to the body.

In Sweden, surgeon Dr. Viking Björk had just proved that it was possible to add oxygen to red blood cells by whirling a film of blood in a stream of oxygen. Björk's system was impractical because whirling shattered too many red blood cells. At IBM, engineers came up with a better idea, cascading the blood over a thin slanted sheet of film while exposing it to oxygen, then collecting the oxygenated blood at the base of the film (later inventive genius Walt Lillehei used the same principle, sending clouds of minute oxygen bubbles through deoxygenated blood). With their new method of oxygenation, Gibbon and the engineers kept twelve dogs alive during open heart surgery for more than an hour.

With oxygenation at least partially solved, IBM remodeled the device to make it appropriate for human use. Gibbon's first patient was a fifteen-month-old baby. Fate decreed that Gibbon would fail. The machine worked, but Gibbon was done in by preoperative misdiagnosis. What he and his cardiologist thought would be a simple atrial septal defect turned out to be far more complex. The atrial septal defect was only one part of the malformation of the baby's heart. Ironically when Dennis had tried his version of the heart-lung machine, he had been done in by the same mistaken diagnosis. Neither surgeon was able to correct more complex congenital malformations, and both patients died.

In May 1953, Gibbon tried again. This time he operated on Martha Cowley, an eighteen-year-old freshman at Wilkes College in Wilkes-Barre, Pennsylvania, about two and a half hours from Philadelphia. When he opened her heart, Gibbon found he was looking at an atrial septal defect about the size of a half dollar. After his prior misdiagnosis fatality, Gibbon breathed a sigh of relief. This was a simple atrial septal defect,

similar in size and complexity to the one Lewis and Lillehei had closed
in Minnesota using hypothermia. Unlike the Minnesota surgeons, who
had repaired an ASD in six minutes, Gibbon was slow, methodical, and
deliberate. Using his heart-lung machine instead of hypothermia, he
could take more time. Gibbon kept Martha on the heart-lung machine for
twenty-six minutes while he closed the defect. Gibbon declared himself
satisfied with his closure. Now history hung in the balance. Would Martha wake up from anesthesia without any brain defect, able to return to
her college studies? Martha woke up feeling fine, and recovered quickly
from surgery.

Only someone with Gibbon's personality could have achieved what
he did. True, he was not an iconoclast in the mold of Harken, Bailey, or
Lillehei, but he shared their persistence in the face of repeated failure, and
their immunity to colleagues' contrary opinions about his work. Gibbon's
nineteen years in pursuit of a single goal stands as a monument to dogged
persistence in cardiovascular research.

The postwar surgeons' serpentine path had entered many blind alleys
and bridged a river of children's blood, but Gibbon had finally broken
through. Amazingly, the period from Harken's D-day shrapnel surgery
to Gibbon's heart-lung machine had been less than a decade, yet as cardiac surgeon Michael DeBakey said, it was "one of the truly great sagas
of medical research in the history of medicine." Two decades later, the
heart-lung machine would play a central role in our attack on coronary
artery disease, the nation's number one killer.

SOME YEARS AGO, radio news commentator Paul Harvey ended his
broadcast with what he called "the Rest of the Story." He would begin
with an intrinsically fascinating story, take a commercial break, then return to relate a dumbfounding final twist that made his tale doubly fascinating. Paul Harvey would revel in telling the Jack Gibbon story. Two
months after his success, Gibbon followed up his landmark achievement
by using his machine for surgery on two more children with congenital
heart disease. Both died. Astonishingly Jack Gibbon, forty-nine years old
and at the peak of his career, quit. Flat out quit. He declared a one-year
moratorium on use of his device. But in fact he was done. At the end of

the year, he gave responsibility for cardiac surgery to a younger colleague. He never again scrubbed, gowned, and gloved for another open heart surgery.

Nowhere in the history of medicine will you find a person who dedicates an entire career to a visionary goal, overcomes seemingly insurmountable obstacles, achieves the goal, and then walks away. Jack Gibbon stands alone.

Two years later Thomas Watson was succeeded by his son as CEO of IBM. Now a dominant company in the emerging computer industry, IBM declared that the heart-lung machine program did not fit its core business, withdrew its team from Philadelphia, and departed from the medical device field.

Having been criticized for all the years he consumed pursuing the heart-lung machine, Gibbon was now condemned by some for abandoning it. Among the critics was Dwight Harken: "All of us who have done firsts and gone on and lost lives and spent a good deal of our own lives to create new things realize what it is like to go through all that. We also know the feeling of triumph as well as the feeling of defeat and we resent it when a man does just one successful case and quits! One patient lives and you can't just sit down and say, 'Now I've done that, that's it, that's my contribution. You are obliged to standardize the technique so as to serve others.'"

Those who knew him, however, knew his decision was quintessential Jack Gibbon. He viewed himself as a scientist and a scholar. He did not even publish a report of the first success with the heart-lung machine until a year later, when he gave an invited lecture at the Mayo Clinic. His report was published in *Minnesota Medicine*, a journal with very limited circulation, rather than in a major medical journal, any one of which would have leaped at the opportunity. Having devoted his professional life to developing the single most important advance in the history of cardiac surgery, Jack Gibbon modestly stepped aside. He had accomplished what he set out to do. But I believe there was another reason. Some, like Harken, Bailey, and Lillehei can tolerate the Pain of the Pioneer, and others cannot. Gibbon could not. I think we can all understand. As his friend George Humphries observed, "The others were taking the risk and killing babies, and he didn't like that." Artistic, sensitive, genial, warm-hearted Jack

Gibbon could not stand the pain. I think that for Jack Gibbon the balance was clear: he would not put young patients at risk even when it meant ceding recognition at the apogee of his life's work to others. Gibbon, always the teacher, went on to write a standard textbook on thoracic surgery.

I have found that medical students and most cardiologists do not recognize John Gibbon's name. As we will see repeatedly in our chronicle, history rewards the person who brings an idea to common use, not the one who has it first. By quitting after one successful use of his device, Gibbon did not pursue the level of surgical immortality that he deserves. *Sic transit gloria mundi* . . . thus passes the glory of the world.

The informal partnership between John Gibbon and Thomas Watson of IBM, however, became an enduring template. Collaboration between physician-scientists and industry would drive virtually all the breakthroughs in cardiovascular medicine that followed. As I tell our research fellows, if you want to go fast, go alone, but if you want to go far, go together.

The final irony is that in Gibbon's time the cardiac risk of smoking was not yet recognized. His heart-lung machine was to become the centerpiece of coronary bypass surgery. But for him it was too late. In 1973, not yet twenty years after his landmark success, lifelong smoker John H. Gibbon suffered a fatal heart attack on the tennis court at the age of sixty-nine.

GIBBON REFUSED TO use his device, and IBM proved a corporate dropout. Was the cardiac meteor that had flashed so briefly across the Philadelphia sky extinguished? What happened to the heart-lung machine? It simply reappeared more brightly at the Mayo Clinic, where Clarence Dennis arose like the phoenix from his transient status in the ashes of surgical history to improve Gibbon's version of the heart-lung machine. Graciously giving credit to the original design that Gibbon had given him years earlier, Dennis and his collaborators called it the "Mayo Gibbon–type oxygenator."

Mayo Clinic cardiac surgeon Dr. John Kirklin and his colleagues used the device on hundreds of patients over the next several years. Kirklin, rigorously intellectual and aloof, and nicknamed The Iceman by one of his biographers, set up a database for long-term follow-up of his operated patients. Kirklin's data illuminates the stunning truth of the birth of open heart surgery. In 1955 their mortality rate for cardiac surgery was 50%. A year later it was 20%, and by 1957 it had fallen to 10%. Today it is a few percentage points, with almost all mortality confined to patients who are at very high risk prior to surgery. Tragedy precedes triumph.

A FEW WEEKS after my last conversation with Sam, Maria and her mother appeared in the lobby of my office. She was small for a twelve-year-old. In a new flowered dress, brown skin, and black hair, she was endearing. A small silver cross dangled from a silver chain around her neck. Eyes downcast, she stood very close to her mother.

A few minutes later in the examining room, Maria still did not look at me directly. I paused to see my examining room as she saw it: narrow, white walls without windows; its only decoration a blood pressure manometer mounted on the wall. Two inexpensive chairs, a small metal desk, and an odd three-piece examining table completed the space in which there was no locus of warmth, comfort, or safety. The examining table was so high she would have to use a stool to reach it.

I got another chair for her mother, and asked both of them to sit close to me in a small circle. I rested my hand on her mother's arm and told her I would like to look at her hands. Then I did the same with Maria, gently opening her closed little fist. Her fingernails had the dusky blue color of tetralogy. Next I told her mother I would like to listen to her heart. I positioned my stethoscope over the mother's heart and listened. Then, with the stethoscope still over her mother's heart, I motioned for Maria to listen to her mom's heartbeat. Her face lit up and she smiled. Young cardiologists sometimes argue that you don't need a stethoscope anymore because you get everything you need to know from the ECG and echo. What's more, the information is far more accurate. But they overlook a critical point: the stethoscope is a metaphor for caring communication, a symbol of the connection between me and my vulnerable patient.

Before having her climb on the examining table, I did a quick sleight-of-hand trick I had done with kids around the world, asking which hand held an object. Kids always choose the wrong hand, and Maria did, too. A smile. I did the trick again. She chose the other hand, and was right.

A big smile of triumph. Now she could look at me. I saw that although Maria had been shy, she did not seem fearful. Maria had already passed through that stage. She had accepted that in this hospital her life lay in the balance. So what I saw was hope. Immense bravery speaking to me from the brown eyes of a frail little girl standing alone in a joyless room, a foreign land, trusting her life to strangers she could barely understand. She touched her cross as I boosted her onto the examining table.

On the exam table, I could feel the outward heaving movement of her hypertrophied right ventricle. She had the typical heart murmurs associated with tetralogy. Alfredo came in. He focused on the chest wall, listened to her heart, and carefully checked the pulses of the vessels to be used during the heart-lung bypass. Imaging of Maria's heart showed no additional congenital abnormalities. Dr. Larry Czer, a member of my cardiology staff who specialized in all of Alfredo's pre- and postoperative care, gave the green light for her open heart surgery. Maria's impossible dream was about to begin.

I slipped in and out of the operating room on the day of surgery. Maria's tiny body was enveloped in a cocoon of four surgeons and an anesthesiologist, backed by what seemed like a second layer of heart-lung machine technicians and scrub nurses. At Alfredo's command, Maria's heart was stopped, and she was "on bypass," her life held in the balance by the heart-lung machine. Alfredo cut open Maria's heart, entering it through the right atrium, so that he could preserve the pulmonary valve and avoid damaging the right ventricle. He easily closed the ventricular septal defect with a patch. Next he turned his attention to the narrowed pulmonary valve. He enlarged the valve's area. Finally he made sure that all blood from the left ventricle would be pumped only into her aorta. The whole procedure took a couple of hours. At the end of the procedure, with the heart-lung machine now turned off and Maria's own heart beating again, Alfredo used echocardiography to check on his repair. The echo showed excellent pulmonary valve function. The pressure in the right ventricle had already fallen dramatically, the two cardinal signs that his fix was going to work.

With Alfredo still in the operating suite, I went to the family waiting area to give her mother the news. She crossed herself as I approached, looking for some sign of good or bad news. Twenty feet away, I gave the universal two thumbs-up sign. Her eyes grew temporarily glassy, but she didn't cry.

On the day following surgery, Maria already looked much healthier. Her blue lips were now pink. Although it is difficult to listen for murmurs immediately after surgery, I heard no murmur of pulmonary insufficiency (backflow across the pulmonary valve). This was the most common complication of tetralogy surgery, created if the surgeon overshoots the mark in correcting the pulmonary valve stenosis. Late on post-op day one, Maria could sit up in bed. The next day she sat in a chair. Soon she walked to the window of her room. In the second post-op week she was ready for discharge.

A few months later I received a letter postmarked El Salvador. It was very neatly written in Spanish.

Dear Dr. Forrester,

Thank you for your kindness and understanding in helping me with the surgery by Dr. Trento. I know that saved my life because I feel strong and healthy now. May God bless you and your family.

Sincerely,
Maria de Silva.

Over the years I lost touch with Sam Bachner. Halfway through writing this book, I called Sam's office to ask if he knew anything about that twelve-year-old child from a decade and a half ago. His secretary set up an appointment for me to call him back.

When I called back a couple of days later, we reminisced for a few minutes.

Then Sam said, "Would you like to talk to Maria?"

Baffled, I wondered if Sam had lost a little over the years. We were both getting older. After a long embarrassed pause, I said, "In El Salvador?"

"No, right now. She's here with me."

The voice of a young woman floated up softly from my speaker phone. "Hello, Dr. Forrester, it's Maria." Accustomed as I am to speechifying, for several moments I found myself without words. Staring at the phone in disbelief. Dumbfounded. Sensing my confusion, her voice filled the uncomfortable void, "I want thank you again for your kindness so many years ago."

Her words recalled a child's letter from years ago, buried emotions now almost two decades old. As that poignant moment passed, I pictured devilish Sam Bachner beaming at the profoundly moving surprise he had dropped in the lap of his old friend. It was time for me to have Maria to tell me the Rest of her Story.

"After the surgery, it took a while for me to recover my strength, so I stayed with my mom at Mr. Bachner's house. But of course after a few months I had to return to my country. When I got home, I felt strong for the first time ever in my life. So I focused on my schoolwork. I was a really good student, good enough to go to college. I graduated with a degree in business."

I beamed as I replied, "I feel just like a proud parent. What a wonderful story."

"But it's not the end of my story, Dr. Forrester. After college, I married my sweetheart, and now we have two children."

"Two kids . . . how lucky can I be to have called just when you came back to LA for a vacation. That's a pretty crazy coincidence," I said.

"Well, not exactly. I came back to be with my mom . . . it's pretty amazing, but she still works for Mr. Bachner. It's been twenty-three years now."

"Sam's a mighty fine boss," I offered.

"He sure is. I am one of his business managers."

I slapped my forehead. "You're kidding" was all I could say. All I could think was thank goodness I was sitting down when I called Sam. My most astonishing phone call ever lasted a quite a while longer as the three of us chatted until finally it was time to say warm good-byes.

When I hung up I leaned back in my chair, closed my eyes, and mused how one life saved created two new ones. I recalled a phrase I had spoken at my mentor's eulogy: "A teacher affects eternity; he never knows where his influence ends." I saw that Maria's life reflected that idea. She was saved by the intuition of Dwight Harken, the inventiveness of Walt Lillehei, and the persistence of John Gibbon years before Alfredo Trento's magical cardiac reconstruction. And, of course, by her own Don Quixote, Sam

Bachner. So different in pedigree, personality, and era, these men shared a uniquely American trait: each had dreamed an Impossible Dream.

TODAY CHILDREN DESTINED to die from a cardiac malformation often have a diagnosis made by echocardiography and have surgical correction while they are still neonates. Given the river of blood with which cardiac surgery began, the mortality rate for congenital heart surgery is now astonishingly low. It has plummeted from 50% in Walt Lillehei's early years to about 2% today. In major centers, the mortality rate for the simplest heart defects is 0%.

John Gibbon's invention had created an outcome far beyond the most fevered imagination of Aristotle, or even Billroth, and Paget, the surgeons who proclaimed the heart was off-limits. Mankind had replaced the function of the heart and lungs given him by nature with a machine so powerful that cardiovascular medicine emerged from its Dark Ages, poised for its own industrial revolution.

PART II

THE INDUSTRIAL REVOLUTION

7

ELECTRIFYING DISCOVERIES

In the event of my Demise when my heart can beat no more,
I Hope I Die For A Principle or A Belief that I have Lived 4.

—Tupak Shakur, American rap singer and poet

THE SUCCESS OF cardiac surgery brought three devastating complications that often caused death on the table: ventricular fibrillation,
complete heart block, and preoperative misdiagnosis. To advance cardiac
surgery to the next level, we had to find a way to cope with these misad-
ventures. But when we did, the solutions created an entirely unanticipated,
electrifying spin-off: our first breakthrough in the treatment of CAD.

Cardiac surgery's single most terrifying complication was the sudden
onset of ventricular fibrillation, the devastating disorder of heart rhythm
that caused Willie the Phillie's sudden death. Ventricular fibrillation,
which claimed many of Harken and Bailey's early patients, is the heart's
electrical system's descent into complete chaos. The simultaneous, synchro-
nized forceful contraction of every ventricular muscle fiber is replaced by
tiny wormlike writhing of the muscle fibers, with the result that there is
absolutely no forward movement of blood. A person with no blood flow
loses consciousness in about five seconds, and is irretrievably brain-dead
in about four minutes.

* * *

IN ENGLAND ON March 17, 2012, in the forty-first minute of the first half, twenty-three-year-old world-class English center midfielder Fabrice Muamba heard his goalie yell for him to pull back to a more defensive position. Congo-born Muamba was a rising English soccer star. He had represented England on its under-21 team, had played briefly for the Arsenal, then moved to Birmingham City where fans voted him the Young Player of the Year. Sold to Bolton for $10 million, he was named as the *Bolton News* Player of the Season in 2010. At just age twenty-one Muamba had signed a new four-year contract. He was now a force on the Bolton Wanderers as they played a nationally televised match against the Tottenham Hotspur before a packed stadium of 30,000 fans in Tottenham. His goalie's voice was the last one he heard that day. With no one near him, Muamba spun and fell face forward on the field. Initial derisive catcalls disappeared as the first players to reach him tried to roll him onto his back and waved frantically for help. Trainers and doctors from both clubs ran out. Someone started cardiac resuscitation. Within seconds, a defibrillator appeared at Muamba's side. The drama escalated further when a fan pushed past guards and raced onto the field. The fan was consultant cardiologist Dr. Andrew Deaner. The stadium fell as silent as a grave as Deaner demanded to take over. Two defibrillator shocks were administered. Players from both teams wept privately; several knelt and prayed.

After six minutes of futile attempts to resuscitate Muamba on the pitch, he was lifted to a gurney and wheeled toward the emergency exit ramp. As he disappeared onto the ramp, every voice in the stadium chanted "Fa-BRICE Mu-AMBA." At the end of the ramp the caterwauling wail of a departing ambulance announced another battle with heart disease. Dr. Deaner accompanied him to the ambulance. In the ambulance he insisted that Muamba be sped to his coronary care unit at the famed London Chest Hospital. Realizing it would be impossible for the teams to continue, referee Howard Webb canceled the game. Bolton's next game, three days later, was also canceled.

SUDDEN UNEXPECTED DEATH. What can one do when faced with such a shocking event? One such moment occurred in 1947 as Cleveland's endlessly innovative surgeon Dr. Claude Beck was operating on a fourteen-year-old boy with a severe congenital inward depression of the breastbone. The proper name of the condition is pectus excavatum, but medicine has nicknamed it "funnel chest." The boy's sternum squashed his heart against the vertebrae like a punching bag. After restoring the normal chest configuration, Beck began to close his surgical incision. Suddenly the boy's pulse disappeared. In a single glance Beck knew he was looking at tragedy. The child's heart was in ventricular fibrillation. Since the invention of anesthesia a century earlier, surgeons were intimately familiar with ventricular fibrillation, the leading cause of death on the operating table. In surgical suites throughout the world "v fib" meant the operation was finished. Ventricular fibrillation meant death. There was no way to bring the patient back to life.

But on that morning Claude Beck had a hunch. He had no painstaking prior research, no study design, no testable scientific hypothesis. He just had an intuition. He immediately began manually squeezing the teenager's heart at sixty squeezes per minute to maintain his circulation. That would keep him alive, but for what purpose? Every person in his operating room, his hospital, his profession knew that no surgeon in the world could bring back the heartbeat during ventricular fibrillation. Nowhere but in Cleveland, Beck was thinking.

As early as 1899 researchers in Geneva had demonstrated that an electrical current could restore normal rhythm during ventricular fibrillation in dogs. The observation meant little to medicine until the development and widespread use of the electrocardiogram in the 1920s. Until the ECG, doctors were unaware that ventricular fibrillation was the rhythm of sudden death. The leader in ventricular fibrillation research in animals in the years surrounding World War II was Dr. Carl Wiggers of Western Reserve in Cleveland. Wiggers had developed a method of defibrillation by delivering an electric shock using two paddles that he applied directly to the heart of his experimental dogs. Beck demanded that Wiggers's apparatus be immediately brought to his operating room. Beck waited. And waited. Imagine squeezing the heart sixty times a minute, with no realistic hope of saving the child. After forty-five minutes, when the device arrived, he could barely open and close his hand. Beck wiped off the paddles—no sense giving his patient an infection—and immediately applied an electrical current directly to the boy's quivering, lifeless heart using

Wiggers's dog paddles. Ventricular fibrillation persisted. For millennia, mankind had tried to restore life to the dead. How grandiose of Claude Beck to imagine that he could accomplish that which was reserved to the gods. It would not be permitted on a Cleveland morning.

But Beck was not one to concede failure. He called for procaine, a drug that suppresses ventricular arrhythmias. He injected the drug directly into the boy's right atrium and continued squeezing to distribute the drug throughout the heart.

Paddles applied again, a second shock, irregular twitches morphing into a few rapid feeble contractions, more regular now, a heart struggling to rise from a knockout blow, as if unwilling to be counted out just yet. Beck returned to squeezing the heart, urging his staggering gladiator to continue this fight, pausing every few moments to see if the heart continued to beat on its own. With each check, the boy's heart seemed stronger, stronger again . . . in about five minutes, it generated a palpable blood pressure with no help from Beck's aching fingers.

Claude Beck had accomplished the impossible. He had miraculously restored life to a boy who was dead. He had proven that the human heart could be restarted after it stopped beating, that the suddenly dead could be restored to life. An Alexander the Great cutting through the Gordian knot rather than untying it, Beck had solved the mystery of cardiac resuscitation with a single definitive slash of his scalpel. Today resuscitation is a commonplace occurrence in hospitals around the world. I can testify that the incomparable profound emotion that engulfed Beck is undiminished today when one is successful. Imagine for a moment my elation, my relief had I restored life to Willie the Phillie on that Philadelphia morning long ago. But Claude Beck was the first, and in that one brief, luminous moment, he had achieved mankind's dream of two millennia, so clearly first given voice in the Christian tradition when Jesus restores life to Lazarus with the words, "I am the resurrection and the life" (John 11).

IN THE AMBULANCE Fabrice Muamba received twelve more defibrillation shocks, as resuscitation continued without success. He was still dead on arrival at the hospital. In the coronary care unit, intravenous lines, intubation with ventilation, and cardiac drugs were given in a more controlled environment, and defibrillation was repeated. Still no response.

At seventy-five minutes after his cardiac arrest, with hope for Muamba's survival nearly extinguished, the resuscitation team delivered another defibrillator shock. Fabrice Muamba's heart started beating. The link between Claude Beck's fourteen-year-old boy to Fabrice Muamba was complete.

In an emotional interview, the soccer club's physician who accompanied Muamba stood astonished at his bedside: "It was forty-eight minutes from when he collapsed to reaching the hospital and a further thirty minutes after that. He was, in effect, dead at that time. We were fearing the worst and didn't think we would get the recovery we had. It's incredible."

In the Congo, Football Association president Omari Selemani said the national hero midfielder had the support of "65 million Congolese." But was the good news really bad news? Would Fabrice Muamba's brain still function? Muamba was put into therapeutic hypothermia in intensive care to let his brain recover.

Dr. Andrew Deaner, the doctor who had come out of the stands, related that moment that as a doctor you can never forget: "Two hours after [regaining consciousness] I whispered in his ear, 'What's your name?' and he said, 'Fabrice Muamba.' I said, 'I hear you're a really good footballer' and he said, 'I try.' I had a tear in my eye."

CLAUDE BECK'S DECISIVE act teaches us one common path to scientific breakthroughs. Revolutions occur when happenstance opens a door just a crack, and a unique individual standing at the door glimpses a shimmering possibility that the rest of humanity has missed. Looking at shrapnel projecting from hearts, Dwight Harken intuited opportunity where others saw hopelessness. Beck's discovery required a thoracic surgeon, an open chest, an open mind, knowledge of Wiggers's research, a defibrillator system near the surgical suite, and the power to demand its instant delivery. When all those factors came together at one moment in time, Claude Beck seized that moment. Louis Pasteur, who discovered that germs are the cause of infection, summarized this profound scientific insight in five words, "Chance favors the prepared mind." Soon after Beck described his experience, every operating room had a defibrillator.

In his own hospital, Beck became enraptured with the combination of manual cardiac massage followed by electrical defibrillation. In June 1955, sixty-five-year-old physician Albert Ransone came to Cleveland's Western Reserve Hospital for a preoperative ECG before his scheduled gall bladder surgery. While in the waiting room he complained of chest pain, then suddenly collapsed and died in the waiting room. Claude Beck and his associate Dr. David Leighninger were nearby. Rushing to his side, without removing his shirt, they immediately slashed through Ransone's chest wall between the fourth and fifth ribs, pried the ribs apart, forced a hand through the incision, gripped Ransone's lifeless heart, and began rhythmic manual cardiac massage. They shouted for someone to bring the defibrillator from the operating room. At the same time others on Beck's team initiated respiratory support. After twenty-five minutes of manual compression of the heart, the defibrillator arrived. Beck was ready. Two paddles delivered an electric shock. It took three shocks, but they restored a normal heart rhythm. But would Dr. Ransone regain consciousness? Would he ever be able to return to the practice of medicine? No one had ever resuscitated a patient outside the operating room, so no one knew. Dr. Ransone completed the miracle. He survived, with his brain intact.

Beck's manuscript recounting this astounding "man-on-the-street" resuscitation struck the medical world like lightning in the midst of a thunderstorm, illuminating the entire landscape of surgery and medicine. He concluded his manuscript with an extraordinarily prescient vision of the future: "This one experience indicates that resuscitation from a fatal heart attack is not impossible and might be applied to those who die in hospital and perhaps to those who die outside hospital." If you could defibrillate a heart in the operating room, you could do it on the hospital ward. If you could defibrillate in the hospital, what about on a busy street or in a crowded stadium?

But resuscitating in the operating room was far different from anyplace else. Only in the operating room did you have an open chest. Beck had a solution for that, too. On threat of being fired on the spot, he demanded that each of his trainees carry a scalpel in their white coat pocket. So, soon around the nation, every surgeon's jacket pocket had a scalpel at the ready. Mercifully this brief fad, which resembled a chaotic Aztec ritual, disappeared suddenly with the arrival of external defibrillators. At Harvard, however, we liked to say that only a fool falls asleep in a cardiology conference with Dwight Harken in the room. Years later, Johns Hopkins Chief of Cardiology Richard Ross's favorite apocryphal story was that he awoke from a fainting spell to see a Hopkins cardiac surgeon with a scalpel poised above his chest. I countered that during an academic turf war with our cardiac surgeon at my hospital, I had the identical experience, except I hadn't fainted.

And the Rest of the Story? Dr. Ransone was hospitalized for eleven days for his myocardial infarction (heart attack), then returned to his practice in Florida. Years later one of the participants in Dr. Ransone's resuscitation decided to track down their original patient. Dr. Ransone had outlived Claude Beck. It was not even close . . . he lived another twenty-eight years, and died at age ninety-three.

BY THE MORNING of March 19, two days after his cardiac arrest, Fabrice Muamba's heart was in a normal rhythm without medication, and he was able to move his arms and legs. By the fourth hospital day his doctors' press release was one of those classic understatements that make Americans so fond of the British. They quite seriously told the waiting press that Muamba had "exceeded our expectations" in his recovery. He received what he affectionately calls his second heart, an implantable cardioverter defibrillator (ICD), and was discharged a day short of a month after his collapse.

His interviews after discharge are emotionally touching even to non-soccer fans. Will he return to the pitch? It is too early to say, but his doctors have not ruled it out. "It all depends on my heart rhythm . . . If it comes back to normality, we'll see what the specialist says regarding me playing again," Muamba said.

Two weeks after his hospital discharge Muamba wended his way, smiling broadly, glassy-eyed, arms raised in gratitude, to the center of

Bolton's home stadium turf, amid the tears and raucous cheers of thousands who knew they were witnessing a miracle. And the opponent that day? Tottenham Hotspur. A life that ended a month earlier face down on Tottenham turf had come full circle. What goes around comes around. Fabrice Muamba, meet Dr. Claude Beck.

8

THE HEART THAT
SKIPPED A BEAT

*Reasonable people adapt themselves to the world.
Unreasonable people attempt to adapt the world to
themselves. All progress, therefore, depends on
unreasonable people.*

—GEORGE BERNARD SHAW, IRISH PLAYWRIGHT

THE OTHER COMMON catastrophic cause of sudden death during the early years of cardiac surgery was surgically induced heart block. Annie Brown, Walt Lillehei's poster child, had a minute of transient heart block, but in many of his early surgeries, it was permanent and ended in his patient's death. In heart block the electrical impulse traveling from the atrium is blocked before it reaches the ventricle. The ventricle's backup electrical system takes over, but at a much slower rate, usually around thirty beats per minute. At this rate the victim typically loses consciousness, and death often follows.

Paul Zoll was a consummate Boston physician, a graduate of Boston Latin School who matriculated to Harvard College and then Harvard Medical School, where he graduated summa cum laude. Slight and wiry, brilliant and inquisitive, he was the quintessential East Coast intellectual, disinclined to suffer fools. Swamped by his white coat, with huge ears, a prominent forehead, and a bald pate, my immediate impression of this intellectual giant was "elfin." Given his stern reputation, I was wise enough to keep that description to myself until today.

During the war, Zoll was the cardiologist for the 160th U.S. Army Station Hospital—the military hospital where Dwight Harken was making his surgical breakthrough. Zoll was the sole coauthor on Harken's landmark publication describing shrapnel extraction surgery. Perhaps Zoll's mind drifted as he stood at the operating table watching the drama of Harken's shrapnel extraction, because it was here that he made the trivial observation which would become the spark that solved heart block. In Harken's operating room, as he stared down aghast at chests ripped open by explosives, Zoll noted that the esophagus, which passes just behind the heart on its way from the mouth to the stomach, abuts on the heart. It was an observation of no conceivable relevance at the time, but as we shall see, it was an image that was critical to Zoll's development of pacemakers, the solution to heart block.

Today we have an entire subspecialty of cardiology devoted to just the heart's electrical system, called electrophysiology. At the end of World War II, however, pacemakers and defibrillators, the yin and the yang of an electrophysiologist's practice, did not yet exist. The pacemaker, like the defibrillator, sprang from cardiac surgeons' despair at seeing heart block suddenly appear in a heart too good to die.

I HAVE SEEN pacemakers save innumerable lives, but I know of no story that compares to the one related by Major Robert Eckart about a thirty-year-old soldier who sustained devastating chest trauma from an improvised roadside explosive device during combat in Iraq. When he arrived at the Ibn Sina 28th Combat Support Hospital (CSH), in Baghdad, his condition was reminiscent of the soldiers Dwight Harken faced sixty years earlier. His upper right arm was shattered, with bone protruding from the skin, and he had an open wound on the right side of his chest wall. In addition he had no detectable pulses in his right leg. X-ray images of his chest and abdomen by computed tomography showed metal shell fragments in his right lung with a pool of blood between the lung and right chest wall, injury to the heart's right atrium, and another fragment in his abdomen in a branch of the aorta leading to his right leg.

Surgeons Robert Stewart and Edward Falta faced mind-boggling challenges. As they opened the pericardial sac which surrounds the heart, blood gushed out. The soldier had not died from the penetrating wound of the heart because, like Wilhelm Justus in Frankfurt a century before him, it had been sealed off by the pericardial sac surrounding it. Stewart and Falta sewed up the tear in the right atrium where a fragment had entered the heart. But where the heck was the shell fragment? It wasn't in the heart! Astonished, they traced the fragment's path. After penetrating the chest wall and ripping into the right atrium, it had blasted its way through the muscular wall that separates the right ventricle from the left ventricle, was then pumped into the aorta, and finally lodged in one of the aortic branches within his abdomen when it could pass no further. As they repaired the hole in the heart and extracted the shell fragment, the soldier's heart rate suddenly fell to thirty beats per minute. Heart block!

Like Claude Beck decades earlier, Stewart and Falta resorted to manual cardiac compression to maintain life. Now with a chest open, a life hung in the balance. They summoned the hospital's cardiologist, Major Robert Eckart, to the operating room. There is no textbook, no article, no manual on how to handle this situation. But Eckart was also a specialist in disorders of the heart's electrical system, and he had an idea on how to pace the heart, how to save the life of a dying soldier. Who could possibly imagine that Major Eckart's soldier's chance of survival traces like a perfectly straight line to the surgeons and cardiologists of a prior war? But it does.

RETURNING FROM THE war to the private practice of cardiology at Boston's Beth Israel Hospital, Zoll was referred a sixty-year-old woman who was suffering fainting spells. Finding a heart rate that intermittently dropped into the low 30s, Zoll diagnosed complete heart block. The electrical impulse that began in the atrium was blocked from passing into the ventricle. Her heart was otherwise perfectly normal—with good heart muscle, good valves, and open arteries. Although she was healthy, Zoll knew she was at risk of sudden death, and worse, that he had no effective preventive therapy. It was not long until she fainted and died under Zoll's care, with him powerless to influence the inevitable event. Zoll reacted to her death as if it was a personal affront to his worth as a cardiologist, hissing, "This should not happen to a heart perfectly normal except for a block of conduction."

Why the image of a soldier's heart lying on top of the esophagus in Harken's operating room rises to one's consciousness defies explanation, but there it was, in Technicolor. Image, imagination, intuition. Zoll knew that before the war someone doing research in rabbits had demonstrated that an electrical stimulus applied directly to the heart could induce it to contract. He knew from reading hundreds of chest X-ray images that the esophagus briefly touched the heart as it passed behind it from the mouth to the stomach. Zoll had a hunch. Perhaps he could deliver an electrical shock to the heart using an electrode positioned in the esophagus just at the point where it touched the heart.

In his mind's eye he saw that electrical stimulus pass through the wall of the esophagus and into the heart tissue, which pressed against it. To test his idea, he advanced an electrode on the end of a wire through the mouth and down into the esophagus of an anesthetized dog, until it reached a position just behind the heart. Since his electrical stimulus needed a target, he put a second electrode on the dog's chest wall. Zoll delivered a brief electrical pulse. Bingo! Zoll's inspired guess was correct. Each time he delivered an electrical pulse, the dog's ventricles contracted.

Zoll's intuition, like all great revelations, was an image that flashed in a receptive mind. After some tinkering, Paul Zoll had a primitive electrical system that delivered a continuous train of electrical impulses, which might be substituted for Nature's malfunctioning pacemaker. But like many of us who entered cardiovascular research in that era, Zoll was not in the animal lab to study electrical systems. His motivation was bedside-to-bench and back to the bedside. He wanted to treat patients. He had only proved a principle. Although he could artificially pace an anesthetized dog's ventricle, his system was impractical for patients because, "in an unconscious patient, quickly passing an esophageal wire down is not the easiest thing in the world. You would have to have a pretty stiff wire, and this might also be traumatic." His invention was dashed on the rocks of impracticality.

Zoll looked again at his dogs, and had a second burst of inspiration: "We realized that dogs have triangular chests . . . the 'brilliant' idea came to me, why not put leads on both sides of the heart externally?" To his delight, his external pacing system also worked, and even more astonishing, "We found that with this new arrangement you could still pace the hearts at about the same thresholds as before."

If he could pace the heart using two electrodes on the dog's chest wall, Zoll asked himself, could he do it in humans? Zoll created a bulky one-of-a-kind system for testing in a patient with complete heart block. Since his device had never been used even once in a human being, the jolts of electricity he would deliver through his patient's chest would result in one of three outcomes. His pacemaker might have no effect at all, it might pace the heart, or it might electrocute his patient. In today's era of fully informed consent, we can imagine Zoll would have faced an uphill climb in convincing a skeptical institutional review board or even a patient to be his first experimental subject. The range of outcomes Zoll would have to describe reminds me of my medical school partner who mocked our ineptitude by imagining saying to our patient, "Well, sir, it's either cancer or the common cold, and only time will tell."

Ironically Zoll's first patient was his neighbor's eighty-two-year-old father, who hovered on the brink of death from heart block, having suffered repeated seizures over a period of four hours. "I ran up the four flights of stairs and attached it to the patient," Zoll recalls to author Allen Weisse. The man's chest looked like he had been hit by buckshot, with puncture marks from thirty direct cardiac injections of stimulants. Primum non nocere forced itself into Zoll's consciousness. "By the time we saw him it was clear that he was going to die, so that it would not be unethical to attempt to stimulate him by a method that in itself might kill him for all we knew," he said. Of course, if Zoll's device did kill the man, it would be an event lost to history. In those days we buried our mistakes. Zoll attached the electrodes and turned on his machine.

"For twenty minutes we drove his heart. He stopped having seizures," Zoll noted. Then his patient's heart simply gave up, and he died. Autopsy revealed a terrible irony. Prior to Zoll's restoration of a normal heart rate by pacing, one of the thirty intracardiac injections had torn the surface of the old man's heart, causing unrecognized bleeding and ultimately death, an echo of the nick on Wilhelm Justus's heart repaired by Ludwig Rehn in Frankfurt, now distant by a continent and half a century.

But Zoll now had proof of principle. Each regular up and down movement of his patient's ECG was a metaphor for a giant step in the history of medicine. Zoll had taken three steps. He had proven electrical stimuli could cause the heart to contract. He had proven that these stimuli could be delivered safely without touching the heart, through the chest wall. And most tellingly, he had proven that the human heart rate could be controlled by a machine. No doctor could miss the implication of this finding. Zoll's little jolt of electricity had done more than pace his patient's heart, it had shocked the world. If his discovery was not resuscitation from death, it was mighty close.

A month later, Zoll got his second patient. Unlike his neighbor, Roger Abrams was only sixty-five years old and was having intermittent fainting spells due to CAD with heart failure. He had a fighting chance of leaving the hospital if he could just survive these acute episodes. Again Zoll's pacemaker restored the man's heart rate to normal: "We stimulated him on and off, interrupting our pacing to see if he might pick up a normal rhythm on this own. We did this for forty-eight hours . . . but his heart did not pick up on its own."

Had brilliant Boston physician Paul Zoll, he who tolerated no fools, failed to foresee that his laboratory work also carried the possibility of a Frankensteinian outcome? Mr. Abrams was conscious, and looked reasonably healthy. And therein lay the rub. His patient was totally dependent on his machine, Zoll had no way to wean him off it, and the machine was not portable. By the fifth day of pacing, it was not hard to imagine that Paul Zoll had condemned his patient and his medical center to a lifetime of immobilization in his hospital bed. "People began to get nervous, 'What are you going to do? You can't let go. You've got to keep going.' Even my cardiac fellow said, 'Maybe we shouldn't be doing this. Maybe you're tampering with the will of God,'" Zoll worried. Had Paul Zoll, like Stevenson's Dr. Jekyll, gone a step too far, had he countermanded the will of The Maker, and would he now pay the Devil's price? After fifty-two hours of bedside angst, providence smiled on his diminutive intellectual subject with the prodigious imagination. Roger Abrams recovered his own normal heartbeat. He soon returned home and survived for another six months.

Zoll published his clinical experiments in medicine's most prestigious journal, *The New England Medical Journal,* in 1952. The electric shocks delivered to Bostonian chests, although sufficient to awaken the entire world of cardiovascular medicine, still led conservative local religious leaders to whisper that Zoll was flouting the will of God. But providence smiled once again, sending Zoll a prominent local monsignor as a heart block patient. Soon thereafter an article appeared in *The Pilot,* America's oldest Catholic magazine, published by the Archdiocese of Boston. Its author had acquired a new level of perspicacity, one that allowed him to imagine celestial approbation for a local Boston physician's groundbreaking efforts at resuscitation. "We should not discourage this sort of thing," the author suggested, because "God works in many wondrous ways, and it is not impossible that he chose this doctor as his instrument."

The person with the first idea is often not the one recognized by history. In 1932 physiologist Albert Hyman described an artificial pacemaker powered by a hand-cranked motor. He paced animal hearts and possibly a human heart, but if he did, he published no human result. Zoll used a large battery as his power source, and maintained that the electrical output of Hyman's device was insufficient for human use. As Charles Darwin's son Francis notes, "In science the credit goes to the man who convinces the world, not to the man to whom the idea first occurs. Not the man who finds a grain of new and precious quality but to him who sows it, reaps it, grinds it and feeds the world on it."

OUR MAN-MADE PACEMAKERS are still a weak sister when compared to the natural pacemaker of the heart, responsible for the heartbeat in every living species. Nature's pacemaker poses an astonishing, you're kidding, how-can-that-be, still unexplained fundamental biologic question. In 1997 Boston cardiologist Dr. Herbert Levine reported that within the animal kingdom, heart rate has a clear mathematical relationship to life expectancy. Species with very rapid heart rates do not live long lives and those with slow heart rates do. What makes this relationship so stunning is that it spans an almost hundredfold difference in heart rate among creatures, and fortyfold difference in lifespan. At one end of the spectrum plods the Galapagos tortoise with a life expectancy of 177 years and a heart rate of 6 beats per minute. Near the other end scampers the common mouse, whose heart beats roughly 500 times per minute. Yet over this massive difference, the relationship between heart rate and longevity remains.

Despite marked differences in body size and heart rate, the number of heartbeats in the lifetime of all species is relatively constant, about 700 million beats. Stated simply, each member of the animal kingdom is endowed with the same number of lifetime heartbeats. No one yet knows the reason for this astonishing secret of Nature. Levine speculated that perhaps heart rate is a marker of metabolic rate, and a creature's metabolic rate in turn determines its lifespan. The candle burning brightest extinguishes first.

There is one conspicuous outlier in the heart rate-longevity relationship. It is we humans, although we did fit the relationship until science nearly doubled our longevity in the past century. The fascinating unanswered question for humans is whether the relationship of lifetime heartbeats to longevity has any medical relevance. Could reduced heart rate prolong lifespan? Although this experiment has never been undertaken in humans, it has been studied in mice. When mice were treated with a heart rate lowering drug, heart rate fell by half, and they survived 21% longer. If heart rate really does influence survival, Levine calculates that a reduction in a human's average heart rate from 70 to 60 would increase lifespan from 80 to 93.3 years. We do know that exercise in humans significantly lowers resting heart rate and also prolongs life expectancy. Levine ends with the provocative question, "Can human life be extended by cardiac slowing?" Disbelievers can hew to astronaut Buzz Aldrin's quip, "I believe that every human has a finite number of heartbeats. I don't intend to waste any of mine running around doing exercises."

Yet there is reason to think perhaps Levine's speculation about slowing heart rate has merit. A drug designed to do just that recently was granted "fast track" status by the FDA, a designation reserved for those drugs that both hold substantial promise and fulfill an unmet medical need. Ivabradine slows the heart rate by inhibiting the current within the heart's natural pacemaker. In a trial 6,500 patients with heart failure and a heart rate greater than 70 were followed for two years, mortality

rate in the group randomized to ivabradine was significantly reduced compared to placebo. The investigators concluded that the beneficial effect of
ivabradine was due to its heart-rate lowering effect.

ZOLL'S BREAKTHROUGH WAS the idea that he could put an electrode on either side of the chest wall of a human being and pace the heart.
Yet this lifesaving treatment had one massive limitation. Zoll's electrical
impulses caused not only the heart to contract—the muscles of the chest
contracted with as much vigor and enthusiasm as the heart itself. If the
heart had to be paced for a long time, Zoll's patient faced an intolerable
choice: live with your chest muscles contracting sixty times a minute or
suffer seizures with a high risk of imminent death. For the rare individual
with the physical and psychological fortitude to surmount this obstacle, a
huge practical hurdle awaited. Outside the hospital the patient needed to
have two electrodes on his chest, and to lug along a portable electrical generator. The solution to these problems clearly required two steps: direct
contact of the pacing electrode with the heart, and a pacemaker battery
that could be implanted within the body.

In Minneapolis, surgeon Walt Lillehei was bedeviled by heart block
of a different origin. He was inducing heart block by his placement of sutures during closure of septal defects. The heart's electrical conduction
fibers traverse the ventricular septum perilously close to the stitches that
Lillehei used to close the hole in the septum. About 10% of his patients
developed heart block, usually caused by transient swelling, following surgery. He now had ten patients who had died due to heart block. It had
become the major cause of his operative mortality. Lillehei knew what he
wanted: a portable, battery-powered device that could deliver enough current to stimulate the heart to contract at a rate of about sixty beats per
minute for at least several weeks. He just did not know where to find it.
But he reasoned that he had one huge advantage: since the chest was open,
at surgery he could actually suture the pacing electrodes directly to his
patient's heart. He could then tunnel these wires out through the chest
wall to a battery, which would provide the pacing stimulus. Nothing that
he imagined existed, but when Walt Lillehei ran into a wall he looked
around for a door. What he found was not particularly promising: a

University of Minnesota electrical engineering graduate student who earned extra income by picking up the hospital's malfunctioning electrical equipment and repairing it in his northeast Minneapolis garage. You play the hand you are dealt, Lillehei must have thought.

Earl Bakken and his brother-in-law needed a name for their little garage business. Since their makeshift repair business could charitably be envisioned as merging medicine with electronics, they came up with Medtronic. Earl, who now lives on the Kona coast in Hawaii, is a gracious host with whom I have had dinner many times during the American College of Cardiology's annual conference held in Kona. Just turned ninety, Earl has large wire-rimmed glasses and a narrow nose that give him the appearance of a benevolent wise owl. With a little urging, he will recount the story of how two guys working in a Minneapolis garage created a revolution in medical technology.

One day Lillehei pulled Bakken aside and explained his need for a small battery-powered electrical stimulator that he could sew directly to his patients' heart. Earl Bakken, the inconsequential shadow that treaded the medical center's halls with broken equipment, the guy who also repaired your TV set because medical equipment repair was not yet a full-time business, had been granted his own Great American Dream. The diffident young repairman segued to medical inventor. Didn't he recall seeing a recent article about new miniature devices called transistors in *Popular Mechanics*? He searched through his stack of back issues to find "Five New Jobs for Two Transistors." One "new job" described how to use transistors to build a musical metronome. Earl Bakken had a hunch, an intuition. A metronome could run at sixty beats per minutes . . . sixty beats! He did not need a metronome, but he did need a portable device that could run at precisely sixty beats per minute, or any other rate within the normal range of the human heartbeat. He bought a metronome, adding some mercury batteries as his power source. Now he could produce an electrical pulse at sixty beats per minute for Lillehei to connect to his wires. Bakken packaged his prototype parts in a device about the size of a paperback book. With no regulatory agency to demand extensive and costly device testing, and no hospital review board to challenge Lillehei's research procedure, Bakken brought the device to Operating Room II.

Within a few days, Lillehei confronted intraoperative heart block. He sutured two wires to the external surface of the child's heart and brought them out through the skin of the chest wall, where he attached them to Bakken's device. As Lillehei's hand rested on the switch, he faced the same three uncertain outcomes as Paul Zoll: no effect, death, or capture of the heartbeat. Switch on! It was a magical moment. The child's heart rate immediately jumped to sixty beats per minute. Within the week, the boy's normal rhythm reappeared. Lillehei removed the wires and the electrodes. Cured of his septal defect and free of heart block, the child went home to live a normal life.

Bakken had created a portable pacemaker, which could be carried in a harness outside the body. But like Paul Zoll's external chest wall pacemaker, it was terribly impractical to carry a battery-powered pacemaker outside the body. In Buffalo, New York, Dr. Wilson Greatbatch and engineer Andrew Gage were collaborating to develop a pacemaker that could be implanted beneath the skin. Financially strapped, Medtronic somehow managed to snap up exclusive rights to this crucial invention.

But even so, they were not to be first with the internal pacemaker. In the summer of 1958, forty-one-year-old Swedish engineer Arne Larsson developed intermittent complete heart block following a viral infection of his heart. During these episodes his heart rate fell to less than thirty beats per minute and he frequently fainted. His wife, who resuscitated Arne by chest thumps as often as twenty times a day, learned that physicians at Stockholm's Karolinska Institute were conducting animal research on an implantable pacemaker driven by rechargeable nickel cadmium cells. She lobbied incessantly for him to be the first to have an internal pacemaker. Arne Larsson's pacemaker was actually put together on a counter in the kitchen of engineer Rune Elmqvist. The finished product was about the size of a thin hockey puck. In October 1958 Swedish cardiac surgeon Dr. Ake Senning inserted the world's first implanted pacemaker. Larsson's pacemaker battery worked off and on for three years before it petered out. During his life Arne Larsson used twenty-two electrical pulse generators and five electrode systems. A billion heartbeats later, Arne Larsson was still going. He died of malignant melanoma in 2002 at the age of eighty-six. Larsson had outlived both engineer Elmqvist, who died in 1996, and surgeon Senning, who died in 2000. In a wonderful touch off irony, the pacemaker designed by Rune Elmqvist was ultimately acquired by St. Jude Medical, where Walt Lillehei would become medical director after his surgical days ended.

The clicking of Earl Bakken's transistor-powered metronome was about to swell into a drumbeat that heralded the emergence of a new medical device industry. In late 1960 Earl's little company manufactured and sold their first fifty implantable devices. Within five years, Medtronic and competing companies were delivering electrical pacing impulses from a battery source implanted under the skin connected to wires that passed into the heart through a vein in the neck. To meet expanding demand for pacemakers, Earl Bakken moved from his garage into a 15,000 square foot facility in 1961. Nonetheless Medtronic teetered on the edge of bankruptcy until 1962, when it stabilized through attracting venture capital, and began a period of innovation and growth which led to it becoming one of the world's most diverse medical technology companies. The company that began in a Minneapolis garage is now the leading corporation in the Fortune 500's Medical Products & Equipment group, with 41,000 employees. On May 19, 2009, Medtronic announced its annual revenue as $14.6 billion.

Earl Bakken had created a revolution in medical technology that not only saved millions of lives, it also skyrocketed the United States into preeminence in the world's burgeoning medical technology industry.

The Medtronic story is highly relevant to today's health care. In its earliest years, Medtronic and its unfettered innovative approach to new technology would not have survived in today's regulatory environment, which requires that devices meet rigorous manufacturing standards, specialists to deal with the FDA, prior approval by institutional review boards, and multimillion-dollar clinical trials. Many years elapse before the first device is sold. If cardiac surgery's early experience with failed oxygenation strategies illustrates the need for regulation, the Medtronic success equally illuminates the need for streamlined regulation. Regulation is essential, but regulators must have the Goldilocks touch: not too hot, not too cold, but just right.

After the first use of defibrillators and pacemakers, we made huge steps forward in our ability to combat the electrical depredations of CAD. Both devices became implantable. Today 100,000 pacemakers are implanted each year. About half a million Americans live today with an

implanted pacemaker, their hearts too good to die. In other patients, pacemakers and defibrillators are combined within a single device for use
in the treatment of heart failure. The pacemaker assures that the heart
contracts in a normal coordinated manner. In appropriately selected patients, it can be very effective in relieving the symptoms of heart failure. The
defibrillator protects against ventricular arrhythmias, which are common
in heart failure, which is, in turn, most commonly a complication of CAD.

IN THE COMBAT support hospital electrophysiologist Major Robert
Eckart delivered devastating news to the surgeons. The hospital had no
electrodes to suture directly to the surface of the soldier's heart. That particular pacemaker-electrode system lay halfway around the world.

Eckart's only available pacemaker system was one designed with pads
that are attached to an intact chest wall. But since the surgeons were rely-
ing on manual cardiac compression to keep their patient alive, they could
not close the chest wall. Eckart thought outside the box. Perhaps he could
cut off the pacemaker pads and expose the wires leading to them. If he
could do this, then perhaps the surgeons could suture the ends of the wires
to the heart's surface. Eckart ripped off the two pads, exposed the wires
leading to the pads, and fashioned two tips that surgeons Stewart and Falta
sutured to the heart's surface. They turned on the pacemaker. Nothing.

Facing death on the table, Eckart tried anew. He got a second set of
electrode pads. This time he stripped the wire from just one pad, and the
surgeons sutured the exposed wire to the heart's surface. Eckart attached
a second intact pad to the chest wall in the way it was designed to be used.
Again he turned on the pacemaker. Capture! They had control of the
soldier's heartbeat at fifty beats per minute. They could cease manual compression and the soldier would at least survive to have his chest closed and
be moved from the operating room to the intensive care unit. But in the
ensuing hours he still needed a functioning pacemaker system. The improvised system was fragile. Until the cavalry arrived in the form of a
permanent pacemaker system, the soldier was skewered to his bed by his
lifesaving device. His life depended on a trivial detail: avoid an inadvertent tug that dislodged one of the wires.

Eckart called the United States and Germany trying to arrange the urgent delivery of a suitable pacemaker system to Baghdad. He could get overnight delivery of a pacing system to an air base forty miles north of Baghdad, but the logistics of travel through the war zone meant that an additional day would be lost in delivery to the combat hospital. Imagine being told, "Do not move. A simple movement could kill you. But don't worry. We are pretty sure we will get a device in a couple of days that could help."

Eckart, desperate for a better solution, called other contacts. Baghdad diplomatic sources sprang into action. They were able to find a pacemaker system, but it was in a civilian hospital miles away. Perhaps for the first time in medical history a pacemaker was given an armed escort. At the hospital, the Iraqi physicians got out the pacemaker system. Then, at great personal risk they trundled it into the armed convoy, winding along hazardous serpentine Baghdad streets until they reached the heavily fortified perimeter of the U.S. combat support hospital to deliver the life-saving permanent pacemaker system.

The convoy arrived at the hospital entrance, and like Olympic relay runners the Iraqis handed the precious baton to Eckart, who rushed to the operating area. He implanted the pacemaker and its battery beneath his soldier's left collarbone. Next he connected the pacemaker to a catheter that he passed into the right ventricle. The moment of destiny had arrived. Like Zoll and Lillehei decades earlier, he, too, flicked a switch. Capture!

In a remote corner of the world, unrecognized and unknown, the life of a young man was saved by a near-miracle of circumstances. Despite his terrible injuries, the soldier now was able to get out of bed and walk. Within days the soldier, with skin staples from his neck to his pubis, was ready to plan for his long trip home. The story ends with Major Eckart offering an understated acknowledgment, capturing an otherwise forgotten act of anonymous, selfless wartime heroism: "The authors wish to express gratitude to the Iraqi physicians who helped this U.S. soldier in a time of need." And I will express our country's gratitude to the brave soldier and his doctors for their heroism.

THE INVENTION OF the defibrillator and the pacemaker was a huge forward step in overcoming heart disease, because within it lay a fantastic new idea: many hearts too good to die could be saved. And yet, it was still only an idea. Disorders of the heart's rhythm appeared suddenly, and more often than not without prior warning. When they appeared they were so lethal that we had no way to bring a defibrillator or a pacemaker to the patient in time. Outside the operating room, sudden death always seemed to catch us completely unprepared. In theory, we could save thousands of lives. In theory there's no difference between theory and practice, but in practice there is. The practical impact of defibrillators and pacemakers, the future savior of patients with acute heart attack, remained minimal. But a decade later, we will see them merge in the creation of the first coronary care unit.

9

SINGED WINGS

When all is lost, ask the I.R.S.—they'll find something.

—Doug Horton, contemporary aphorist

IN THE SEARCH for medical cures and scientific breakthroughs, we always encounter both triumphs and failures. Human beings who seem superhuman exhibit faults. No failure is, perhaps, as heartbreaking as that of Walt Lillehei.

Let's follow Walt Lillehei's career. With his pioneering role in hypothermia, cross-circulation, methods of oxygenation, pacemakers, and later prosthetic heart valves, Lillehei stood as a modern Thomas More, a Man for All Seasons poised to challenge every assumption of a deeply entrenched establishment. In the late 1960s, passed over for the position of chief of surgery at the University of Minnesota, he was recruited with great fanfare to become the chief of surgery at the prestigious New York Hospital-Cornell Medical Center. That was when I first met Walt. His lymphosarcoma was now a distant memory, but as the years passed, scarring of the tissues in his neck caused his head to tilt to one side. With his bald head tilted precariously on his narrow neck and an enigmatic smile, he reminded me of Steven Spielberg's E.T. By now, people who knew Lillehei fell into two camps. Those who liked him because he was true to himself whatever the cost, and those who disliked him for the same reason. The flip side of being a creative iconoclast is lack of respect for convention. I saw Lillehei as a maverick with compassion. So I liked him.

When Walt Lillehei came east, his wife, Kaye, elected to stay in Minneapolis so that their three younger children could remain in local schools. Before he left, Walt was returning home from dinner in his powerboat with Kaye. Roaring at high speed in low light along the Mississippi River, he was risk-taking Walt being Walt. In the evening darkness he failed to see a sandbar. He ran suddenly aground. Kaye was launched into the boat's dashboard, sending a part of the rearview mirror into her skull and the ignition key into her nose. Beautiful Kaye survived but required hospitalization for facial reconstructive surgery.

After he arrived in New York, as Kaye observed, "Walt went a little crazy." Single in Manhattan, he acquired a four-bedroom apartment with a split-level living room, recreation room, and spectacular city view on the swanky Upper East Side. He hired an interior decorator. He threw lavish parties and continued his pattern of assignations with local nurses that he had begun in Minnesota. He became a denizen of a nearby local bar, the Recovery Room, got in a barroom fight, and ended up with a black eye.

Lillehei's antics shocked Cornell Medical Center's conservative power elite. The aggressively self-confident entourage of Minnesota surgeons that trailed in his wake on hospital rounds seemed like the hospital's own Macy's Day Parade. His over-the-top expensive redecoration of his office, including a flamboyant fabric on the wall of his private bathroom, was seen as creating an aura of arrogant superiority. Within the medical center, he skipped executive committee meetings, implying that he was above the petty concerns of the local power structure. As a newcomer whose every action was scrutinized and judged, he seemed hell-bent on proving both entitlement and his disdain for the norms of his new Manhattan community.

Frustration boiled into outrage when Walt sent a letter on Cornell stationery to all New York state physicians urging them to donate in support of Minnesota's Senator Hubert Humphrey's candidacy for the Democratic presidential nomination. Cornell had had quite enough of Walt Lillehei. The Minnesota maverick was a misfit in Manhattan society. Cardiac surgery's Caesar was surrounded, the long knives emerged, and Walter Lillehei, uncrowned Father of Open Heart Surgery, past president of the American College of Cardiology, Lasker Award recipient, and Nobel Prize nominee was summarily fired as chairman of the department of surgery.

He would be allowed to continue operating and to retain his title as professor. At age fifty-one, just sixteen years since Annie Brown's VSD repair during cross-circulation had brought him international fame, many were saying Walt Lillehei was a modern-day Icarus whose reckless lifestyle had carried him too close to the sun. What his critics could not possibly imagine was that Lillehei's spiraling descent was about to become a pure vertical fall.

Less than two years after his demotion at Cornell, a St. Paul Minnesota grand jury indicted Walt Lillehei on the charge of tax evasion. The charge carried the possibility of twenty-five years in prison and loss of his medical license. As always Walt Lillehei emerged as the sole architect of his torment. He had first attracted the attention of the Internal Revenue Service in 1964 by completely failing to file income tax returns for two consecutive years. When challenged, he paid his taxes and penalties; then with stunning Lillehei chutzpah, did not pay taxes for the next three years. Such behavior irritates the IRS. When the IRS again contacted him, what did he do? He raised the stakes. He simply ignored them. Walter Lillehei's lifelong contempt for entrenched authority, the fount of his brilliant innovations in surgery, had become his Achilles' heel. The IRS relished destruction of high-profile tax cheaters. Walt Lillehei, the world-famous doctor with the tawdry personal history, had single-handedly, almost magically levitated himself to the status of their perfect foil. The IRS initiated a savage public attack. Recalling those days, the ferocity of the IRS take-no-prisoners attack seemed equal to those launched on mobsters like Al Capone years before, or John Gotti years later.

Lillehei's case went to trial with broad media coverage. His billing records consisted of a messy assortment of file cards stored in shoe boxes. The IRS matched every shoe box card he submitted to the hospital's records of his actual operations. His file cards failed to show $250,000 of income from 318 operated-on patients. That was a lot of tax evasion. But the IRS then rolled out tax deductions, which were so ridiculous that they were hilarious. Under the category drugs and pharmaceuticals, the IRS research revealed that Lillehei had deducted veterinary expenses for his family cat. Under business expenses he had deducted the cost of his parents' fiftieth wedding anniversary. The IRS completed their dissection of Lillehei by publicizing lubricious tidbits that made Lillehei a subject of ridicule: as a married man, he had deducted gifts to three girlfriends as professional expenses. One of the three testified that they had an intimate relationship. The prosecutors then presented the jury with their salacious slam dunk, perfect for jaded New York tabloids even today. The good doctor had deducted a payment to a Las Vegas call girl as "typing expenses." The call girl was brought to court to testify that she had no particular talent for typing. She did not do shorthand. In fact, she testified with a coy smile, that typing was not really the service she provided.

In response to the missing bills on 318 patients, Lillehei then found a water-damaged shoe box in his basement. He had not evaded taxes, really . . . he had just misplaced the box of file cards. These just-discovered records, however, quickly mired Lillehei deeper in legal quicksand. The IRS prosecutorial team subjected the ink on the index cards to infrared forensic examination. Their expert testified that some of the original billing amounts on the cards had been later altered with different ink. Now in addition to tax evasion, the cloud of criminal fraud hung over Walter Lillehei. By the end of the four-week trial, prosecutors had overwhelmed his defense with 164 witnesses. In exposing the darker side of "work hard, play hard," the IRS lawyers had decimated both the career and the personal life of the best that cardiovascular medicine had to offer.

Lillehei's lawyers rose to his defense. They argued that his failure to file returns was the understandable mistake of a dedicated surgeon too busy to attend to life's details. His errors in tax deductions came not from an intent to deceive, but from poor memory combined with sloppy record bookkeeping. As for back taxes, the defense had its own bombshell. The defense claimed that the IRS actually owed the good doctor Lillehei $53,000, because he had donated the proceeds from a prosthetic valve he had invented to the University of Minnesota without claiming a charitable donation. Independent of guilt or innocence, however, the defense was pilloried with the evidence that Walt Lillehei was incredibly cavalier with his personal finances, and the impression his sins emanated from a philosophy of life that few jurors endorsed.

The Day of Judgment arrived. After two days of deliberation, the jury delivered its verdict: Dr. C. Walton Lillehei, the pride of the University of Minnesota, was guilty, resoundingly guilty on all five counts.

At sentencing, Lillehei's lead lawyer Jerry Simon begged for leniency, based on his service to his country in war, his generosity to patients who could not afford his services, and his remarkable contributions to the advancement of medicine. "Society is indebted for what he has done, and perhaps this is the time for society to recognize and perhaps in some measure repay him for the contributions he has made," Simon pleaded.

Judge Phillip Neville confronted a personally wrenching decision. Should Lillehei go to jail? He seemed flagrantly guilty. Yet Lillehei's unique strength had been his willingness to challenge conventional wisdom, combined with the intense focus he brought to a single problem. Gazing down on his frail, guilty defendant he could see a modern Greek hero whose strength became the source of his demise. Lillehei's flaw did not seem to be greed; his failure lay in his deliberate disregard of the rules that governed other men's behavior. In the final analysis, Lillehei generated not contempt, but astonished disbelief in his reckless conviction that he could ignore society's rules and pay no price. Judge Neville could not bring himself to send this flawed genius to jail. He fined Lillehei $50,000, the maximum amount allowed, and added six months of community service.

Perhaps Neville also knew that Lillehei's greatest punishment for hubris and recklessness would lie outside the courtroom. His professional career was finished. The state of Minnesota revoked his license to practice medicine. The American College of Surgery suspended him indefinitely. In cardiology's inner circles I am sorry to say I sensed schadenfreude far more often than sympathy. To add to his misery, his mother and his father both died before the end of the year.

On the last day of December 1973, C. Walton Lillehei performed his very last surgery at the young age of fifty-five. His vision now impaired by cataracts, a side effect of his radiation therapy two decades earlier, Walt Lillehei was an academic pariah. There were no invitations to lecture, no prestigious visiting professorships, no colleagues calling him forward to rhapsodize about his accomplishments or to drape a beribboned medal around his neck. He was ostracized in Minneapolis society. His long-standing friend Dr. Daniel Goor recalls in his Lillehei biography being seated with Walt and Kaye at a Minneapolis country club dinner. Among about twenty people who stopped to chat with Kaye, not a single one spoke to Walt. The Minnesota Silent Treatment must have withered his soul. To his critics, Lillehei's life stood as a parable of a man supremely gifted yet unable to recognize his own fallibility, prone to flawed judgment, shattered by the very hubris that had originally carried him to the pinnacle.

WALT LILLEHEI, AS in the days and months surrounding his diagnosis of cancer, remained outwardly strong, the living embodiment of Ernest Hemingway's phrase for courage: "grace under pressure." Loyal Kaye stayed with him. And then years later, Walt Lillehei was granted a heart-wrenching epilogue. John Kirklin, his former intellectual foe from the Mayo Clinic, had succeeded Lillehei as one of the world's most respected cardiac surgeons. In 1979 Kirklin was elected president of the American Association for Thoracic Surgeons. We may recall that his biographer nicknamed him The Iceman, reflecting both his scintillating intellect and aloof persona. Speaking at his presidential inauguration ceremony, Mayo Clinic's Kirklin spotted his old University of Minnesota surgical rival in the audience. The Iceman gestured toward Lillehei, and then spoke from his heart: "He was and still is a great hero of mine; because of his enormous ability . . . he was one of cardiac surgery's greatest innovators. Dear colleagues, may I depart from my text to ask this great and pioneering surgeon to stand to your applause. Walt Lillehei may we see you?" Walt Lillehei—brilliant innovator, savior of hundreds of children, iconoclast, consummate risk taker, showman, press charmer, reckless carouser, and finally Dead Man Walking—was himself resurrected in that glorious moment, as he stood glassy-eyed to a standing ovation of a thousand hands.

Viewed through my own retro scope of history, I like to imagine that Walt Lillehei rose from the ashes, and was reborn on that day. Buoyed by a thunderous wave of heartfelt applause, his deeply painful ignominious isolation was over. The last years were good to Walt and Kaye. He served as medical director of St. Jude Medical, the Minnesota manufacturer of pacemakers and one of the world's most successful artificial heart valves, which we used for many years at our medical center. Walt again became a respected sought-after lecturer.

And the Rest of the Story? At his eightieth birthday party the former Minnesota Queen of Hearts, Annie Brown now Janakowski, once a four-year-old dying with a VSD and now a healthy forty-seven-year-old, joined him in celebration of his life and hers.

Six months later Walt Lillehei encountered his old surgical nemesis, pneumonia, but this time it was personal. He passed away quietly in his home. In his obituary Denton Cooley, one of his students, who had become one of the greatest surgeons of the next generation, wrote that the unique innovative genius of the American heartland had outlived his humiliation. He had regained the respect and affection of his surgical brethren, and been levitated to the pinnacle . . . he had earned a legitimate claim to the title of Father of Open Heart Surgery.

10

HOW TO WIN A
NOBEL PRIZE

*You see things; and you say, "Why?" But I dream things that
never were; and I say, "Why not?"*

—THE SERPENT IN GEORGE BERNARD SHAW'S PLAY,
BACK TO METHUSELAH

AS SUDDEN AND shocking as can be imagined, neither ventricular
fibrillation nor heart block was the most psychologically devastating complication of early heart surgery. It was death on the table due to preoperative misdiagnosis. Because early surgeons and cardiologists had to
base their preoperative cardiac diagnoses on their stethoscope, the heart's
X-ray silhouette, and the ECG, their diagnoses were imprecise. Surgeons,
thinking they were operating on a simple hole in the heart, opened it to
find additional complex abnormalities of valves for which they had no surgical solution. Desperate children died on the operating table or soon
thereafter as surgeons tried to explain the mistaken diagnosis to grieving
parents. Cardiac surgeons needed preoperative images of the chambers,
valves, and the inflow and outflow vessels. And so it was that another tragedy of cardiac surgery stimulated the development of X-ray suites called
catheterization laboratories, devoted solely to analysis of the heart.

The origin of cardiac catheterization is the most improbable story in
all of cardiology, maybe in all of medicine. It begins just before World

War II in a small German hospital less than an hour's drive northeast of Berlin in the forest town of Eberswalde (literally, "Forest of the Boars").

In 1929 unknown twenty-four-year-old resident-in-training Dr. Werner Forssmann became obsessed with an idea. He reasoned that the concentration of drugs acting on the heart would be much higher if they were delivered directly into the heart's chambers rather than being diluted by injection into a peripheral vein. He could push a tube from an arm vein all the way into the right atrium. No one had ever tried this, or if they had, never admitted it. Conventional wisdom held that like surgery on the heart, pushing a tube into the heart carried a great risk of inducing ventricular fibrillation and certain death. Forssmann's support for his idea was gossamer-thin: he had read that seventy-five years earlier some Frenchman had conducted this very experiment in a horse. Nonetheless he proposed his idea to Dr. Peter Schneider, the hospital's chief physician.

Schneider's answer was swift, appropriate, and unequivocal.

"I cannot possibly allow you to carry out such an experiment on a patient."

Forssmann's response to his rejection suggested a touch of insanity. He countered that his commitment to his idea was so profound that he would accept the risk by passing a catheter on himself. Schneider, shocked by the young doctor's absurd and grandiose response, countered with the finality of the Kaiser.

"My no is final and absolute." Forssmann was absolutely prohibited from pursuing his crazy idea further.

Forssmann pretended to be humble, accepting his rejection. After all, he was completely boxed in because he had no catheter. He did not even have access to the necessary surgical supplies, which the hospital kept under lock and key. But he had one asset that Schneider had failed to consider. Werner Forssmann was an eligible young doctor in a sea of nubile nurses. He hatched a scheme of headstrong defiance.

"I let a few days go by and then started to prowl around Nurse Gerda Ditzen like a sweet-tooth cat around the cream jug . . . it was easy to find something to gossip about and she'd invite me back to her little office . . . So little by little I won over my essential disciple," he said. She was indeed essential. Nurse Gerda was the keeper of the keys to the hospital's closet of sterile supplies.

After two weeks of Forssmann's amorous charm, Nurse Gerda Ditzen was so thoroughly smitten that she seemed bereft of all judgment. What followed is almost beyond imagination. She walked to a cabinet, unlocked it, and extracted a scalpel, a vial of local anesthetic, and a catheter designed to empty urine from the bladder. Nurse Gerda and Forssmann then strolled to an isolated empty hospital room and closed the door behind them. Nurse Gerda lay down supine and helpless before Forssmann. He had convinced her to be the first subject in his mad scheme. With Nurse Gerda willingly defenseless, Forssmann moved with the alacrity of an obsessed scientist.

"With the speed of light I strapped her down so tightly that she couldn't reach the buckle. Then I tied down her hands. Amazingly enough she accepted my explanation that I had to take all these precautions against her falling off the table since I had no one to assist me. I had pushed the instrument table behind her head so she couldn't see what I was doing," he said.

Did Forssmann possess the charm of Rasputin, able to separate an apparently well-adjusted nurse from her most basic impulse of self-preservation? Having mesmerized his prey, was he actually going to proceed with an unthinkable assault on a healthy young woman? Every doctor, regardless of his native language, knows primum non nocere. First do no harm. Was Werner Forssmann really prepared to sacrifice his career, and even worse, endanger the life of an infatuated woman, possibly kill her, just for his idea? What happened next made medical history.

"In the twinkling of an eye I had anesthetized my left elbow . . . I quickly made an incision in my own skin . . . and pushed the catheter about a foot inside. I packed it with gauze and laid a sterile splint over it. Then I released Gerda's right hand and loosened the straps around her knees."

With the urinary catheter protruding from his arm like an emerging snake in a horror movie, he and a pale and speechless Gerda hustled past disbelieving nurses all the way to a fluoroscopic X-ray suite in the hospital basement. The X-ray technician, wanting no part of what was happening, bolted from the room. Moments later, Forssmann's drinking buddy, Dr. Peter Romeis, awakened from an afternoon nap by the terrified X-ray technician, barreled into the room screaming at Forssmann to terminate his rendezvous with death. Forssmann, always stubborn and reckless but now deeply invested in his plot and righteous in his crusade, was adamant. He turned on the fluoroscope.

"As I'd expected the catheter had reached the head of the humerus (the tip of the shoulder). Romeis wanted me to stop at this point and remove it. But I wouldn't hear of it. I pushed the catheter in further, almost to the two foot mark . . . Romeis tried to pull the catheter from my arm. I fought him off, yelling Nein, Nein, I must push it forward. I kicked his shins and pushed the catheter until . . . the tip had reached my heart."

And . . . nothing happened. No sudden arrhythmia, no ventricular fibrillation, no collapse to the floor. The catheter just curled up and went to sleep.

Forssmann ordered, "Take a picture." The X-ray image showed the catheter in the right atrium. The tube was too short to be advanced further.

Now Forssmann had to face Dr. Schneider. Schneider flew into Teutonic rage when he learned of Forssmann's rank disobedience. Yet his fury abated as he stared in astonishment at the young doctor's X-ray images. Forssmann had put a catheter in the heart and suffered no problem whatsoever. Schneider was of two minds. Did Forssmann's act of disobedience represent a medical curiosity or an important advance? Could a tube within the heart itself be of value in treating a deathly ill patient?

Forssmann's boss Schneider had to admit he did not know, because no one had ever been treated in this way. So he actually allowed Forssmann to catheterize a young woman dying from a botched abortion. In an era before antibiotics her condition appeared to transiently improve with intracardiac drug therapy before she died. The result was inconclusive. Schneider decided the risk of continuing the experiment exceeded the benefit. He terminated Forssmann's studies on patients. Forssmann, his immunity to criticism so similar to the postwar American surgeons he preceded, was entirely undeterred. He puttered around further, injecting X-ray contrast dye to outline the chambers of the heart in dogs, and he continued his own self-experimentation. According to legend Forssmann only quit his research on himself when he used up all of his veins after cutting into his blood vessels seventeen times.

Forssmann published his results in Germany's premier medical journal *Deutsche Medizinische Wochenschrift* in 1929. The medical establishment's reaction covered the spectrum from an indifferent shoulder shrug to intense scorn. A catheter in the heart provided no conceivable value and carried huge potential risk. Forssmann's image among his colleagues transmogrified from stubborn misfit to dangerous madman, a misfit who had disregarded the norms of his profession. His research summarily dismissed by the medical establishment, Forssmann discovered that the doors of German cardiology were firmly and irrevocably closed to the Eberswalde troublemaker. He could go no further in cardiology training.

In Berlin he found a different specialty. Forssmann had used a urologic catheter to probe the heart, and now in a bizarre twist, he entered training as a urologic surgeon. He never looked back, never returned to cardiovascular research. Forssmann had proven that right heart catheterization could be safe and could be used to create primitive images of the heart's chambers. For the next ten years, however, the judgment of the medical establishment was outright contempt. A pigheaded fool in a small German town had provided no useful scientific insight about the heart. Forssmann had performed a dangerous parlor trick, nothing more.

As the storms of war engulfed Europe, American investigators Drs. André Cournand and Dickinson Richards at Bellevue Hospital in New York reasoned that they could marry Forssmann's ridiculed catheterization method to their methods of recording pressure, flow, and images of the heart chambers. Richards focused on pressures and flow; Cournand made images by injecting an X-ray-dense dye, a process dubbed angiography. As war erupted, their arcane research was suddenly transformed into a medical imperative. Measurement of intracardiac pressures and cardiac output guided treatment of soldiers dying of traumatic shock. War had transformed Forssmann's primitive technique into a practical tool.

After the war, with the birth of cardiac surgery, misdiagnosis became a plague. Clarence Dennis in Minnesota and John Gibbon in Philadelphia both failed on their very first attempt to use their heart-lung machines because their cardiologic colleagues had misdiagnosed the nature of their patient's heart defect. Tragically in both cases the child died on the operating table. To visualize the anatomic abnormalities of a child's heart prior to opening the chest, surgeons needed detailed images of its four heart chambers and the major vessels. In response cardiologists reached for the techniques that Cournand and Richards had used on the battlefields of Europe.

At Johns Hopkins in Baltimore, at the behest of cardiac surgeon Dr. Alfred Blalock, Dr. Richard Bing opened the nation's first cardiac catheterization laboratory. In Boston, Dr. Lewis Dexter, working with Dwight Harken, also opened a lab. The early cardiac angiographic images, however, were desperately primitive. The heart was in constant motion, yet images could only be acquired one at a time. The surgeons needed movies, not photographs. Industry quickly responded by creating automatic film cassette changers that produced a stack of photographs in rapid succession, and trumped that the following year by recording images on movie film. The first films were recorded at a paltry two images per second. It wasn't a movie, but it was a start. Today we manipulate digital images of the heart and its vessels in colorful three-dimensional displays. Our early images were Charlie Chaplin silent flicks compared to today's *Star Wars*. When I entered cardiology, we spent hours debating diagnosis; today we know the diagnosis: we debate treatment.

AND THE REST of the Story? In 1932, three years after his Eberswalde escapade, Forssmann joined the Nazi Party. When war erupted in Eastern Europe, he joined the troops as a doctor on the Russian front. As the Wehrmacht collapsed in the snowfields of Leningrad, he fled before the onslaught, ultimately reaching the river that separated Russian and American forces. Fearing imprisonment in the notorious Russian prisoner-of-war camps, Forssmann dove into the bone-chilling water and swam to the opposite bank, to be captured trembling and humiliated by American forces. He had reached the low point in his life. Released at war's end, Forssmann returned to the private practice of urology. In later years, he repeatedly apologized for his involvement in the Nazi party.

In 1956 Werner Forssmann, with no other important contribution to medical science in the years that followed his act of youthful duplicity in the Forest of the Boar, shared the Nobel Prize in Medicine with Cournand and Richards. Only eight years after Charles Bailey's first mitral valve surgery, the world of medical science had completely reversed its opinion about the events on that day in the Forest of the Boar. History had decreed that the German youth who defied authority, tricked a smitten nurse to provide forbidden supplies then strapped her to a bed, and proceeded with a potentially lethal experiment on himself was right, and the rest of his world was wrong. He had, the Nobel Prize proclaimed, made a monumental contribution to science.

Some have diminished Forssmann's glory by sniping that he is the least intellectual person ever to win the Nobel Prize in Medicine. Perhaps, but who among us would have done what he did? Werner Forssmann is certainly our boldest winner.

IN JUST A decade, Dwight Harken's challenge to conventional wisdom when he clamped a hemostat onto a shard of shrapnel on D-day had precipitated the evolution of closed heart surgery, open heart surgery, and the development of the heart-lung machine. The complications of open heart surgery led to the invention of pacemakers and defibrillators, and to the development of the catheterization laboratory. For the first time we could see the heart's secrets during life. We could see malformed structures, analyze their effect on the heart, and see how surgery restored heart function. And yet the greatest prize remained beyond our reach. We could not see the disease that caused most cardiac death and disability, the disease that lurked in the coronary arteries. We could not see CAD until our patient was on the autopsy table. We were like jewelers trying to fix a watch wearing a blindfold. And so the proscenium was set for our emergence to today's modern era.

PART III

THE PAST CREATES
THE PRESENT

11

ONE MAN'S DISASTER IS ANOTHER MAN'S BREAKTHROUGH

Serendipity is the faculty of finding things we did not know we were looking for.

—GLAUCO ORTOLANO, BRAZILIAN-AMERICAN WRITER

TO DIAGNOSE AND evaluate CAD, we needed to see the coronary arteries. X-ray dye injected into the heart itself outlined the chambers, but the dye was far too diluted by the time it reached its coronary arteries. Everyone knew that a catheter could not be inserted directly into a human coronary artery because it might completely obstruct the small vessel, depriving the heart of blood and causing sudden death. Even if the catheter allowed some blood to flow past, the nonoxygenated angiographic dye would fill the coronary arteries, obstruct oxygen delivery, and end in fatal ventricular fibrillation. There was no solution. Cardiologists were stumped.

In mid-1958, Portland Oregon radiologist Dr. Charles Dotter challenged this conventional wisdom. He devised a special catheter with a balloon near its tip. He positioned his catheter just above the aortic valve, then inflated the balloon for a few seconds to completely obstruct blood flow from the left ventricle into the aorta. At the same time he injected X-ray-opaque dye through the catheter. The only egress for his injected dye was into the two coronary arteries that originated in the small space between the inflated balloon and the aortic valve. He created spectacular images of the coronary arteries in dogs, and all his dogs survived. Dotter had shattered the myth that injection of X-ray dye into the coronary arteries would induce ventricular fibrillation, and had set the stage for one of cardiology's greatest breakthroughs, coronary angiography.

Three months later, in his Cleveland Clinic basement catheterization laboratory, cardiologist Dr. Mason Sones prepared to perform a routine catheterization procedure called aortic angiography, in which X-ray dye is injected into the aorta. Since the dye disappears in a heartbeat or two, he placed the catheter tip just above the aortic valve, and injected a large volume of X-ray dye (20 to 40 cc) over a very short period of time (two seconds). This flow rate is vastly greater than is possible with a human hand, so Sones was using a specially manufactured mechanical "power injector."

Staring intently at the image of West Virginian Abner Darby's heart, Sones gave the command to his cardiology fellow Dr. Royston Lewis to inject. The sudden surge of the dye through the small diameter catheter whipped the catheter tip like a garden hose. No problem there, that was typical. But this time, Sones watched transfixed in horror as the thrashing tip flipped into Darby's right coronary artery, and the power injector blasted away with its lethal load. In that two seconds Sones had the sudden agonizing realization that like the captain of a firing squad, he was watching a man killed at his command. For a doctor there is no more devastating experience than to be the sole, unequivocal mechanism responsible for a patient's sudden death. Sometime in their career, this happens to every interventional cardiologist and every cardiac surgeon. Sones saw that his own moment of searing self-recrimination had come. In a few seconds, twenty-seven-year-old Abner Darby would be in ventricular fibrillation.

Abner Darby's heart stopped beating. Sones shouted, "Cough, Goddammit," and yelled for Lewis to yank back on the catheter. He grabbed a scalpel . . . the Claude Beck strategy of direct cardiac massage and direct defibrillation still held sway. Then as quickly as it began it was all over. Abner Darby's heart . . . straightlined for a few agonizing seconds . . . and then slowly began beating again. It was so fast that the briefly terrorized Darby coughed and never lost consciousness. A decade later when I learned coronary angiography, we knew that Darby's heart rate response is common following direct injection of contrast dye into a coronary artery. But this was the world's first time. In a mini-tribute to Mason Sones's theory that coughing somehow helped to clear the dye from the coronary vessels we still shouted "cough" when the heart paused. Although I have remained suspicious about the totally unproven effect of the lowly cough for dye-clearing and heart-starting, my Harvard mentor Dr. Richard Gorlin assured me the cough represents the art, not the science of medicine. My view is that the cough gives us something to do while Nature bails us out of trouble.

The door of serendipity opened just a crack to give Mason Sones a transient but perfect image of Darby's right coronary artery. Rather than let it close, he tore that metaphorical door off the hinges. Within minutes of what he briefly imagined was a horrifying doctor-induced death, Sones stormed triumphantly back to his office to announce to all within earshot that "We just revolutionized cardiology!" Legend has it that his long-standing secretary, Elaine Clayton, dryly retorted, "Again?"

Mason Sones had discovered the way for us to see CAD. In science the difference between fame and failure, between preeminence and mediocrity, can be how one deals with a mistake. The discovery of the wonder drug penicillin came from a lab mistake. Now Mason Sones was poised to turn his mistake into a turning point in cardiology. That afternoon Mason Sones did not explain away his mistake, he embraced it. Just hours after his roller-coaster ride from precipitous descent into despair and ascent to exhilaration, he made a quick instinctive leap. He realized that he could insert a catheter directly into a coronary artery, and inject contrast material. He could provide an incandescent image of the disease that was now the nation's number one killer.

Mason announced to his fellow cardiologists that he would begin scheduling patients for angiographic study of their coronary arteries. As his friend Dr. William Proudfit recalled, "He recognized right away that this would revolutionize medicine. I thought it was amazing that instead of just being thankful that the patient hadn't died, he recognized immediately that this was a tremendous advance."

Until a disease has a name, medicine stands idle. Once it has a name, we define its symptoms and its physiognomy at autopsy and under the microscope. This information helps to define its cause, and finally its treatment. For most of mankind's history CAD did not even have a name, its symptoms only becoming clearly recognized in the 1700s. Even so, it took another hundred years for pathologists to clearly define its features. Then another century passed before we began to define CAD risk factors, like smoking, blood pressure, and cholesterol. World War II hero Dwight Eisenhower, who suffered a heart attack during his presidency, for instance, had been a four-pack-a-day smoker during the war, unaware of its risk. After the war, images of obstructions in coronary arteries linked symptoms and cause, and stimulated the first creative treatments. We could see the cause of CAD. Cause precedes cure. The coronary angiogram marks the beginning of the end for CAD.

Let's pause to credit dumb luck—serendipity—in science. History credits serendipity for the Greek mathematician Archimedes' discovery of buoyancy and the English physicist Isaac Newton's discovery of gravity. Perhaps our serendipity champion is Christopher Columbus, who according to author Dr. Morton Meyers "did not know where he was going, where he was when he got there, or where he came from when he returned." A visit to Barcelona convinced me. His statue points not across the Atlantic toward the New World, but across the Mediterranean toward Libya.

But serendipity still requires an innovator. Sones and his constant cath lab companion Dr. Earl Shirey became the Tweedledum and Tweedledee of coronary angiography, meshing like the perfect fit of a torn bill. Sones created a catheter with a tapered tip and multiple side holes like a garden sprinkler so that the catheter would neither recoil nor obstruct the vessel. Together they found the perfect concentration of X-ray dye for coronary arteries, developed ways to manipulate the catheter into the openings of the right and left coronary arteries, and figured out the best body positions for separating the images of the coronary arteries from ribs and vertebrae. Demand for Sones's catheter created an entire new industry around Glens Falls, New York—nicknamed Catheter Valley—and in a few years the company that fabricated his catheter sold its millionth device. Like many physician-scientists in his time, Sones made millions in profits for corporations, but not a penny for himself.

In those years *Reader's Digest* magazine had a monthly feature called "The Most Unforgettable Character I Ever Met." Were I asked to contribute, Mason Sones would be my choice. As a child Mason had struggled as a short, tubby unathletic kid with glasses. He resorted to outrageous, often hilarious behavior, which carried into his adult life. My first encounter with Mason occurred when I was a visiting professor at the Cleveland Clinic. Mason was now a legend, the world's most recognizable name in cardiology. Eight years after he described it, I had learned the "Sones technique" of coronary angiography at Peter Bent Brigham, where his name was held in reverence. As he approached to welcome me, everything about Mason said unpretentious. Round-faced with glasses perched far down his nose, Mason was a short, stout, shambling sartorial disaster in a tie-less shirt. The shirt appeared to bear splotches from his most recent cath procedure. A bespectacled Homer Simpson. He clutched his constant companion, a cigarette. Even before speaking, Mason Sones's appearance had announced to his young starched white shirt visitor, "I am a maverick."

But as we strolled the halls, Mason became a force of nature: constant energy, exuberant with patients, nurses, doctors, and—on this day—me. He was endlessly talkative, colorful in language, curmudgeonly, unpretentious, feisty, outrageous, daring you to argue, cursing like a sailor. He threw all aspects of his complex personality at you at once. Mason was determined that you see it all. With his abundant talent and self-evident flaws, Mason Sones was quintessentially human. His biographer David Monagan describes him as "storming through the hallowed Cleveland Clinic's corridors in a sweat-stained white T-shirt that made him resemble the lowliest janitor. Ruddy-faced, he bellowed, cursed, and cajoled, and left trails of assistants and nurses recoiling and guffawing by turns. When desperate to dictate case reports, he was known to kick in the ladies' room door and roar that it was time for some secretary to get off the pot. 'Type, type, type!' was his only half-self-mocking staff greeting in the morning." Mason was legendary for his extraordinarily long workdays and his hard-drinking nights. Unpretentious Mason Sones was an unforgettable one-of-a-kind lovable misfit to everyone he encountered in life.

Possessed by a vision, Mason Sones was Steve Jobs in a lead apron, a man who took responsibility for developing every small detail of his discipline. He worked with engineers to create catheters, larger imaging devices, and wider movie film. And in the end, like Jobs, he transformed his world. Sones changed the unseen to the obvious, the unobservable to the observable. For the first time, we could actually see our enemy in every patient. The lurking atheroma, the cholesterol plaque in the blood vessel, the cause of angina, heart attack, and sudden death, had finally been exposed.

AND THE REST of the Story? Sones's coronary angiography completely eclipsed radiologist Charlie Dotter's idea of visualizing the coronaries by transiently obstructing the aorta with a balloon. But Charlie still had the last word. He sent his radiology trainee Melvin Judkins to Cleveland to learn Sones's new technique. Judkins saw the one flaw that Sones overlooked. Manipulating a catheter into the tiny orifices of the two coronary arteries required consummate technical hand-eye coordination, precise knowledge of the anatomy of the aortic root, and the ability to translate a two-dimensional image into three-dimensional reality. In Boston, it took me a full year to learn the Sones technique. Judkins reasoned that since the coronary artery origin was always in the same anatomic location, he could develop a set of special J-shaped catheters for aortas of different diameters. With Judkins's catheters, a virtual novice could now catheterize the coronary artery, with minimal catheter manipulation, and markedly reduced X-ray exposure time. The Judkins catheter replaced the Sones catheter in a matter of a few years. Melvin Judkins, like Sones, never patented his invention and never profited from it.

Late in his career, Sones was showered with awards. He loathed the pomp and pretension of black-tie banquets, especially those with honorees. His biographer David Monagan relates a quintessential Mason Sones moment, told to him by William Proudfit, which occurred in the early 1980s. Cleveland's Stouffer Foundation had selected Mason as the honoree for their annual black-tie affair, which brought together the city's most prominent citizens in a once-a-year spare-no-expense gala. The previous year, Spain's Queen Isabella, the namesake of the Queen who launched Columbus's exploration of America, had been the honoree. Mason being Mason sought refuge in the bar. After the speeches extolling Mason's humanitarian virtues, scientific brilliance, and place in history, the Great Man was called to the stage. Mason wobbled to the podium, gripped the lectern, and paused. A hush filled the room as the crowd awaited the insights of their most accomplished citizen.

"You know, it's the environment," said Mason. A long pause.

The multitude sat baffled. What in the world could that mean?

"It's the environment for sure. If anybody thinks you're an asshole, they call you an asshole." And with that, Mason Sones began his long staggering stroll back toward his seat. For a long moment, the audience looked at each other in stunned disbelief. Then someone stood to clap, and in a moment the whole room stood to applaud Mason Sones. The man is an eccentric genius, but he's one of our own. And that is why his boss Dr. William Sheldon called him, "the stormy petrol of cardiology."

It was not the first time Mason had appeared drunk in public. We in cardiology had seen him stagger across the stage at medical meetings. But when you looked at Mason Sones you had to see the whole man: brutally honest, self-critical, unpretentious, hilarious, generous, hardworking, innovative, bombastic, lovable, imperfect Mason.

Mason died as he had lived, with a cigarette in his hand, of lung cancer.

WHEN I LEFT the academic confines of my internship at the University Hospital to drive cross-country to Los Angeles in the mid-1960s I had not yet seen a coronary angiogram. In my three-year Los Angeles County Hospital internal medicine residency were profound lessons in both humanity and medicine. I had far fewer supervisors. In contrast to my university years, many of my patients had hit financial, medical, and psychological rock bottom in their struggle to survive. Responsible for these often-desperate souls, I became deeply immersed in every daily detail of their care. A segment of my fellow resident physicians looked down on these people, contemptuously calling them "gomers," allegedly short for "go home." I saw the opposite: when treated with respect for their inherent humanity instead of implied disgust with their failures, you discharged a deeply grateful patient. At the university I had been immersed in facts, in the country hospital I learned humanity. Near the end of my residency when I finally became aware of the potential power of coronary angiography, I knew what I had to do. Mason Sones had proven that coronary angiography was feasible. I wanted to be part of the new generation poised to attack CAD. I had to return to academia, to Harvard's Peter Bent Brigham Hospital.

Back in Boston, I devoted two years of my life to learning every intricacy of cardiac catheter manipulation in the lab of world-renowned cardiologist Dr. Richard Gorlin. Harvard medicine captured the quintessential Boston of that era, where the Lowells talk only to the Cabots and the Cabots talk only to God. I had entered a formal society stratified by rank, with a medical history of tremendous intellectual achievements. When your medical superiors spoke, it was taken as truth. We did not imagine aggressively challenging authority. Sometime during that first frigid Boston winter, I concluded that when finished with my training in the "Sones Technique" I must return to hurly-burly Los Angeles with no tradition, no social stratification, no "establishment." I wanted a medical environment fully open to new thinking, to challenging the old ideas, to being a misfit.

SONES'S DISCOVERY-BY-SERENDIPITY—WHAT his eulogist Dr. Robert Hall calls "a, if not the, most important advance in cardiology in the 20th century"—stands as an enduring lesson that chance favors the prepared mind. For the first time we had a full diagnostic tool kit. We could assess chamber structure and function with angiography, valve obstruction by pressure drops across a valve, and now we could see the coronary arteries. We could describe the number, location, and severity of coronary obstructions in each patient. We could correlate this information with a patient's risk of a cardiac catastrophe.

Because knowledge is power, coronary angiography revolutionized our thinking. The new idea was simple enough: if we could see the obstructions that caused angina and precipitated heart attack, perhaps we could find a way to treat them.

The idea was liberating, but still, it was only a concept. Seeing the problem does not mean you can fix it. Mason Sones would need a partner. How Mason found his cardiologic soul mate, what they achieved together, and their subsequent fates is hard to believe and yet it is all true.

12

WHEN THE PAMPAS CAME TO CLEVELAND

You can imprison a man, but not an idea. You can exile a man, but not an idea. You can kill a man, but not an idea.

—BENAZIR BHUTTO, PAKISTANI LEADER ASSASSINATED IN 2010
DURING HER RETURN TO HER COUNTRY

THE FULL IMPACT of coronary angiography finally burst like July Fourth fireworks over cardiology in mid-1967 as I drove west to return to Los Angeles. As a treatment solution to CAD, coronary artery bypass graft surgery (CABG) would stand as the pinnacle achievement of surgery's glorious century that had begun with the discovery of anesthesia. It is tempting to imagine that CABG was so obvious that surgeons only needed the proper tools. No idea is more off the mark. For two decades after Harken's battlefield breakthrough, surgeons pursued highly innovative surgical solutions to CAD. All failed.

In Philadelphia, the indefatigable Charles Bailey found that he could strip out atheroma from the inside of large blood vessels in the leg. So he reasoned that the same procedure would work in coronary vessels. Whereas the large diameter vessels of the leg tolerated this surgical insult, the smaller diameter vessels of the heart turned out to be far less forgiving. Bailey's results were disastrous. Tearing of a vessel's surface almost immediately led to the formation of an obstructive blood clot in the coronary artery, and a heart attack immediately followed. Not unfamiliar with disastrous innovation, Bailey abandoned the procedure.

In Cleveland, defibrillator developer Claude Beck reasoned that he could stimulate blood flow to the heart by irritating its surface. So he cracked opened the chest, sliced a hole in the pericardium, and poured in talcum powder. Yes, talcum powder. Sure enough, his supposition was correct: in the animal lab a complex mesh of tiny new vessels soon ran from the pericardium to the surface of his dogs' hearts. But when he performed the same surgery in humans, he discovered to his dismay that the volume of additional blood flow was trivial, and completely ineffective in relieving angina.

Beck next hypothesized that he could circumvent coronary artery obstructions by pumping in oxygenated blood through the veins. So he connected the aorta directly to the heart's largest vein, calling the procedure "retroperfusion." When his patient died one day after surgery, he abandoned the procedure. In modern surgery, we often use retroperfusion from a heart-lung machine to support the heart during cardiac arrest. And what solution is pumped through the heart? A chilled nutrient solution, the child of Lillehei's hypothermia surgery, preserves the heart in hibernation during the surgical procedure. Men die, but their ideas live on.

In Canada cardiac surgeon Arthur Vineberg had a different intuition. If delivering blood to the surface of the heart was insufficient—Beck had tried with talcum powder—why not deliver it directly to the heart muscle? Why not tunnel a nearby artery to the heart muscle itself? The internal mammary artery (IMA) lies an inch or so from the heart and it runs down the inner surface of the sternum (breastbone), from the level of the collarbone to the bottom of the rib cage. There are two IMAs, one on either side of the sternum. Vineberg clamped off the left IMA at its origin, freed it up from the length of the sternum, cut off its side branches, burrowed the vessel into a dead-end tunnel within the heart muscle itself, and released the clamp on the IMA. Blood surged down the vessel and, like a garden sprinkler, spilled out of its many open side branches into the tunnel within the heart muscle. Vineberg imagined that the IMA implanted within the heart muscle would grow new side branches that would become a source of nutrient blood flow to the heart.

Vineberg's procedure did ameliorate angina in many patients, but cardiologists were deeply skeptical. Charles Friedberg, author of the era's leading cardiology textbook, joked of surgeons that "if the heart has a hole in it, they want to close it, if the heart doesn't have a hole they make one." Skeptics claimed that angina relief by the Vineberg procedure was nothing more than the placebo effect, possibly augmented by cutting nerves that carried pain sensation from the chest. But when Mason Sones reported that his own angiographic evaluation of over a thousand IMA implants showed open IMA vessels in 92% of patients and communications between the IMA and the coronary artery in 54%, the procedure was more widely accepted. I recall, however, my own experience looking at similar angiograms in our Harvard cath lab as a fellow. We would all gather around our boss, the famed Dr. Richard Gorlin, who was an enthusiastic advocate of the procedure, as he reviewed our angiographic films. "There it is boys . . . see the dye perfusing that heart muscle?" he would say. Standing behind him, most of the time we would look blankly at each other with raised eyebrows. We would see dye coming down the IMA, and then . . . nothing more. "That man is a wizard," we would say when out of earshot, "he can see things that escape the vision of the average man." Looking back, I believe that relief of angina after the Vineberg procedure was predominantly due to the placebo effect. Whether the Vineberg operation was effective is irrelevant today, because at that moment in time, the Canadian's procedure stood at the base of another Cleveland avalanche.

IN 1967, NINE years after his first serendipitous coronary angiogram, Mason Sones's discovery paid off on its promise. The world of cardiac surgery was turned upside down by an unknown Argentine surgeon named René Favaloro who had spent years collaborating with Sones at the Cleveland Clinic. René Favaloro reported that he had surgically restored blood flow beyond an obstructed coronary artery. Most dramatically, the patient's disabling angina disappeared and did not return.

I admired René Favaloro. His personal story for me stands as the most inspirational in all of cardiology. He was born to Italian immigrants in a dusty rural town about thirty miles south of Buenos Aires. His father, a carpenter, was barely able to provide for the family. As Favaloro told oral historian Dr. Allen Weisse, "[My father] was really an artist . . . He did

very fine carving with very delicately constructed pieces . . . I began working with my father at the age of 10. I could have made a living doing
carving." His mother supplemented their meager income working as a
seamstress. With free schooling throughout the country, both René and
his brother Juan José merged their genetic endowment of fine carpenter
and seamstress. Both became surgeons.

René was in medical school during World War II when revolution
brought fascist Juan Perón to power. Perón sent his military to train in
Germany, creating Argentina's bizarre dichotomy in which its government
was pro-Axis, but its population supported the Allies. An idealistic pop-
ulist, Favaloro's opposition to Perón cost him. He was jailed twice by the
government for his participation in anti-Perónist rallies. When he graduated first in his class, he refused to sign a document stating he did not
oppose the Perónists. In retaliation, he was denied the coveted academic
job traditionally reserved for the school's top graduate. As he recalled, "all
doors were closed to me." When opponents of the government began to
disappear by the hundreds and thousands, "I exiled myself within the
country, going to the southwest, to the dry Pampas. It's an area very similar to the southwestern United States, Texas or Arizona." He spent twelve
years there as a country surgeon.

Yet during those years in exile, Favaloro never lost his dream of what,
in another time and place, might have been. His passion was to contribute
something new to his society. Over his years of exile, he envisioned learning the spectacular cardiac new surgery techniques in the United States
and bringing them back to his homeland. In 1962, with little money, no
promise of a job, very limited English skills, and now middle-aged,
thirty-nine-year-old René Favaloro traveled to Cleveland where he introduced himself to Dr. Donald Effler, the chief of thoracic surgery at the
Cleveland Clinic. After interviewing Favaloro, Effler was blunt: "You don't
have the qualifications. You can only be an observer. We won't pay you
for anything."

Favaloro replied, "Look, I saved some money. I can live on my own
money. Don't worry about it."

What could Effler say? He took on Favaloro as an unpaid laboratory
technician.

René was both intellectually and surgically gifted. Over the ensuing months, Favaloro's dedication and technical skill shone through his fractured English. Favaloro assisted the surgeons by day, and when he finished he spent countless nights with workaholic Mason Sones, studying coronary angiograms and visualizing ways to cure CAD with surgery. Effler was deeply impressed. When Favaloro passed the U.S. Foreign Medical Graduate exam, Effler took the unprecedented step of offering him a cardiac surgery training fellowship. He dedicated those years to his new profession: "Living just across the street I was at the Clinic all the time." Paraphrasing Gabriel García Márquez, he worked when others stopped and rose while others slept. In his training years, Favaloro emerged as Effler's star pupil.

In 1966, four years after he arrived as an unknown immigrant, Favaloro's transformation was complete. Effler offered him a full-time staff position in thoracic surgery. To Effler's astonishment, Favaloro replied that he could not accept the position. He had come to Cleveland with a dream. His destiny was to create the first heart surgery program in Argentina, one that would serve the rich and poor alike. He had to return home.

At home, however, Buenos Aires sent the dreamer packing: no one was interested in supporting a country surgeon with a grand delusion. With Effler begging him to return to the Cleveland Clinic, Favaloro abandoned his quest after several months.

On his return to the Cleveland Clinic group, Favaloro and his boss, Effler, collaborating with Sones and Proudfit in cardiology, set out to find a surgical solution to coronary disease. Favaloro did not practice in the animal lab. Most animals' coronary arteries were too small, and there were no animal models of CAD. Like the first generation of cardiac surgeons, Favaloro simply worked on intuition, and like them, he was condemned to endure the agony of a string of deaths without knowing if he would ever succeed. Initially he tried slicing open the coronary artery along the length of the obstruction, then enlarging it with a patch cut from the pericardium. It seemed like a logical idea. The pericardial patch, however, was a stimulus to blood clot formation. Favaloro logged a devastating 70% mortality rate before he admitted defeat. Self-critical like Harken before him, Favaloro talked openly about his pain as a pioneer, labeling his first outcomes "terrible" and "tragic."

But for Favaloro, failure was fuel. Then he set rules to reduce risk until he succeeded. He would only bypass completely obstructed coronary arteries, theorizing that if a clot formed, there would be no additional loss of blood flow through the vessel. He chose the right coronary artery because it supplied less myocardium (heart muscle) than the left coronary artery. Finally, he chose patients whose Vineberg procedure had failed, and had no other options.

In early 1967, he dissected the coronary artery free from the heart, then cut out the diseased segment of the coronary artery. In its place he patched in a vein he had removed from his patient's leg. More clots. He decided to abandon patching the vessel. Years of failure surrounded him. Retroperfusion had failed. Extracting the atheroma had failed. Replacing the vessel segment had failed. Patching it had failed. Tunneling was doubtful at best. Was there still another way? Why had not anyone thought of the highway planner's way: when traffic on a main artery becomes congested, bypass it?

Favaloro decided to use the leg vein, but now to connect one end of the vein to the aorta and the other end to the obstructed artery just beyond the obstruction. Eureka! No clot. He had "bypassed" the coronary obstruction. His patient survived bypass of the obstruction in good condition. The miracle was complete when their patient strolled the hospital's halls without a trace of angina. Now came the moment of truth. Sones performed a postoperative angiogram. The two men stood transfixed as they watched blood flow briskly through the vein graft directly into the coronary artery segment. It entered the heart and spread throughout the muscle. Short, irrepressible Mason and tall, serious René, as unlikely a pair as one might imagine, had restored coronary blood flow in a patient with intractable angina. It was an incomparable moment in the history of surgery. Favaloro and Sones had wandered through a maze filled with tragic blind alleys, to emerge with a stunningly simple and thus brilliant solution. They had restored blood flow to a starving heart. The year 1967 was a very good year. America had its first African American Supreme Court Justice and its first Super Bowl; cardiology had its first bypass surgery and its first heart transplant.

I still recall the first time I saw a before-and-after angiography on a CAD patient who had vein bypass surgery in 1968. Compared to our usual tunneling procedure, which required both faith and a vivid imagination, the Favaloro procedure showed blood charging down a previously obstructed vessel, followed by an obvious transient "blush" in the heart muscle. It seemed miraculous: seeing blood flow restored to a floundering heart muscle was like seeing a gasping fish thrown back into water. The images were so convincing it seemed almost absurd to question whether the procedure worked. The only question we had was if the benefit justified the risk. Although he was not the first to perform coronary artery bypass surgery, by the end of 1968, Favaloro had the largest series of bypass surgeries in the world, 171 cases, and by June 1970, just three years after his first surgery, he had an astonishing 1,086 cases. After his disastrous beginning, Favaloro's surgical mortality rate with his bypass procedure was only 4%, incredibly low for a new procedure. Today he is universally recognized as the surgeon who fathered coronary artery bypass surgery (soon called CABG, and pronounced cabbage), which clearly relieves angina. Since CABG carried an immediate 4% operative mortality, we knew that many more years of follow-up would be required to demonstrate that CABG reduced long-term mortality rate, but no one could reasonably doubt that the inscription of this final exclamation point was only a matter of time.

Favaloro's publication was like Cortez's legendary proclamation to "burn the boats" after landing on the coast of the Yucatán peninsula. There would be no turning back. Although most of us devoutly believed in the efficacy of the bypass surgery, some annoying naysayers persisted. New Orleans's renowned old guard, crotchety cardiologist Dr. George Burch, claimed CABG was new wine poured into an old bottle, snorting, "If you were offered an anti-angina pill that cost $10,000 and had a 5% chance of killing you, would you take it? Of course not. Well, that's bypass surgery." But the younger generation of cardiologists ignored the adamant claims of Burch and his calcified old guard. As physicist Max Planck observed, "A new scientific truth does not triumph by convincing its opponents and making them see the light, but rather because its opponents eventually die, and a new generation grows up that is familiar with it."

In New York cardiac surgeon Dr. George Green, building on a report by Albert Einstein's cardiac surgeon Dr. Robert Goetz, championed the idea that if a vein extracted from the leg could bypass the coronary obstruction, an artery might be even better. Once again, prior failure informed future success. Green freed up the internal mammary artery (IMA), the same vessel Vineberg had used to tunnel into the heart. But when Green got the IMA free from the chest wall, he connected its free end directly to the side of the coronary artery, again just beyond the obstruction. He was performing bypass surgery with an artery instead of a vein.

Green's reasoning proved to be resoundingly correct in a way we never imagined. Follow-up studies of Favaloro's vein bypass surgery showed that at one year after bypass surgery, about one in five veins were occluded. In contrast, 95% of IMAs were wide open. Clearly the thicker walled artery, nature's vessel for transporting blood under high pressure, was superior to a thin walled vein. In the decade following Favaloro's landmark saphenous vein bypass surgery, cardiac surgeons began using the IMA as their first choice vessel. They did not abandon the leg vein; rather when more than one vessel was needed, they used the leg vein on the less important coronary artery. The left anterior descending coronary artery typically has first dibs on the IMA.

It took another decade, however, before a completely unanticipated, massive limitation of vein bypass surgery became apparent. When angiograms were repeated at ten years after surgery, half of the vein grafts were closed, clogged with an accelerated form of atherosclerosis. We had logically assumed that transplanted veins would behave just like arteries. But in the short space of a decade, the veins fell victim to a virulent form of atherosclerosis far worse than that in arteries. We had been too quick to believe in our magical solution. Once again our humanity was showing. We were desperate for a solution to this new problem.

In the mid-1990s as a Principal Investigator on a National Institutes of Health–funded multicenter trial of the long-term effects of lowering cholesterol levels in patients after CABG, my colleagues and I found that aggressive lowering of LDL (low-density lipoprotein) cholesterol ("bad cholesterol") levels with a statin drug reduced atherosclerosis in bypass grafts, with a 30% reduction in the need for new revascularization procedures over seven and a half years of follow-up. Our research proved that long-term cholesterol lowering therapy is mandatory following bypass surgery. Bypass surgery had given us a powerful answer to the problem of chest pain caused by coronary obstructions. On the other hand, we had to admit that surgery alone had little effect on the progression of disease.

FOUR YEARS AFTER his landmark surgery in Cleveland, Favaloro again heard the call of his lifetime dream, his commitment to his people. He would again return to Argentina, possessed as always by his vision of creating Argentina's own Cleveland Clinic. But this time he returned not as an unknown hat-in-hand exile from the Pampas begging for support, but as an Italian Caesar, marching home as a conquering hero. René Favaloro had become, and remains today, Argentina's most famous citizen. Sones begged him to stay, but to no avail. When word began to circulate that he was leaving the Clinic, offers of jobs poured in. From Miami he was offered a starting annual income of $2 million, an unheard of doctor's salary in the 1970s. But Favaloro was unmoved. His philosophy of life is captured and preserved in a lecture he delivered to students in Israel at that time. "I would like to ask especially of the younger people to understand that material things are temporary, only ideals last forever . . . the battle cry should be education and scientific development for a society in which social justice is the priority."

On his return to Argentina, Favaloro used his status as national hero to raise both private and government support for the Favaloro Foundation, which in 1975 became one of the largest dedicated cardiology programs in the American hemisphere. The foundation's mission statement describes its founder's core philosophy: "advanced technology at the service of medical humanism." The Favaloro Foundation, like the Cleveland Clinic, offered the full spectrum of treatment, education, and research. Although he was the world's most famous surgeon, throughout his career Favaloro referred to himself as a "country doctor." True to his days in the Pampas, he made certain that those who could not pay were not turned away. Despite the cost of bypass surgery, Favaloro operated on indigents on a daily basis. When I met him on my trips to lecture in South America, he struck me as a person of such genuine integrity and goodness that he might have arrived directly from having delivered the benediction from his window in St. Peter's Square

Ten years after Favaloro left Cleveland to build his foundation into one of South America's leading medical institutions, chain-smoking Mason Sones fell ill with metastatic lung cancer. Four months before Sones's death, Favaloro and his wife made a special trip back to say good-bye to Mason, whom Favaloro loved like a brother. "Finally we embraced and said goodbye for the last time in this world . . . I will always thank God for giving me the opportunity to share with Mason many years of common work, understanding and deep friendship," Favaloro recalled.

Of Sones and Favaloro, we can say each needed the other, and together their work constitutes one of the greatest milestones in our story.

A YEAR BEFORE his death, René Favaloro spoke about his pride in the Favaloro Foundation's accomplishments to author Dr. Allen Weisse. "We have over two hundred full-time members on our staff. . . . We have published over one hundred peer-reviewed papers in international journals. Our people are [collaborating with investigators in Germany, Italy, France, Poland, Canada, Belgium, and the United States]. Latin America was once far behind the rest of the world in cardiovascular research. I don't think that anyone could say that this is true today."

But within a year Argentina's economy collapsed amid projections that it might default on its public debt and that the currency would be devalued. In December 1999 Fernando de la Rúa was elected president, campaigning on the promise to save the Argentine economy and end the corrupt ten-year rule of President Carlos Menem. Six months later, La Rúa announced massive spending cuts. Two days later 20,000 protesters took to the streets.

The Favaloro Foundation, dependent on government support, fell progressively into debt, reaching $75 million (USD). As the foundation appeared to teeter on bankruptcy, federal subsidies cut off completely. Favaloro desperately sought relief. Every door was closed. In a note to President de la Rúa, he expressed his dismay at "being a beggar in his own country." As his foundation's default and collapse became imminent he wrote seven letters, recalling his dream and recounting his foundation's accomplishments. In one, he said: "We insisted on the admittance of a number of beds for the poor. This meant that hundreds of patients were treated completely free of charge . . . At this moment and at my age, it is incredibly difficult to break off with the ethical principles that I got from my parents, my teachers and my professors. I can't change; I would rather disappear." Letters written, the beloved idealist who had performed bypass surgery on over 13,000 patients closed his bathroom door forever, and in a final symbolic act, shot himself through the heart. It was July 29, 2000. Remarkably, the foundation weathered the storm and remains a beacon of hope today. I can only fathom the tragic, operatic denouement of René Favaloro's illustrious career in the context of his mission, as the final poignant expression of his soaring idealism. I must believe this, and so I do. I am not alone.

The United States had provided the fertile ground for invention, and a country doctor from Argentina possessed by a vision had found the solution. His nephew Roberto Favaloro, director of the Favaloro Foundation, summed up his uncle's life: "Despite his greatness he had humility . . . He was a great man who was able to be charming and be a normal person. In the end he always carried on being a country doctor in his way of life." Favaloro was a man of a different generation, a different time, with values rooted in a bygone era that no longer exists, and perhaps never did. A decade after his death, in *The Argentina Independent* article "Shot Through the Heart: The Life and Death of René Favaloro," reporter Hannah Vinter summarizes his vision by quoting from one of his speeches: "I have always believed that in the future, reality will be constructed on the foundations of ideals and utopias." René Favaloro, the Don Quixote of the Pampas, lived and died that dream.

THE EVOLUTION OF CABG from the early days has been dramatic. Today we have surgical alternatives. The surgical incision may be made through the breastbone or the ribs. The latter, called minimally invasive surgery, is more technically challenging but often has more rapid postoperative recovery. A third alternative is beating heart surgery, which is even more technically challenging but eliminates the need for a heart-lung machine. Robotic surgery, in which devices are inserted through small incisions in the chest wall, is also being tested in some institutions.

During my years as chief of cardiology the cost of bypass surgery escalated. To counter rising costs, we initiated a sea change in the concept of postoperative care. Our emphasis went from gradual recovery to early ambulation. We were successful beyond our imagination. Not only did we reduce costs, but our patients' recovery was less eventful. In the earlier years, patients were hospitalized for two to three weeks; today we discharge most patients in three to seven days. Our patients typically resume driving at two to three weeks, and return to work by one to two months.

The risks and benefits of bypass surgery are very well defined. The risk of serious complications during hospitalization is small: heart attack 1%, stroke 3%, and mortality 2%. CABG relieves angina chest pain in about 95% of patients, and postoperative survival is 90% five years after the procedure.

13

EXPANDING HORIZONS

Don't be afraid of new ideas. Be afraid of old ideas. They keep you where you are and stop you from growing and moving forward. Concentrate on where you want to go, not on what you fear.

—Anthony Robbins, American motivational speaker

AS MASON SONES and René Favaloro pursued surgical solutions to CAD, surgeons cast their eyes on heart failure (severe reduction in the heart's pumping function). The two most common causes of heart failure in adults are diseases of the heart valves and scarring of the heart muscle after a heart attack.

Today it is hard to imagine the era before the spectacular developments in surgical treatment of heart failure. Cardiologists relied on digitalis, a foxglove-derivative handed down from the prior century, which sometimes provided a spectacular relief of symptoms. One of the toxic effects of digitalis is distortion of visual shape and color. Vincent Van Gogh's obsession with yellow and his distortion of perspective has been alleged to be the result of digitalis intoxication. Even if the story is apocryphal, his paintings do capture how digitalis's toxicity affects vision. In 1785, English physician William Withering first described giving foxglove to a forty-year-old lady, a "Mrs. H. of A. near N" who was "nearly in a state of suffocation, her pulse extremely weak and irregular, her breath very short and laborious, her countenance sunk, and her arms of a leaden color. She could not lie down in bed and had neither strength nor appetite, but was extremely thirsty. Her stomach, legs, and thighs were greatly swollen." Within a week these signs disappeared. A century later the father of pharmacology, German chemist Oswald Schmiedeberg, isolated the first pure digitalis crystal from foxglove, launching the modern pharmaceutical industry. Despite its efficacy in relieving symptoms, however, digitalis had little effect on the progressive downhill course of the heart failure. Could surgeons offer a better solution?

Dr. Albert Starr was only sixty-three years old when he abandoned the comfortable confines of East Coast academia to create the University of Oregon Hospital's brand-new program in cardiac surgery.

Starr's mandate was to achieve results comparable to those of Lillehei and Kirklin in Minnesota, and to do it as soon as possible. Soon after his arrival a fragile sixty-year-old retired engineer with early Parkinson's disease dressed in crumpled slacks and a sports shirt without a tie made an appointment to see him. Lowell Edwards did not walk into Starr's office with a heart murmur, he came with a proposal.

Edwards was a hydraulic engineer who held sixty-three patents on a spectrum of inventions from a hydraulic lumber-debarking system to a fuel injection system for World War II aircraft. The patents provided royalty income to support his Edwards Laboratories in Portland. Edwards wanted to propose that he use his knowledge of fluid dynamics to create an artificial heart. His motivation was personal. In his teens, Edwards had two harrowing episodes of rheumatic fever, the cause of most of the heart valve disease in that era. As he grew up, for years he feared that he would develop valve disease and die in early adulthood. Starr admired Edwards's vision of creating a pumping device to help people with heart valve disease. But he had a different vision. Cardiology did not even have a satisfactory artificial valve, he told Edwards, let alone a whole heart. The first step in helping the failing heart was not an artificial heart, but an artificial valve. Asking the heart muscle to endlessly pump against the tremendous resistance offered by a severely narrowed valve was like trying to pump the Hudson River through a storm pipe. Conversely, when a valve failed to prevent backflow, the heart muscle was like a sailor trying to bail out a boat with a huge hole in its hull. Both tasks were ultimately impossible, and the heart failed. Starr proposed a direct solution for Edwards's greatest fear. Instead of an artificial heart, they would create an artificial valve. Like Harken before him, Starr chose the mitral valve as his first target.

Edwards and Starr confronted three critical initial questions, each with the potential to consume years of research. Was it possible to design a valve simpler than Nature's impossibly complex mitral valve with its two leaflets and attached cords? Could they find a material that could be flung back and forth sixty times a minute, twenty-four hours a day without respite for an entire lifetime? How could they possibly attach their device within a vigorously contracting and relaxing heart?

Edwards and Starr made their first critical decision. They would not use Nature's sheets and cords design. In its place Edwards's first valve consisted of a circular ring into which he inserted two thick semicircular "leaflets" hinged on a metal crossbar. For his materials, Edwards chose Teflon for the ring and Silastic (a portmanteau of silicon and plastic) for his leaflets. Starr inserted the valve in place of the normal canine mitral valve apparatus. His dogs survived the operation with good cardiac function. Their collaboration had proven that a rigid valve could function in place of Nature's more flexible living structure.

But their design was still an abject failure. All the dogs died within two to three days from congested lungs. Puzzled, Starr performed autopsies. He found two devastating complications. First, the circular ring housing the valve partially detached from the heart, and second, the exposed metal hinges were covered with fragile blood clots waiting to be dislodged to the brain and other organs. Edwards went back to the drawing board. He returned with a thicker, more compliant sewing ring. He had solved the problem of valve detachment. But they made no progress on eliminating clotting on the central crossbar and the animals continued to die. Two bars sitting in the middle of a flowing bloodstream was too tempting a target for platelets to build fatal clots.

Starr and Edwards had to admit that their leaflet design was a failure. Their new design, although not original, certainly reflected outside-the-box thinking. They created a free-floating spherical poppet inside a cage. When the heart contracted the ball leaped forward, to be limited in its forward excursion by the arms of the cage. When the heart relaxed the ball fell back into its circular seat, preventing backflow. They hoped that the constantly moving, spinning ball would not induce clot formation. Their new design had the short-term effect of lengthening animal survival to about a month, but the clotting problem reemerged. Over time blood clots formed on the cloth sewing ring that attached the valve to the heart. The clots ultimately became huge, blocking blood flow.

Then in the spring of 1959, while bounding up the stairs to his research laboratory, Starr glanced outside at the cherry blossoms emerging from their sheaths. Intuition flashed: "All of a sudden I had a Eureka moment . . . my mind wandered, and suddenly I thought of the solution to the thrombosis problem. Why not create a Silastic shield that could be retracted during implantation of the valve, and then snapped into place covering the entire zone of tissue injury?" Edwards created a retractable shield. Starr sewed the valve in place, and then pulled the shield over the sewing ring. The "cherry blossom" refinement resulted in 80% long-term animal survival.

Starr soon had a kennel full of happy dogs, which he planned to follow for the next few years looking for late complications. Early in the summer of 1960 Starr's vision of logical and progressive scientific development evaporated in an instant when Dr. Herbert Griswold, Oregon's chief of cardiology, stopped by the lab. What Griswold saw was a kennel full of healthy dogs with prosthetic mitral valves clicking away. One of the dogs licked his hand. Griswold had many patients in the hospital in the terminal stages of heart failure with mitral valve disease. He insisted that Starr treat his patients. As Starr recalls, "we were suddenly thrust into the real world of informed consent, liability, and the need to separate manufacturing from scientific assessment, with the first potential patients already in the hospital."

NORMA FORBES HAD rheumatic fever as a child, and it damaged her heart valves. When she became incapacitated by mitral stenosis years later, a surgeon had treated it by opening the valve using the closed heart technique pioneered by Harken and Bailey. The surgeon opened the stenosed valve, but left her with a new complication. Now the mitral valve did not prevent backflow when the ventricle contracted. She now had the opposite of mitral stenosis: mitral insufficiency. Her lungs were flooded with back flow. At just thirty-three years of age, she lay in a University of Oregon Medical Center oxygen tent continuously gasping for air, dying of heart failure in the prime of her life.

Norma Forbes posed a wrenching ethical issue for Starr. Should he use the unshielded ball valve that achieved long-term survival in only one of fifty dogs, or the shielded valve that provided predictable long-term survival in 80% of the dogs? The answer seems obvious, but now uncertainty made its usual appearance. The much simpler unshielded valve was also much easier to implant. In addition, the human coagulation system is far more forgiving than the dog's. Perhaps the simpler device would be sufficient. But since Starr had never used either valve in a human being, which should he choose?

"I grappled with it myself and decided on the simple device for the first implant. The thinking was this: If we started with the simple device and it worked, we would not have to use the more complicated valve. If it did not work, we could then go to the more complicated valve. However, if we started with the more complicated valve and it worked, how would we know whether the simple valve might also have worked?" he thought. Starr had set his own stage for the Pain of the Pioneer.

With Norma on the heart-lung machine, Starr opened her heart, and cut out all of her scarred mitral valve. In its place he sutured in the un-sheathed valve that he and Edwards had created. He felt confident, having performed the same surgery with the same valve in many dogs. As he closed the chest, he mused how Norma's surgery proved to be quite a bit easier than his operations in the animal laboratory because Norma's heart was larger.

Postoperative care was a different issue. "We had no intensive care unit and had to create one for this project. We literally mobilized the whole medical school faculty for this project," Starr wrote. Norma awakened from anesthesia in the late afternoon. By evening was she able to sit up in bed for a portable X-ray of her chest. Starr was elated. On his first case, he had succeeded far beyond what he could have imagined when he and Edwards first met two years earlier.

Later that night, tired from lying on her back all day, Norma asked for help in rolling onto her right side. Hovering beside his patient's bed, Starr immediately reached out to help.

"While I was helping her, she gasped and died suddenly in my arms," he wrote. Again imagine yourself as the young surgeon at that moment. For Starr, the devastating experience was almost beyond endurance. This could not be. How could this possibly have happened?

The cause of Norma's death, Starr would learn at autopsy, was massive air embolism. Her change in body position had released a large air bubble trapped in her left ventricle. As he closed the heart, Starr had allowed air to remain within the ventricle. He had actually seen the air quite clearly on Norma's post-op X-ray, but assumed that he was looking at air trapped between the heart and the pericardium, a finding that carried no risk, since the air would be absorbed without symptoms over a couple of days. Instead, Starr had joined Bailey and Lillehei as a surgical pioneer done in by the same, simple, avoidable technical error. Just ten hours after the miraculously return of life's simplest function, a breath of fresh air, youthful Norma Forbes's vitality had been snatched away by the simplest of human errors. How stupendously unfair. But tragedies precede successes. He pledged to himself, "I will never let that happen again." He never did.

Starr's second patient was a fifty-two-year-old truck dispatcher who had two prior surgical procedures on the mitral valve using the Harken and Bailey's finger-fracture method. His second patient became his first survivor. Starr and Edwards had gone from design to implementation in just two years. But he had hardly solved his problems. Starr would have to endure the wrenching learning curve that I have seen plague all the great new cardiovascular interventions. His operative mortality in the first year was a devastating 50%. Five years later it was less than 10%. Starr had learned from his repeated failures. Starr's experience represents an eternal, inescapable truth I know too well. In medical innovation, if we are unwilling to fail, we rarely succeed.

After Starr presented his results at the American Surgical Association in the spring of 1961, surgical programs around the country began demanding heart valves. The new field of prosthetic valve surgery exploded. Lowell Edwards, who had made Starr's early valves by hand, formed a company in Santa Ana, California, to meet the demand, and to continue valve development and testing. At the same time, Starr and Edwards modified their mitral design to make it suitable for aortic valve replacement. The first aortic valve was implanted just a year later. In California, Edwards Laboratories conducted accelerated fatigue tests that demonstrated the durability of the ball to beyond forty years without damage. From one of my many visits to Edwards Laboratories a few years later, I still recall the bizarre experience of seeing and hearing a chamber full of Silastic balls, like caged crazed drummers, each whacking away their rhythm at sixty times a minute into eternity.

TODAY BOTH THE diagnosis and treatment of valve surgery bears little resemblance to the early Starr-Edwards years. In those halcyon years, I focused on the intricacies of physical diagnosis, hoping to discern the correct diagnosis by palpation (touch) and listening for murmurs with my stethoscope; today I am a cardiovascular dinosaur: my trainees get an irrefutable answer from the echocardiogram.

We also have abandoned the bulky ball-in-cage structure for valves with synthetic leaflets strikingly similar to Starr and Edwards's first failed designs. But in addition we fashion leaflets from pig, cow, or even human tissue. And in some patients with aortic valve disease, we use a cadaver aorta with intact valves. Best of all, in selected cases surgeons can "resculpt" the diseased valve without even replacing it. When we come later to the future of valve surgery I will show you the most amazing feat of all: restoration of valve function without surgery.

Among the many valve types how do we choose which one to use, what are the pros and cons? Valve resculpting is appealing because we preserve the strength of the heart muscle and do not need to use blood thinners after surgery. Pig or cow tissue valves also eliminate the need for long-term blood thinner treatment, but they deteriorate over ten to fifteen years and must be replaced. Synthetic valves have greater durability but require blood-thinning therapy. So when a valve cannot be repaired, in a younger patient we favor a synthetic valve to avoid repeat surgery, whereas in an older patient we may recommend a tissue valve.

We recommend surgery based predominantly on a patient's symptoms and evidence of progressive deterioration of cardiac function. Fainting, angina, or shortness of breath is an indication for surgery for patients with aortic stenosis, since with medical therapy, survival after the appearance of these symptoms is only two to four years. I seldom see mitral stenosis since the virtual eradication of rheumatic fever in the West, but would choose surgery with these symptoms or with coughing blood. For insufficient or incompetent aortic and mitral valves, we use the same criteria, always juggling the uncertainties: the risk of the disease, the risk of surgery, and the benefit of therapy.

In the earliest days, assistants gave the head cardiac surgeon a clear view of the heart by continuously vigorously spreading the ribs with a metal device shaped like a curved hand (now we have mechanical devices). A half century after medical school, I still wince at the memory of "rib retraction," which required neither brains nor skill, and was assigned to the lowest person on the totem pole. After surgery we hospitalized our surgery patients for two to three weeks, treating them as if they were the human equivalent of expensive, fragile Dresden china. Today, our nurses remorselessly insist on postoperative day one that patients cough, blow into a resistant tube to reinflate their lungs, flex their legs to prevent blood clots, and start walking to restore vitality. If all goes well, we aim for hospital discharge on postoperative day three to five.

Each year we do about a hundred thousand heart valve surgeries in the United States, about a quarter of a million worldwide. Today we operate on patients in their nineties. Despite accepting people who were inoperable in earlier years, we have reduced the operative mortality from 50% in Starr's first year to about 3% today. In otherwise healthy patients, our surgical mortality rate is less than 1%. For this reason it is often a fool's errand to compare mortality rates among surgeons. In major medical centers, a surgeon's mortality rate is more a reflection of the number of desperate, high-risk patients she accepts than her surgical skill. Yet despite all these advances, we are poised to enter a brilliant new era of treating valve disease. As we will see in our chapters that deal with the future, many procedures that began in the operating rooms of cardiac surgeons will be performed in the catheterization laboratory.

ALBERT STARR AND the cardiac surgeons had proven that we could completely reverse one form of heart failure. Restoring valve function allowed a grateful heart to return to work without facing an insurmountable resistance from a stenosed (narrowed) valve or volume overload from an incompetent valve. The impact of artificial heart valves on the thinking of surgeons was profound. With the heart-lung machine, it seemed, anything they could imagine, they could do. Some began to imagine the inconceivable: that one day an intrepid surgeon might replace a heart itself, not with an artificial one, as Lowell Edwards had imagined, but with a real one. Was the heart-lung machine so effective, so mind-bendingly potent, that it could sustain life in a patient who had no heart at all?

14

"THE SHIP HAS WEATHER'D EVERY RACK, THE PRIZE WE SOUGHT IS WON"

It is infinitely better to transplant a heart than to bury it to be devoured by worms.

—CHRISTIAAN BARNARD, SOUTH AFRICAN CARDIAC
TRANSPLANT PIONEER

AS WE ENTERED the mid-1960s, buoyed by Al Starr's spectacular valve surgery at the beginning of the decade, a few hundred miles south at Stanford University, surgeon Norman Shumway focused on the other major cause of heart failure: damage to the heart muscle, most commonly caused by CAD. After a third heart attack, the heart often has so little remaining muscle that no amount of supportive treatment is possible. In those years, the patient was doomed. We had nothing more to offer. Shumway aspired to the most impossible surgical feat of all time: replacing the whole heart in patients with severely damaged heart muscle. For those of us who lived through it, there is no more shocking, more memorable story in cardiology than the development of the cardiac transplantation.

* * *

WHEN THE SANTA Ana winds of October suddenly arrive in Los Angeles, you do not need a weatherman to tell you. The winds that blow off the desert to the east tear relentlessly at every window and door, demanding entry; dry and hot, they scorch your face like a suddenly opened oven. Riding on the gusts of the Santa Ana is an unspoken fear. Is this wind the killer, the one that brings wildfires that man cannot control? It was on such a day in the mid-1990s that I received a call from a valued friend from across the country, the past president of the American College of Cardiology. The call had an unusual provenance. In academia, an "endowed chair" refers to a philanthropic donation, which supports in perpetuity the salary or the research of the so-honored professor. Our patient comedian George Burns created the George Burns and Gracie Allen Endowed Chair in Cardiovascular Research, and I was its first recipient. My cardiology friends around the country referred to me simply as "the George and Gracie." So I was not surprised to learn that the patient was one of George's professional colleagues.

"Jim, I've been taking care of a Hollywood personality." I recognized the patient's name immediately. I will call him Marcus Stuart. "He's seventy years old, but he is still working. He has severe congestive heart failure, which I've managed for a few years. He is in otherwise very good health, but his heart has brought him to the end of the line. It's sad because he's over sixty-five, so we cannot consider him for a cardiac transplant. He is in bad shape and I expect that he'll die in the next year. But between now and then he is going to require multiple hospitalizations. He and his wife are going to need someone to shepherd him through the final days. He has homes in both Manhattan and Los Angeles, and he's returning to LA now. Can you help?"

I thought about congestive heart failure (CHF), a disorder as smothering and potentially lethal as that Santa Ana wind. CHF has many causes, but the most common are valve disease and death of cardiac muscle, the latter from a heart attack or from an infection. The volume of blood that the left ventricle ejects on a single beat, called ejection fraction, is normally 60 to 70%, whereas in CHF it falls to 40% or less. In severe heart failure the ejection fraction is much less than half-normal. The resulting symptoms are weakness and fatigue because of diminished flow to vital organs, and shortness of breath because blood backs up into the lungs.

CHF is now one of society's most pressing public health concerns. About 5 million Americans now have CHF and over half a million new cases appear each year. About a quarter of the patients with CHF are less than sixty years of age. CHF is a high-risk disease, with a mortality rate over 50% within five years of first diagnosis. The sudden death rate in CHF is about nine times that of the general population. CHF ranks at the very top of the nation's health-care issues, because it is an exceptionally high-cost illness and patients require repeat hospitalizations—now more than all forms of cancer combined.

The medical treatment of a patient dying of CHF has much in common with caring for terminal cancer. Today, a very good specialist can reduce emergency room visits and hospitalizations by careful adjustment of potent drugs with different modes of action. A great doctor goes a step further, recognizing that the primary goal of treatment subtly morphs from prolongation of life to maximizing the quality of remaining life. Doctors who are able to do this focus equally on the physical and the metaphorical heart, supporting the patient on every step of the downhill descent to death. Because this requires both time and empathy, many doctors are not able to find that exquisite and ever-changing balance between honestly answering a question and never relinquishing hope. In my medical school years, when we had virtually no effective therapy to offer a patient with terminal heart failure, my professors quoted the great nineteenth-century physician Oliver Wendell Holmes, who taught us to "beware of how you take away hope from another human being." It is a life lesson that I pass on to my own students in an era of statistical probabilities.

A few days later Mr. Stuart stood in the doorway of my office. Tall, slim, and distinguished in a black open-neck sweater, with a gray beard and mustache, he cut the perfect image of a distinguished Hollywood personality. We chatted amiably about our mutual friend who had referred him to me. In the process we discovered that we shared the same beach in Malibu. He lived about a ten-minute walk north along the Pacific. In his medical history I clicked off all the causes of congestive heart failure. He seemed to have none of them . . . certainly none of the most common causes like CAD, hypertension, or valve disease. I diagnosed Mr. Stuart's problem as idiopathic cardiomyopathy. Although it sounds profound, the term disguises abject ignorance. Idiopathic cardiomyopathy simply means heart muscle malfunction of unknown origin.

As I examined Marc, I focused on assessing the severity of his heart failure. His thin frame was due to muscle wasting. His mouth opened slightly with each breath. His neck veins were distended, reflecting the inability of the heart to pump out all the returning blood. The muscles between his ribs pulled in hard with every breath. Listening to his lungs I heard the cardinal finding of congestion, the crackling sound of fluid in his airways. By tapping on his chest to outline the border of his heart and lungs, I found that Marcus's heart was markedly enlarged, the result of its inability to effectively pump blood to the rest of the body.

The echocardiographic image spoke a thousand words: his heart looked more like it was twitching than contracting. My assessment confirmed every detail I had been given on the phone. Marcus Stuart had a heart so damaged that he very likely had less than a year to live. He had passed the point at which we had an effective medical therapy to offer. He needed a new heart. I asked him to get some routine lab work and to come back to see me again in about a week. I got the lab results back the next day. The function of his other organs, including his liver and kidney, was remarkably normal. I sat looking at the results for a few minutes. Marc was a man with a body too good to die, but with a heart beyond repair. I walked across the hall to plop down in a comfortable chair in the office of our cardiac surgeon Alfredo Trento, who years before had found a way to treat Maria, our child with tetralogy. Alfredo is also one of the nation's leading transplant surgeons.

"Alfredo," I said, "I have a seventy-year-old man, otherwise highly productive, with end-stage idiopathic cardiomyopathy. He's otherwise in good health, and I feel that he is physically able to withstand the trauma of heart surgery. If you were willing to consider an age exception, is it even possible?"

Alfredo gave me a big smile. "Sometimes people get lucky, Jim. It turns out I'm initiating a heart transplant program for otherwise healthy patients over sixty-five. Mine will be one of the first in the country. My idea is that since people over sixty-five have a shorter natural lifespan, we could use hearts from older potential donors that would be rejected for a young person. So yes, I'd consider him. But he's gotta have very good insurance. A heart transplant costs about three hundred thousand dollars."

When Marcus came to see me the following week, I gently told him my honest assessment of his prognosis. "I knew that you would say that, Jim," he said. "My body tells me that, too. I have no strength and I can barely breathe."

"Marc, I want to offer a ray of hope," I replied. "Would you consider a heart transplant?"

Marcus Stuart's reaction was as profound as any I can recall in any patient over my forty years of cardiology. I was looking at a man who had recently passed through the stages of denial, anger, depression, and acceptance of death. In the space of a single sentence, he was being asked to discard those months of wrenching adaptation. Marcus sat there, self-consciously searching for an emotionally safe place within himself where he might be allowed to hope. His eyes turned glassy. His mouth opened as if to reply but he couldn't speak. He rubbed his eyes. He held up his right hand in the universal stop sign. For a moment I thought he was telling me to stop, until I realized he was signaling that he needed a few moments before he could speak.

I reached out to rest my hand on his arm. "I understand what you're going through," I said. "I have as much time as you need." I waited quietly. Marcus did not need to hear my words. He needed to listen to his own heart.

Finally he cleared his throat and said, "Of course I want a transplant. But you forget I am seventy. Everyone knows I am seventy years old. I can't just claim I am sixty-five and get a transplant. Hearts are so scarce. They have to go to younger people." Reassurance had to precede hope.

I explained Alfredo's new over-sixty-five transplant program, which used hearts that were deemed too old for younger patients. After he realized the reality of potential transplant, I tried to caution him about the ordeal of multiple cardiac biopsies and the side effects of immunosuppressive drugs. It was not an easy road, even for a young man. I had the impression I'd scarcely been heard as he brushed aside these concerns. The white-hot radiance of reprieve from death blinded him to lesser concerns. Then I delivered the sobering reality. Even if both he and Alfredo decided to proceed, he still had to have a willing insurance company. The company could easily refuse to pay, arguing that the current standard of care was that transplants were not done in people over sixty-five years.

"I have insurance through the Guild," Marc replied. "They take very good care of us. But this is a huge, one-of-a-kind request that no one has ever made before. So I have no idea what they'll say. Plus they may take a month or two to decide and I might not live long enough to find out. So don't let the cost slow us down. Madeline and I will find the money," he said, "and I will deal with the Guild."

Alfredo saw Marcus and agreed that he was a suitable candidate for his over-65 transplant program. Marcus had one stipulation: "I want all my records to be in an assumed name. In the movie business the people who finance the movie require a completion bond on the stars, to protect them from loss if the movie does not get made. If everybody knows I had a transplant, insurance companies might refuse to issue a completion bond, and I would never work again." I arranged the assumed name, and promised I would tell no one his secret. I passed the baton of Marcus's care to the cardiologists who worked with the transplant team. It typically takes about six months to a year to find a heart. Selection of a heart depends on a waiting list stratified by both risk of imminent death and duration of waiting. The donor heart is then tested against each potential recipient's profile until a compatible match is found.

Marc's ordeal had just begun. His would have an agonizing wait, knowing that he had to be constantly available to race to the hospital on short notice, and that about a third of those on the recipient list die before their match is found. Then in the ninth month after his name was entered on the transplant list, we received the call. His new heart would arrive by plane from a northern city in an ice container hardly more sophisticated than the one used for soft drinks on the beach. Marc swallowed hard in both anticipation and fear as he raced from Malibu to the hospital for his gamble with destiny. Would this be the end of life, or a new beginning?

THE IDEA OF surgically replacing a diseased heart had percolated in the musings of surgeons since the early 1900s when Nobel Laureate surgeon Alexis Carrel took the first step in demonstrating technical feasibility when he transplanted the heart and lungs of a small cat into the neck of a larger cat. Carrel reported that "The lungs became red and after a few minutes effective pulsation of the ventricles appeared," and although it must have been a grisly scene, the recipient cat survived for two days. After World War II, eccentric Russian surgeon Vladimir Demikhov set the stage for future research when he succeeded in replacing one dog's heart with another. His dog actually climbed the Kremlin steps on the sixth postoperative day, but soon thereafter died of cardiac rejection.

The development of modern cardiac transplantation, however, is the story of two men, a Tortoise and a Hare. Whereas most scientific developments follow the path of investigators building on the work of those who preceded them, the foundation for human cardiac transplantation was largely the work of one man, the Tortoise, Dr. Norman Shumway of Stanford University, who for more than two decades devoted his life to solving this tremendous challenge. In the 1950s Shumway, with his associate Dr. Richard Lower, initiated his program. Shumway had been inspired to pursue cardiac surgery research as a trainee of the great Walt Lillehei, whom we met during his tumultuous years in Minnesota. Shumway later said that Lillehei changed the course of his life.

Shumway was the most relaxed, irreverent, witty surgeon I have known. His humor turned on himself as often as it did on others. His endearing personality made him my favorite person among all the cardiac surgeons, and my feelings were shared by his colleagues, trainees, and patients. My favorite irreverent Shumway quip came at a get-together honoring his mentor Lillehei many years after Walt's bout with the Internal Revenue Service and his subsequent resurrection. Lillehei, Shumway said, reminded him of Al Capone. "He killed a lot of people but the government could only get him on taxes." Those training years at Minnesota set Shumway's life's course. "The atmosphere at Minnesota was unbelievable, it was electric," he told his biographer David K.C. Cooper. "We used to say you had to invent an operation to get on the operating room schedule."

As he set out on the long journey to human cardiac transplantation, Shumway faced three unknowns. The first was basic: would a heart, highly sensitive to both nervous and hormonal stimuli, be able to function normally after it had been separated from all its surrounding supportive tissue? Over a period of several years, he proved the long-term feasibility of the surgical procedure by auto-transplant, i.e., removing a heart from a dog and then transplanting it back in the same animal. Shumway's dogs survived without a problem for several years.

Shumway's answer led to a new question. How do you attach the donor heart to the recipient? The logical technical approach would seem to cut out the entire heart including a stump of the aorta and the major veins. This approach, however, performed in an era long before modern techniques of bleeding control were available, resulted in blood spurting from the aortic anastomosis (the site where two vessels are joined together by a surgeon). On each heartbeat, cells ejected into the aorta ripped at his suture line like an Oklahoma tornado, relented, then attacked again on the next beat. He needed to find a way to make his anastomosis under low pressure. Shumway finally found an ingenious solution. He cut out the donor heart leaving a cuff of right and left atrium behind. He did the same with the recipient heart. He then sutured the atria of the donor and recipient together. Because the pressure within the atria is only a tenth of the pressure in the aorta, he was able to create a stronger, leak-free anastomosis. Shumway had mastered the technical details of heart transplantation, but his dogs still died after a few weeks. He had arrived at transplantation's greatest barrier, tissue rejection.

Rejection of transplanted tissue occurs when a recipient's immune defense attacks the transplanted organ. It is the same process the body uses against foreign invaders like germs and poisons. The body's immune system is activated when it recognizes proteins in the transplanted tissue called antigens. No two people, except identical twins, have identical tissue antigens. The more different antigens between donor and recipient, the more violent the rejection response.

Shumway soon discovered that suppression of the immune system using the few drugs then available to him created vulnerability to devastating infection. So he devised electrocardiographic methods for identifying the onset of rejection, and saved his powerful pharmaceutical guns for these episodes. Even so, immune suppression was desperately inadequate. Shumway had consumed a decade conducting research in the animal laboratory defining the best strategies for transplantation technique and for immune suppression. His was a lonely pursuit, since no one else seemed crazy enough to invest their entire career with the real possibility of eventual failure. He could perhaps take some consolation that if nothing else, he was the world's acknowledged leader in cardiac transplantation research. By 1967 Norman Shumway announced that he was prepared to culminate his life's work by attempting the world's first human cardiac transplant. But now, with his moment of final achievement so palpably near, Shumway encountered a problem he could not solve.

In his animal research, Shumway had removed a beating heart from a donor dog, and immediately plunged it into an iced solution to preserve it until the moment of transplantation. But he could not use this method in humans. In the United States death was defined as absence of a heartbeat and respiration. Although physicians now recognized the irreversibility of brain death, it was not part of the legal definition of death. Hospital administrators were unwilling to allow him to remove a beating heart, even from an obviously brain-dead patient. Shumway was skewered on a catch-22. Shumway could hardly gather a group of surgeons at patient's bedside watching for the last spike on a dying patient's ECG, then plunge in to remove the heart.

On Sunday morning December 3, 1967, Norman Shumway and the world awoke to the stunning news that Dr. Christiaan Barnard, a cardiac surgeon in Cape Town, South Africa's Groote Schuur Hospital, had performed the world's first cardiac transplantation. As I sat flabbergasted over morning coffee at the death of Norman Shumway's lifelong dream to be the first to successfully perform a human cardiac transplant, my thoughts flashed to the excruciating juxtaposition of victory with the agony of defeat, expressed by Walt Whitman's poem on the death of Abraham Lincoln: "O Captain! my Captain! our fearful trip is done; / The ship has weather'd every rack, the prize we sought is won;" . . . "But O heart! heart! heart! / O the bleeding drops of red, / Where on the deck my Captain lies, / Fallen cold and dead." Norman Shumway had weathered every storm during ten long years of research, and had victory snatched from him at the last moment. He had seen the triumph of cardiac transplantation, but someone else would receive the world's accolades for what was the culmination of his life's work.

* * *

WHO WAS CHRISTIAAN Barnard? Not one of us knew. Intrigued, I did a quick search of the published literature that revealed he had one publication dealing with a different topic in cardiac surgery and one publication on experimental renal transplantation. He was a complete academic unknown. Some cardiac surgeons knew him because he had served as chief resident on Walt Lillehei's service at the University of Minnesota soon after Shumway left for Stanford. At the end of his training the chief of surgery Owen Wangensteen thought enough of Barnard's skills to offer him a position on the surgical staff, but he chose to return to Cape Town to establish his own open heart surgery program. Wangensteen had used his connections within the U.S. government to get a heart-lung machine for Barnard. As part of his desire to remain current with the latest trends in cardiac surgery, Barnard had returned frequently to the United States and to England for medical meetings. He had visited surgeon Donald Ross during his last stop in London before his landmark surgery. Ross told a historian, "He had just seen some experimental work (in the United States) involving heart transplantation and said 'Christ, Donny, I'm going to do that!' I thought nothing more of it until, soon after, his historic operation was announced on the radio . . . I know he got the idea there during that visit . . . I'm not taking sides on this issue . . . but he had just seen Shumway or Lower's group transplanting hearts in animals, and he came back determined to do it himself."

Back home in Cape Town, Barnard had mixed reviews. His surgical outcomes in the new Cape Town program were quite good, so he had earned the respect of his fellow South African physicians, although his detractors carped that he had only average technical skills for a surgeon. He was the opposite of the relaxed, self-effacing Shumway. Barnard was legendary for his frequent angry operating room outbursts in which he blamed others for his surgical difficulties. Years later, fair or not, I flashed on Christiaan Barnard when a cardiac surgeon in a movie exploded: "I have an M.D. from Harvard, I am board certified in cardiothoracic medicine . . . So I ask you; when someone goes into that chapel and they fall on their knees and they pray to God that their wife doesn't miscarry or that their daughter doesn't bleed to death . . . who do you think they're praying to? . . . You ask me if I have a God complex. Let me tell you something: I am God."

When he returned to Africa to focus on being the first to transplant a human heart, Barnard prepared himself by practicing the procedure in the animal lab. When he was satisfied, he then performed a human kidney transplant, the only one of his career. When the kidney transplant patient survived, Barnard deemed himself ready to transplant a human heart. Why not? He was familiar with heart surgery and now he knew transplantation. His recipient would be Louis Washkansky, a fifty-seven-year-old diabetic who had sustained several prior heart attacks. Washkansky was undoubtedly a legitimate candidate. His heart failure was so severe and unmanageable that he could not leave the hospital. With a patient at the ready, Barnard attacked the barrier that had stopped Shumway: the definition of death.

South African law held that a patient was dead when declared so by a physician. Barnard consulted a medical ethicist, who informed Barnard that he was quite happy with brain death as a criterion. Barnard then wisely stipulated that to avoid subsequently political turmoil in the racially charged milieu of South African apartheid, both the donor and the recipient should be white. He turned down a suitable heart from a dead young male black donor. Two weeks later a woman in her mid-twenties who had sustained a devastating head injury in an automobile accident was brought to Groote Schuur Hospital. Shortly after arrival Denise Darvall was declared brain-dead. She had the same blood type as Louis Washkansky. Barnard would wait no longer.

Barnard placed Darvall in one operating room, with Washkansky in an adjacent one. Barnard wrote afterwards that as he entered the operating suites he thought, "I am not terribly religious, but I must pray today . . . I couldn't say 'Let me be a brilliant surgeon' because I'm not a brilliant surgeon. Please help me to do this operation as well as I'm capable of doing it.' I decided I would not take out Denise's heart while it was still beating. I was scared I would be criticized . . . I disconnected the respirator myself. She didn't breathe. After five or six minutes her heart went into ventricular fibrillation [in ventricular fibrillation the heart does move, but we define it as the absence of heartbeat]. I then said to my colleagues to open the chest and remove her heart." Although Barnard gave this version of events many times, his brother Marius, a surgeon present at the operation, recalled this episode quite differently. Marius insisted that the heart was removed while still beating. I have wondered which version is correct, and I have wondered if Barnard's anxiety about public reaction to him removing a beating heart explains this difference in their recollections. On the other hand we transport nonbeating hearts packed in ice, and restart them after transplantation, so either account is credible.

Although Barnard had practiced the technique of cardiac transplantation in his animal laboratory, his two assistants had never seen a transplant performed. The removal of Washkansky's heart followed by the attachment of Denise Darvall's to the remaining stump of recipient heart, using Shumway's technique, consumed nine hours. When they were ready to come off the heart-lung machine, however, the donor heart would not start. "I was horrified," Barnard recounted. He tried again. The heart was not doing well. "But on the third attempt, the blood pressure kept rising." They had successfully completed the world's first human heart transplant.

Barnard had told no one, neither the hospital supervisor nor the head of surgery, that he was about to perform the transplant. So there were no photographers memorializing the procedure, and when he emerged exhausted from the hospital, there were no reporters waiting. "I left the hospital at about 6 o'clock in the morning . . . sat down for breakfast, and "it was only an hour later when phone calls came in from all over the world . . . I don't know how they got the information," Barnard wrote. "On Saturday, I was a surgeon in South Africa, very little known. On Monday, I was world renowned." I was so shocked that I still recall precisely what I was doing when I heard the news that Sunday morning.

Louis Washkansky recovered well after surgery. But late in the second postoperative week he developed pneumonia. Barnard and his team thought they were dealing with rejection. Their aggressive immunotherapy may have led to an accelerated spread of the pneumonia throughout his lungs. Washkansky died on the eighteenth postoperative day.

Barnard followed his initial technical success in cardiac transplantation with a second transplant twelve days after Washkansky's death. Philip Blaiberg, a fifty-eight-year-old white Cape Town dentist, received the heart of twenty-four-year-old Clive Haupt, a black man who had died suddenly the preceding day on a Cape Town beach. The cross-racial transplant precipitated an almost comical debate. Author Marius Malan's contemporary recounting of the debate includes this different-era insight from a white politician: "The relief of suffering knows no color bar . . . The heart is merely a blood-pumping machine and whether it comes from a white, black or colored man—or a baboon or giraffe, for that matter—has no relevance to the issue of race relations in the political or ideological context."

In London reporters asked the South Africa House whether Dr. Blaiberg was classified as white or black now that he possessed Haupt's heart. Blaiberg survived hospitalization to become an international celebrity. He lived for nineteen and a half months after the transplant.

Around the world, I witnessed the ethical barrier to human heart transplantation crumble in the face of the media reaction. Three days after Barnard's announcement, Dr. Adrian Kantrowitz transplanted a human heart in a child at Brooklyn's Maimonides Medical Center. Kantrowitz's patient died within the first twenty-four hours.

Several days after Blaiberg's surgery, Norman Shumway was allowed to perform his first cardiac transplant at Stanford. In proving the technical feasibility of heart transplantation, the Washkansky and Blaiberg surgeries had somehow also dismantled the ethical and administrative barriers surrounding the definition of death.

The intense publicity stimulated virtually every leading cardiac surgery program to perform cardiac transplantation. Drowned out in the clamor were the voices of nonsurgeons like renowned cardiologist Helen Taussig who hoped that "surgeons will proceed with extreme caution until such time as a cardiac transplant will not announce the imminence of death but offer the patient the probability of a return to a useful life for a number of years." I shared Taussig's deep skepticism. Over the next year ninety-nine heart transplants were performed around the world.

The stampede to perform cardiac transplantation devolved into a catastrophic embarrassment.

In the year that followed Washkansky, almost every patient died in the postoperative period because the surgeons had little knowledge and few tools to monitor or treat tissue rejection. In cardiology our past informs our present. I would like to say that from this experience we learned that even potentially great advances must be analyzed carefully before widespread implementation. As the deaths accumulated, most surgical programs abandoned heart transplantation. In 1971, just three years after the initial furor, only seventeen transplants were performed in the entire world, and only four cardiac transplant programs remained; all the rest had quit. Those four programs stood as testimony to the power of mentors: all four were directed by surgeons who had direct ties to Walton Lillehei.

Barnard, the Hare in the race to cardiac transplantation, performed only nine cardiac transplants in the next six years. The handsome, charming forty-five-year-old son of a poor Dutch Reformed minister was drawn like a moth to the incandescent flame of public adoration. He was more often seen in nightclubs than in operating theaters. He toured the world, his clean-cut features and dazzling smile adorning magazine covers in every language. Paparazzi pictured him with a different beautiful woman on his arm at each public event. Although married, he gloried in a much-publicized torrid love affair with 1960s iconic sex symbol Italian actress Gina Lollobrigida, and often dated actress Sophia Loren. The new rage became not the surgery, but the man himself. Photographed, interviewed, fawned over, and lionized like no other physician in modern times, he was received by the Pope in Rome and entertained by President Johnson in the United States. Barnard's wife of twenty-one years, a nurse who had helped support him in his early years, divorced him within two years. After a few years of gallivanting, Barnard married a glamorous teenage daughter of a multimillionaire.

Cardiology reacted badly as Barnard donned the media-bestowed mantle of father of cardiac transplantation. Although part of our reaction, particularly in the United States, reflected loyalty to Shumway, much of the reaction was a direct response to Barnard's own behavior. He traveled to the United States as an invited honored lecturer soon after the Blaiberg surgery. Richard Lower told historian David Cooper, about Barnard's lack of political savvy: "I felt terribly sorry for Chris because he was smart in a lot of ways but he was really stupid when it came to this transplant thing. All the early pioneers of heart surgery and heart transplantation were in the audience. Chris could have shown a little humility, and said . . . 'we built on what a lot of you had done.' But he never once acknowledged anybody except himself. Every other word was 'I' . . . I don't think anyone talked to him until he went out of the front door of the hotel and was mobbed by the press and the teeny-boppers. I thought 'Gosh how stupid he was. He could have had the whole thing. Besides being so extraordinarily popular with ordinary people, young people and beautiful girls, he could have had the profession too if he had just turned that corner. But he couldn't do that." He left the nation's cardiac surgeons with the impression that he was cardiology's quintessential narcissist.

To me, the difference between Barnard and René Favaloro, which was profound, is captured in how they dealt with a surgical death. Here's Barnard:

> I have stood at patients' beds when they died, and I've been upset
> with everybody around me . . . but I realize what I'm really upset
> about is that when I write up my series of operations, I have one
> more mortality. It wasn't really the death of the patient . . . it is
> the ego that is hurt. I should not have a death . . . I'm too good
> for that.

Favaloro experienced a patient's death quite differently:

> I suffer with every single death of my patients . . . The day that I
> don't feel the sensation that I am the guilty one, then I will drop
> the knife and I won't operate anymore. I don't mean "guilty" but
> "responsible" for the life of the patient. That is the feeling . . . The
> deaths associated with surgery are personal and the surgeon must
> endure their burden as long as he lives.

Narcissist vs. Humanist? Barnard showed me how ambition and acclaim could obliterate compassion; Favaloro held fast to benevolence and humility in spite of fame. Favaloro's country doctor values transported me back to my reverence for a doctor's humanity as a child in the cocoon beneath my father's living room table, helping me find the balance between ambition and compassion.

Cardiology began to give Barnard the silent treatment that had engulfed Lillehei after his indiscretions. But Christiaan Barnard was not intimidated by his colleagues' rebuff. He was a different breed. The more cardiology rejected Barnard, the more he stuck his finger in the profession's eye. Here's Barnard again:

I have heard the Americans say in front of me that I stole the idea from Shumway. As far as that is concerned, after all that these people had published, I ask, "Do they publish it so other people can learn from it or is it a secret after they have published it?"

In the spirit of science, Barnard was absolutely correct. All scientists stand on the shoulders of those who went before them. Ideas are free. But the Americans were right in a more subtle way. Barnard had taken the final relatively straightforward technical step in an incredibly difficult ten-year quest pioneered by another man. Any competent cardiac surgeon could take that last step (and, as soon as the ethical barrier was lifted, many did). Yet Barnard seemed unwilling to express the generous, magnanimous gesture of recognition for Shumway's groundbreaking research that had made his own success possible. And so, neither side bent an inch.

Barnard found other ways to tarnish his persona. He endorsed Glycel, an "anti-aging" skin cream, which most physicians considered quackery. The cream made him wealthy, but terminally smeared his image. It was withdrawn from the U.S. market in 1987. By that time Barnard's charisma had run dry. He was ostracized as a snake oil salesman. But Barnard had chosen his course, and was disinclined to apology. He countered by writing a sensational autobiography, *One Life*. The book was widely criticized as self-indulgent. With the help of a professional ghostwriter, Barnard also wrote several quite passable thrillers which involved skulduggery in organ transplants.

His second marriage failed after twelve years and two children. He married for a third time, this time to a model forty years his junior. When this marriage failed, also after twelve years and two children, Christiaan Barnard returned full circle, back to the Karoo region of his youth, to live on his 32,000-acre game preserve among the springbok and wildebeest. His implausible, complex, controversial, storybook life ended in a final touch of drama, with a sudden fatal asthma attack while on vacation at age seventy-nine.

SHUMWAY PERSEVERED. IN the 1970s his program stood virtually alone as the only center undertaking cardiac transplantation. The worldwide failure of cardiac transplantation had exposed an intimidating number of flaws in the system. Shumway and his team attacked each flaw. He worked out methods for selecting compatible donors and recipients. He stimulated a program to increase the donor pool. He worked out methods to improve organ preservation so that hearts could be transported between centers. He worked out a schedule of heart biopsies. He tested drugs to prevent rejection. Eventually Shumway found the path to more effective immunosuppression when Switzerland's Sandoz Laboratory discovered the potent immunosuppressive agent cyclosporine. In December 1980, thirteen years after Barnard's first heart transplant, Shumway introduced cyclosporine for the first time in cardiac transplantation. While it did not prevent either rejection or infection, the severity of these two deadly complications was sharply reduced.

In 1981, Shumway headed a team that performed the world's first successful combined heart-lung transplant on a forty-five-year-old advertising executive, Joan Brand, who lived five more years and wrote a book about her experience. As his success rate with cardiac transplantation combined with immune suppression with cyclosporine became public, cardiac transplantation was reborn in the mid-1980s. Norm Shumway, the Tortoise, had indeed won the race to be the Father of Cardiac Transplantation. Cardiology, like all of science, awards the man who convinces the world, not the one who got there first. I first experienced that surprising insight when Dwight Harken repeated a surgery first performed by Ludwig Rehn a half century before him. And how did Norm Shumway feel about Barnard's hopping past him on the stairway to immortality? His view was typical laid-back, generous Norm. He never bought into the resentment expressed by others; rather he found merit in Christiaan Barnard: "We were having a heck of a time trying to get our people to come around to accept brain death as diagnosis and confirmation of death. Had it not been for his December 1967 surgery, I don't think our people would ever have submitted to acceptance of brain death . . . Within a year of Barnard's case, the Harvard committee came out with the criteria of brain death. That's the contribution I see from Chris that really helped all of us." That remark, repeated to me personally as well, captures the essential beneficence of Norm's character, and explains why he is my most admired surgeon.

* * *

ALTHOUGH "EVERYONE KNOWS" that Christiaan Barnard performed the first heart transplant in man, they are all wrong. In January 1964, three years before Barnard, University of Mississippi surgeon James Hardy, renowned for having performed the world's first lung transplant, reached for further glory. He performed the world's first human cardiac transplant by transplanting the heart of a chimpanzee into sixty-eight-year-old African American Boyd Rogers. A recent amputee, Rogers was semi-comatose, attached to a mechanical ventilator, and responsive only to painful stimuli. Compared to today's documents, the consent form captures the ethics of a different era. It was a single paragraph, signed by the family since Rogers was unable to comprehend. The form does state that human heart transplantation had never been done, but does not mention the use of a chimpanzee heart. Hardy succeeded in the technical procedure of transplanting the heart, but the chimpanzee heart was too small for Rogers's large body, and he died on the operating table. In an era of civil rights turmoil, the response of the nation was hardly positive. Hardy was invited to describe his experience at the meeting of the Transplantation Society in New York City a week later. Hardy described his reception to historian David K. C. Cooper: "When I got up to talk, the chairman William Kolff (inventor of the artificial kidney) said, 'I want to ask Dr. Hardy a question before he begins. Dr. Hardy do they keep the blacks in one cage and the chimpanzees in another in the Southern states?' . . . I gave my presentation, reporting exactly what we had done, and at the end of it, there was not one single hand raised in applause . . . It was a bad day." Years later, Shumway would see the chance for another bon mot. "Hardy was an unbelievable enthusiast. But there was absolutely no evidence to suggest that the darn thing would succeed. If you'll pardon the expression, we called it a fool-Hardy procedure."

MARCUS STUART SAILED through the cardiac transplant procedure like he was a sixty-year-old. He started a battery of immunosuppressive drugs that are unpronounceable even to cardiologists. Each month for the first six months he had a cardiac biopsy for early detection of

beginning rejection. As the months progressed and he did well, the biopsies became less frequent. A few months after surgery Marc remarked
proudly to me, "I've had a heart replaced and a knee replaced, and believe
me the knee was harder."

A few months later, I got a worried phone call on the weekend. "Jim,
I am having a lot of chest pain, on the left side."

"How bad it, on the basis of one to ten?"

"It's pretty severe, say seven on the basis of ten. It is not going away.
I am worried that it's my new heart." It certainly sounded that way. Rejection is the feared disaster of transplantation. It is treatable, but it can
be lethal. What terrible luck, I thought.

Except . . . otherwise he felt fine. Marc had no other symptom. No
fatigue, no shortness of breath, no cough, no pain on exercise. Absolutely
nothing. "Nothing at all? No tenderness? Nothing?" I repeated, looking
for an alternative explanation.

"Well, actually, the skin itches in the same area where the pain is."

"Marc, I could walk up the beach and put a stethoscope on your chest,
but it's not enough. You need to get to an emergency room and have an
ECG. But don't panic . . . there's an excellent chance that this is nothing
serious."

Marc's ECG in the emergency room was perfectly normal. It was that
little throwaway end-of-the-conversation remark about itchy skin that gave
the clue to his diagnosis. The next day a rash appeared, a track of blisters
limited to the precise area of his chest pain. Marcus Stuart had shingles,
an intensely painful viral infection of the nerves that lie between the ribs.
The medical term for shingles is herpes zoster, the virus that causes chicken
pox. It is more prone to infect the elderly and patients taking immunosuppressive drugs. Marc had both risk factors.

Marcus recovered from the shingles. With his new heart, he was vastly
energized. About a year later I got a call. "Jim, I am sitting here taking a
rest on some God-forsaken railroad track out in the middle of nowhere.
Shooting a movie. Not much for my wife and me to do at night here. I
am wondering, can you prescribe me some Viagra?" I chuckled. His new
heart was able to love just like his old one.

Before his movie opened, Marcus invited my wife and me to a special
showing of his new film. It was a terrific movie. When it ended, Marcus

stood in the packed theater to a standing ovation. In the glow of the moment our eyes met for an instant as, like an Oscar winner, he graciously thanked all those who had made this moment possible. I beamed at this image of a healthy seventysomething, his secret intact.

AND THE REST of the Story? At a more recent annual Academy Awards ceremony, Marcus Stuart was called to the stage to receive the Lifetime Achievement Award, the Academy's highest honor. After expressing his gratitude, he said, "I'm here under false pretenses . . . Eleven years ago I had a heart transplant, a total heart transplant. I got the heart of, I think, a young woman who was about in her late thirties. By that kind of calculation you may be giving this award too early because I think I've got about forty years left." As the audience sat uncertain how to react at this most personal of revelations, he added advice to others with terminal heart failure. "Your doctors know what they're doing. I mean, they really know what they're doing. While you're in their hands, you just have to say, 'I'll do my part.' As much as you can. You do your part." Eleven years from our first meeting, Marcus Stuart had turned the tables. I was the speechless one, looking at my feet, glassy-eyed.

Although he made a public revelation of his heart transplant as millions watched on television, Marcus Stuart never released me from my promise to never mention his name, so I honor that promise today. Marcus passed away in his eighties from a blood disease.

SINCE THAT VASTLY overhyped December 1967 morning in Cape Town, over 100,000 patients have received cardiac transplants. Last year, about 3,600 cardiac transplants were performed in 225 centers worldwide. We perform about 2,000 cardiac transplants each year in the United States. My hospital has the world's largest annual volume, about 100 per year.

Cardiac transplants are reserved for people knocking on death's door, unlikely to survive a year, or at most two years. In fact, a substantial number of candidates pass away before a suitable heart is found. Ironically, the most common cause of death in the years after successful transplantation is accelerated atherosclerosis, a problem that stands a reasonable chance of substantial resolution as we reduce mortality from CAD. For those who receive a transplant, the improvement in quality of life is dramatic.

Today if you or a family member is a transplant candidate, here are some things to know. Assignment of transplants in the United States is managed by the nonprofit United Network for Organ Sharing (UNOS). Recipients are matched to donors using two major principles: the sickest patients are given first priority, and patients are selected based on tests that assess the likelihood of rejection. Since we have a shortage of available hearts, the wait for a suitable heart varies from days to many months or even a year.

Donors and recipients are typically in different hospitals and different cities. When a match is made, the recipient is summoned to the hospital. At the donor hospital, the donor heart is stopped with an injection of potassium chloride, removed, and packed in ice for transport to the recipient's hospital. Since the ice only preserves the heart for four to six hours, the logistics of rapid transport are critical. When the heart arrives, it is transplanted and then shocked back into a normal rhythm. With a new heart, the recipient begins a lifetime of drugs that suppress his/her immune response to the new heart. Depending on the recovery from surgery, our patients return home in one to two weeks, and then come back for periodic checks of their immune system. Most recipients can return to work within six months of surgery.

How much have we improved since the year following Barnard's groundbreaking surgery, when almost no one survived for a year after surgery? About 90% of our transplant recipients now survive the first year, and 70% are alive five years after the procedure. The average survival following cardiac transplantation currently is fifteen years.

And what about quality of life after cardiac transplantation? It can be pretty darn good. Most recipients can return to work within six months of surgery. Southern California transplant recipient Kelly Perkins travels the world with her husband promoting awareness of organ donation through her blog *The Climb of My Life*. She has climbed the peaks of Mount Kilimanjaro, the Matterhorn, Mount Fuji, and Mount Whitney. Edmonton, Canada's Dwight Kroening runs marathons and became the first recipient to complete an Ironman completion in 2009, twenty-two years after his cardiac transplant. Norwegian-American golfer Erik Compton qualified for the Professional Golfers' Association (PGA) tour at age thirty-two after his second heart transplant. The longest survivor after cardiac transplantation, Ohioan Tony Huesman, received his heart from Norman Shumway way back in 1978, before the discovery of our primary immunosuppressive drug cyclosporine. Huesman survived thirty-one years, dying of cancer in 2009. In Shumway's era an advertisement for Virginia Slim cigarettes, a prime cause of heart attack, boasted, "You've come a long way, baby." In treatment of "end-stage" heart failure, indeed we have.

CARDIAC TRANSPLANTATION GAVE us an answer to another of CAD's most devastating complications, chronic heart failure caused by extensive muscle damage. It was a technical tour de force beyond imagination. And yet, although it is a lifesaving answer for an individual, it is impractical as a solution for society. Transplant requires two teams of cardiac surgeons and prolonged hospitalization, intensive follow-up, and expensive medication. It costs hundreds of thousands of dollars, and consequently is a therapeutic option for only to a few thousand people each year. As I completed my cardiology training in Boston and moved to Los Angeles, the world was initiating cardiac transplantation. Even with the euphoria that surrounded Barnard and Shumway I knew that we were reacting long after the horse had left the barn, that we needed more effective treatment for a heart attack as it was happening.

15

MERGING STREAMS

Our Lord has written the promise of resurrection, not in books alone, but in every leaf in springtime.

—Martin Luther, sixteenth-century German priest

WHEN I FINISHED my cardiology fellowship training at Harvard, and returned to Los Angeles, my generation was questioning the wisdom of our fathers. In my own world, I found I could hardly speak to my father—a staunch Iowa Republican—about the Vietnam War. The world of cardiology mirrored society. My new mentor in Los Angeles was Dr. Jeremy Swan. Born in Sligo, Ireland, Jeremy had been both an amateur boxer and a thespian in his youth. Now middle-aged with a square face and flowing white hair, he was one part quick Irish temper, one part Irish creativity, and every inch charismatic Irish leader. He had come to create Cedars of Lebanon's (now Cedars-Sinai) first academic division of cardiology, devoted to teaching and research. Starting with a program that was largely unknown, he began by hiring six young cardiologists, among them me. Jeremy came from the Mayo Clinic Catheterization Laboratory, where he had worked with John Kirklin and the other Minnesota surgeons who had pioneered cardiac surgery. Jeremy's passion was to improve the outcomes of patients who had suffered a heart attack.

I was surprised to learn that Jeremy wanted to employ my catheter skill in the CCU, not the cath lab. Jeremy opened the topic by asking me, "Jim, what do you think are the three most important problems in treating heart attack? I want you to pick one and solve it." The biggest problem, we quickly agreed, was acute heart failure, and Jeremy thought he knew how to solve it. But he had started by asking me to think independently. He wanted me to question authority. Even if I was about to pursue his idea, he still wanted me to feel it was my own.

Jeremy appointed me director of our Myocardial Infarction Research Unit, funded by the National Institutes of Health (NIH). I secretly felt, although I did not admit, that I was not qualified for this role—my two years of specialty cardiology training were spent in the cath lab. Although I knew cardiology, I had little direct experience managing patients with a heart attack. But Dr. Swan had no one else to take the role. He must have thought that in some sense I looked the part since I was from Harvard and had published a manuscript in *The New England Journal of Medicine*. So I spent the first few months in fear of being exposed as a fraud. Oddly none of the doctors on the staff noticed. Maybe they had the same affliction and were too caught up in it to notice my uncertainty. I was reminded of that time recently when singer Barbra Streisand said in an interview that she had refused to do public performances for twenty-three years, fearing public failure and humiliation. She finally overcame the fear and so have I. But if you have ever known the feeling, that makes three of us.

Contrary to my expectation, as I traversed the country from Boston to Los Angeles I spent the next seventeen years in clinical research directed at improving the care of patients with acute myocardial infarction (heart attack), and had a role in the development of CCUs.

ALEXI KROON, A thirtysomething guitar-playing member of a music group, was admitted to our unit. His scraggly long-haired scruffy look identified him as a committed member of the post-Woodstock counterculture generation. He wore the universal avatar of the cocaine user, a silver chain with tiny silver spoon around his neck. After his group's evening performance, Alexi had spent the night and early morning hours drinking and snorting cocaine. He first noticed chest pain while he was having sex with a younger woman he had met backstage after the concert. The pain, he said, felt like an elephant sitting on his chest, and it radiated upward to his jaw. He graded the pain as eight on a ten-point scale. In our emergency room, he was sweating profusely and was gulping air in short, rapid breaths. His blood pressure was 110/82 and his heart rate was one hundred. His ECG showed signs of a "massive" heart attack. A heart attack or myocardial infarction (literally, heart muscle death) occurs when a segment of the heart muscle dies because it has suddenly been deprived of blood supply from its coronary arteries. The size of the heart attack is determined by how much muscle is supplied by the obstructed arterial segment. Alexi's ECG indicated the obstruction was in the left anterior descending artery, close to its origin from the aorta. So we knew that the amount of heart muscle not receiving blood flow was about 30% of the entire left ventricle. Soon after arriving at our unit Alexi deteriorated further. His blood pressure fell to 85/60 (normal: 120 to 130/80 to 85), and his heart rate increased to 120 (normal: 60 to 100). When blood pressure falls into the 80s in patients with a heart attack, we call the condition cardiogenic shock. I took a deep breath. Alexi's risk of mortality had now risen from 30% to 80%.

WHEN I BEGAN at Cedars, coronary care units (CCUs) were in their infancy. The paradox of the first appearance of the CCU is that it was unanticipated, yet absolutely logical in retrospect. As the newly minted cardiac surgeons battled heart block, ventricular fibrillation, and misdiagnosis in their 1950s operating rooms, not one of them imagined they were working toward a treatment of heart attack. Why should they? The business of cardiac surgeons was heart surgery; cardiologists treated heart attacks. In historical perspective, however, we can see that the development of the CCU was inevitable, because cardiologists caring for patients with acute myocardial infarction battled precisely the same disorders of cardiac rhythm. Unlike the brilliant intuitive leaps of the cardiac surgical revolution, the CCU simply required good organization. Someone had to figure out how to efficiently deliver defibrillators, pacemakers, and drugs to a patient who died suddenly. It is the difference between the brain's right hemisphere and its left, between creativity and logic, between the Greeks and the Romans.

The critical breakthrough that triggered the subsequent emergence of the CCU illustrates how chance favors the prepared mind. While re-

searching defibrillation in dogs, Johns Hopkins engineer William Kouwenhoven and Dr. James Jude noticed that when they forcefully applied
the defibrillation paddles to the dog's chest, it induced a pulse in the dog's
leg artery. From that observation came the technique of chest compression. In 1960 they tried chest compression in people who had died suddenly, then defibrillated the heart. When fourteen of twenty patients
survived until hospital discharge, they had proven that sternal compression combined with artificial respiration could maintain life until they were
able to accomplish external defibrillation, that resuscitation outside the
controlled operating room environment was feasible.

The Hopkins group breathlessly announced in their publication, "Anyone, anywhere, can now initiate cardiac resuscitative procedures." But it
was simply not true. For the next few years, hospital physicians attempted
resuscitation with absolutely dismal results. The reality was the precise opposite from the Hopkins team's assertion: no one, nowhere was successfully initiating cardiac resuscitation. I had my own personal proof in my
nightmare experience with Willie the Phillie. Cardiology had failed to
recognize the huge chasm between the results of a few dedicated Johns
Hopkins researchers and routine clinical practice.

As we compared their success to our failure, we discovered that we
had ignored three huge practical limitations. Patients with acute myocardial infarction were scattered throughout the hospital so the resuscitation
team was often starting CPR minutes, not seconds, after sudden death.
More delay was caused by the lack of available devices at the site of the
cardiac arrest to support advanced CPR. Macabre cynics suggested that
if you want a defibrillator to save you, go stand beside it as you conk
out. Finally few doctors or nurses were trained in the fundamentals of
CPR. Our programs bore the universal hallmarks of failed enterprises: too
disorganized, too little, and too late.

Londoner Dr. Desmond Julian's frustration boiled over into print:

Many cases of cardiac arrest associated with acute myocardial
ischemia could be treated successfully if all medical, nursing and
auxiliary staff were trained in closed chest cardiac massage and if
the cardiac rhythm of patients with acute myocardial infarction
were monitored by an electrocardiogram linked to an alarm

(sounded and recorded) at the onset of an important rhythm change . . . The appropriate apparatus would not be prohibitively expensive if these patients were admitted to special intensive care units. Such units should be staffed by suitably experienced people throughout 24 hours.

We had the tools, but we did not have the system. This was not a problem requiring a flash of intuition. It was a problem of organization. We needed a Henry Ford to come in and set things straight. Henry Ford's revolutionary outside-of-the-box idea had been to bring his cars to the workers rather than workers to cars. Desmond Julian was proposing to do the same for heart attack victims.

Two years later, like the goddess Athena emerging from the forehead of her father Zeus, Julian's imagined unit suddenly burst forth full grown from the convergence of four separate streams: defibrillators, pacemakers, new TV monitors, and CPR. In the United States, a single determined individual in a small private hospital in Kansas City acquired a grant from the Hartford Foundation to create a coronary care area, then cajoled his hospital's administrators to dedicate the space for the first functioning CCU with a mobile crash cart with emergency supplies and drugs, a defibrillator, and an external pacemaker. An unthinkable preposterous idea, that sudden death due to heart attack could be a routinely treatable condition, was slouching toward Kansas City to be born.

Dr. Hughes Day opened the first CCU in small private 200-bed Bethany Hospital. The unit consisted of four private rooms adjacent to a seven-bed intensive care unit. At almost the same time as Day established his CCU in Kansas City, Londoner Desmond Julian, thoroughly frustrated in his attempt to establish a unit in England, moved to Australia to establish a CCU there. Within a few years Dr. Bernard Lown at the Peter Bent Brigham Hospital in Boston, Massachusetts, initiated a critical shift in emphasis, from resuscitation after cardiac arrest to monitoring for precursors of cardiac arrest. Other centers around the country began to report huge declines in the heart attack mortality rate after the opening of their CCU.

Nonetheless our greatest advance in treatment of heart attacks was met with the naysaying establishment's holier-than-thou hostility, just like the days when the establishment condemned the innovators of cardiac surgery. Julian's first report of his CCU experience was briskly dismissed by the prestigious *British Medical Journal* with just the right whiff of Anglican condescension, saying it was "irresponsible to suggest that all patients with myocardial infarction should be admitted to wards in which they could receive intensive care." Harvard professors Bloom and Peterson complained that randomized trials were needed to prove the efficacy of CCUs. But to those of us on the firing line, we had ample, firsthand experience that CCUs saved lives, and you don't need a randomized trial to know if a parachute works.

With resuscitation becoming routine in every town across the nation, Woody Allen could offer a twist on our miraculous new capability, saying, "I don't want to achieve immortality through my work. I want to achieve it through not dying."

We finally had our first major breakthrough in the treatment of the nation's number one killer. But as we reduced death from electrical complications in the CCU, a new problem emerged. Many of my patients that we saved from the electrical complications of heart attack survived with such extensive damage to the heart muscle that they died of heart failure. We now needed a way to assess and treat heart failure at the bedside.

IN THE MAYO Clinic cath lab, my mentor Jeremy Swan had been an expert in measuring cardiac function. We can quantify the function of the heart using two measurements. We measure the volume of blood the heart ejects in a minute, called cardiac output. Cardiac output tells us how well the heart is doing in supplying oxygen to vital organs. Our second measurement is pulmonary capillary pressure, which tells us the effect of heart failure on the lungs. When this pressure rises, it causes lung congestion and shortness of breath. In a failing heart, cardiac output falls and the pulmonary capillary pressure rises. Jeremy wanted to make these two measurements at the bedside of heart attack patients so that we could continuously assess the effect of our treatment of heart failure.

Jeremy knew that he could use X-ray imaging to help him insert a catheter into an arm vein, advance it to the right atrium, cross the tricuspid valve into the right ventricle, cross the pulmonary valve into the pulmonary artery, and then push it out to its capillaries. Although it sounds complex, a first-year cardiology fellow learns the procedure easily if the catheter is visible on an X-ray monitor. In the CCU, however, there was no X-ray system to illuminate the path through this cardiac catacomb, and catheters pushed blindly simply coiled up sleepily in the right atrium. Maneuvering a catheter into the pulmonary artery was an impossible, insoluble problem.

One weekend, pondering this dilemma as he sat on Santa Monica beach watching sailboats, Jeremy had a fit of Irish intuition. He wondered if a catheter equipped with a tiny sail could bob along in the current of blood flowing from the right heart out into the pulmonary artery. Why not? He knew he could pass the catheter into the right atrium. Then if he could unfurl the sail, it would be like those sailboats . . . the sail would capture the force of the blood, and flow like a Mary Poppins umbrella out into the pulmonary artery.

As a consultant to Edwards Laboratories, he took his idea to their engineering group. The engineers took no time to agree: constructing a catheter with wires and sails was virtually impossible. But as the discussion wandered, someone made a second intuitive leap: maybe the same result could be accomplished with a balloon. "Balloons will float, used to do it when I was a kid," one of the engineers said.

Edwards Laboratories knew exactly how to put balloons on catheters. They were inflating balloons on the ends of catheters to keep them from pulling out of the urinary bladder, and to drag clots out of blood vessels. Jeremy Swan's intuition, put into highly improbable juxtaposition with a completely unrelated technology, had created an entirely new idea.

Edwards Laboratories Director of New Product Development David Chonette got some infant feeding tubes, affixed an inflatable balloon to the shaft, and delivered it to newly arrived Czechoslovakian immigrant Dr. Willie Ganz in the cardiovascular animal laboratory research laboratory. On his first try the catheter shot instantly into the pulmonary artery, carried by the force of blood flow behind the inflated balloon. In a few seconds that afternoon, Jeremy's vision had morphed from laughable fantasy into feasible possibility.

When I arrived from Boston, our first-year cardiology fellow and I decided to try it in our Myocardial Infarction Research Unit. We chose

Samuel Bernstein, a comatose eighty-year-old man in shock following a heart attack, who we felt would not survive the day.

In those days there was no institutional review board to approve our testing of the new catheter. Like Lillehei with Bakken's improvised pacemaker, we just walked up to his bedside and did it. When my fellow and I advanced the catheter into Mr. Bernstein's right ventricle, his heart reacted with intense fury, ventricular tachycardia (literally, very rapid beating of the ventricles). In a sick heart, ventricular tachycardia often degenerates into ventricular fibrillation, the rhythm of sudden death. Terrified, I imagined that my decision to test the new device might cause our patient's sudden death. After what seemed an interminable period—I am guessing maybe fifteen seconds—his heart reverted back to normal rhythm. Mr. Bernstein passed away from his disease late that evening, never aware of the brief, ultimately inconsequential episode at his bedside.

My decision to use the catheter more than forty years ago, however, still haunts me. In the guise of advancing science and our understanding of managing heart failure at the bedside, I had put a patient at immediate, life-threatening risk. That afternoon, like Dwight Harken, I went home, got into bed, and cried. In those fifteen seconds of panic, I had experienced an epiphany. Yes, by the ethical standards of that era I had done nothing wrong. Yes, my patient was near inevitable death, and suffered no adverse consequence. Yes, I had noble intent. And yet, should I really have sole authority over whether or not to use an untested device in my research? Should not a group of peers independently assess risk vs. benefit in advance, and as my research proceeded? Worse, my patient had not participated in the decision to use the new device; he had not given his consent. My experience illuminated the terrible flaws in the professional ethic of that era. My personal penance has been to serve on our Institutional Review Board since its inception, the obligation of those who dedicate their career to clinical research.

I went back to the animal laboratory. I wanted to use a continuous X-ray to see what happened when the catheter entered the right ventricle. What I saw amazed me. The balloon was mounted about an inch or more from the catheter tip. When I inflated the balloon, the segment beyond the balloon began to thrash about in the flowing blood just like a balloon in a wind tunnel, whacking away at the heart's inner surface. Each impact of the catheter tip on the heart's inner surface induced an extra beat. In a sick heart, one of those extra beats would induce the ventricular tachycardia, the common predecessor of ventricular fibrillation and sudden death. So we asked the Edwards Laboratories' engineers to move the balloon all the way out to very tip of the catheter. Now when we inflated the balloon it actually bulged around the tip. The bulging balloon was a perfect soft cushion, a pillow, which hid the catheter's rigid tip and eliminated ventricular arrhythmias.

That little technical tweak turned out to be a huge breakthrough in bedside management of acute heart failure. We found that we could measure the severity of lung congestion, and we could also assess the effect of our cardiac drugs on the congestion. We discovered that our measurement was far more sensitive than either our stethoscopes or the chest X-ray, which often did not reflect the benefit of our therapy until the following day. Equally important, nurses could make the continuous measurements in our absence, and immediately notify us of important changes.

Now we desperately wanted that second measurement: cardiac output. The solution to our problem emerged from Communist Czechoslovakia. In Prague, at about the same time that Jeremy was sitting on Santa Monica beach, cardiac physiologist Dr. Willie Ganz was pondering how to escape. He had a lot of experience in survival, first as a youth in the World War II Budapest underground and later as a survivor of incarceration in a Nazi labor camp. In 1966 at age forty-seven, Willie, his wife, and their two small sons made a daring escape across the Austrian border, finally wending their way to the Jewish community of Los Angeles. Willie brought with him no worldly goods, but he did have one possession of inestimable value: he had developed a method of measuring cardiac output.

Incorporating Willie's method into a catheter presented huge technical problems, but after two years of alternating exhilaration and frustration, I could measure cardiac output in critically ill patients. I found that my patients' prognosis depended on these two measurements. When both were normal, the mortality rate was 1% whereas when both were abnormal 60% died. When only one of the two was abnormal, the mortality rate was 10% and 20% respectively. Four years later, after treating hundreds of patients in our Myocardial Infarction Research Unit, I was able to describe the effects of all the then-available therapies for disordered cardiac function. My mentees and I had created a solid basis for treating heart failure in acute myocardial infarction, which I described in *The New England Journal of Medicine*. The method, dubbed the Forrester classification, revolutionized critical care medicine.

ALEXI KROON'S HEART muscle was failing to deliver sufficient output to maintain the function of his vital organs. His heart was failing. In its most severe form, when the heart cannot even maintain a normal blood pressure, the condition is called cardiogenic (literally, heart-caused) shock. When a sudden obstruction of a coronary artery causes cardiogenic shock, the mortality rate skyrockets. I was looking at a young man with no prior symptoms who was dying of heart failure before our eyes. We needed a way to continuously monitor his heart muscle function as we used both drugs and a mechanical pump to supplement his cardiac output.

As Alexi moved in and out of consciousness we passed the balloon catheter into his heart. His cardiac output, the volume of blood the heart pumps out in a minute, had fallen to less than half normal. His pulmonary capillary pressure, the pressure in the small blood vessels of the lungs, was elevated into the range that causes severe pulmonary congestion. With about 30% of his heart muscle damaged, his brain compromised by diminished blood flow, Alexi was dying in front of us. Without effective treatment his chance of dying within the hospital was 80%. But unlike my days in Philadelphia, this time I was not helpless.

I started an infusion of dopamine, a drug to increase blood pressure, which raised the systolic blood pressure back over 100. An anesthesiologist inserted a tube into his trachea to supplement his breathing, and we added a drug to diminish his pulmonary congestion. To supplement his cardiac output we inserted a temporary pumping device into his aorta. My measurements showed that Alexi's cardiac function improved substantially. I knew I was headed in the right direction, and I could adjust the dose of each drug to maximize his heart's function.

Over the next forty-eight hours, Alexi's damaged heart and congested lungs struggled to bring his body back from the looming chasm of death. I tested his recovery by turning off his circulatory assist device, nervously watching to see if his heart function collapsed. It did not . . . his measurements stayed stable. So I left the machine turned off. By the early afternoon of his third hospital day, I could see clear signs that Alexi was on his way to recovery. I disconnected his respirator from his tracheal tube, and again watched his response. He remained stable. Next we discontinued his dopamine infusion and still his blood pressure remained stable. When he remained stable overnight, we removed the monitoring catheter from his heart. It was an inspiring day. In the years before our ability to manage severe heart failure during myocardial infarction, Alexi would have had virtually no chance of survival. We had pulled a young man back from the brink.

By the end of the week, we were able to send Alexi to a room on the hospital floor. He began walking. A few days later, I was stunned to learn that after a visit from a friend, he had dressed, and walked out of the hospital. Not even a good-bye note. Over the years, I have often wondered about Alexi after he left. He was as irreverently off-kilter as the lyrics of one of the songs he admired: "I don't give a damn about your greenback dollar, spend it fast as I can." I never saw him again. When the Internet emerged at the turn of the century, I knew if he were alive, he would be my age. I googled his unusual name. Not a trace. So we will always be two ships that passed briefly in the night during our journey through life.

IN THOSE EARLY days of heart attack management, when my fellows and medical students took me to the bedside of a man in his thirties with a premature heart attack, I would always ask, "How many packs a day does he smoke?" Most young men with a heart attack were smokers. Nowadays I ask another question: "Have you done a 'tox screen'?" That's a urine screen for the common recreational drugs. My clinical impression is that the cardiac risk from cocaine, or the current drug du jour methamphetamine, is vastly greater than cigarette smoke. Alone or combined with heroin as a "speedball," cocaine claimed the lives of Hollywood celebrities John Belushi, River Phoenix, Jim Morrison, Chris Farley, and sports figures like National League MVP Ken Caminiti and Boston Celtics forward Len Bias. Cocaine users quickly become aware that it increases heart rate, blood pressure, and respiratory rate, but their two big cardiac risks are virtually unknown to them. Cocaine causes coronary arteries to constrict, diminishing blood flow. At the same time it increases the stickiness of platelets, the disk-shaped cell fragments that initiate clotting of blood. These two factors can come together in the sudden catastrophic development of an occlusive clot in a coronary artery. I suspect this was the cause of Alexi Kroon's heart attack. The final blow is that chronic cocaine and methamphetamine use predisposes to the early development of plaques in coronary arteries. So even if you don't have a sudden heart attack the first time you use the drug, you greatly increase your longterm risk.

The irony of Alexi Kroon's case is that he found one more way to increase his risk. With his young first-time partner, he exercised vigorously immediately after snorting cocaine, adding further the release of a hormone called norepinephrine that mediates the biologic response to exercise, and also potentiates the effect of cocaine on coronary constriction and clot formation.

What about sex causing heart attacks? It's overrated. The heart attack part. It is true that there are occasional tabloid headlines about a celebrity having a heart attack during sexual encounters, the most famous of which is former potential presidential nominee Nelson Rockefeller, who allegedly collapsed during sex with his twenty-seven-year-old mistress. Panicked, instead of calling an ambulance, she called a girlfriend, who then called the ambulance about an hour after he first collapsed. Rockefeller allegedly died in the ambulance on the way to the hospital. The world's most famous victim was Attila the Hun, who history tells us died of heart attack in his wedding bed.

Although suffering a heart attack during sex is extremely uncommon, about 75% of men experience sexual dysfunction after a heart attack, predominantly related to fear. Here are some facts. In controlled laboratory studies of sexual activity, volunteers have a significant increase in heart rate, breathing rate, and blood pressure pulse. The magnitude of increase approximates that of a moderate workout. But what about married couples in their own bedrooms? Twenty-four-hour heart rate monitors show that heart rates don't increase, and remain lower than those recorded during normal daily activities. This is the reason that sexual activity rarely is identified as a precipitating factor in a myocardial infarction. An analysis of fourteen studies on the risk of cardiac death during sexual activity, from the Tufts University Center for Clinical Evidence Synthesis and the Harvard Department of Epidemiology in *The Journal of the American Medical Association*, concluded that the risk of death was 2.7 times more likely to occur during sexual activity, but only in the subgroup of people who rarely exercised or rarely had sexual relations. So if you have had a heart attack, a frequently quoted rule of thumb is that it is safe to have sex with your partner six to eight weeks after a heart attack, if you are able to walk up two flights of stairs without chest pain or feeling out of breath. For those who cannot pass that test, cardiac rehabilitation programs can assist in the return to normal daily activities.

IN THE YEARS that followed, I could not have imagined the profound effect my role as director of the MIRU would have on my life as a doctor. Until that time I had always had a one-to-one relationship with my patients and families. Throughout my years in medicine, I had been fully immersed in the care of each of my patients. I took a detailed history from each patient, did a complete physical examination, read the chest X-ray and ECG myself, decided on appropriate treatment, and monitored each step in my patient's return to good health. In my new role, three or four cardiology fellows who reported to me did all this before I saw the patient, and described their findings to me. My new role, while I was still in my early thirties, became that of a gray eminence. I still saw our patients, but now I would ask a few questions, listen to the heart and lungs, then step away from the bedside to discuss our patients' care with my younger colleagues. As my relationship to patients became less tactile, my sense of fulfillment increasingly came from being a mentor. Our authority structure was transforming me from hands-on physician into a role model for other doctors.

When we won a huge new National Heart Institute grant called a Specialized Center of Research in Ischemic Heart Disease (known colloquially as a SCOR) with me as its director, my relationship with patients with heart disease was modified further by my responsibility for creating and supervising groundbreaking clinical cardiovascular research. I had to identify the most important problems in cardiologic patient care, then design and test potential solutions. The lessons I learned from living with several great mentors was fundamental: get a young colleague to discuss the critical unsolved problems in clinical care, get him/her enthused about solving it, get him/her the resources, and get out of the way. It was oddly similar to my direct patient care years: I was deeply committed to encouraging and supporting others, but now both doctors and patients. I'd get up every day looking forward to improving patient care. With $20 million to spend on cardiovascular research, a number of the young physicians in our previously unheralded Cedars of Lebanon Hospital advanced patient care and emerged as world leaders. I am deeply fulfilled today by their success in the dominant roles they played in bedside hemodynamic monitoring, nuclear stress testing, imaging inside the coronary arteries, heart disease in women, and interventional cardiology. I did not do the work, rather I created the environment where new ideas flourished and were translated into patient care. As I told my mentees, ideas are free: it's the one who does the work that deserves the credit. Like so many others of our generation, we challenged established thinking. Yes, we, too, were misfits.

ONE OF MY favorite mentees, Dr. Neal Eigler, has taken my research, in which I used a catheter to measure the pressure in the lung vessels during a heart attack, to a spectacular new level. Neal asked, "What about the patient after she leaves the hospital?" It's a critical question because rehospitalization for symptoms of heart failure is today's most expensive health-care problem. The symptoms of heart failure are due to backup of blood into the lungs. The resulting increase in pressure within lung vessels forces fluid across the exquisitely thin membrane that separates the blood from the air sacs in the lung. Fluid in the air sacs causes the patient to experience acute shortness of breath, precipitating an emergency room visit and hospitalization. Neal wondered if the rise in lung vessel pressure that precedes symptoms can be detected using modern technology and treated at a presymptomatic stage. He invented an implantable device that measures the pressure in the lungs. His device instructs the patient to take a dose of medication previously programmed into it by his/her doctor. The dose of drug varies with the pressure. Other devices send the pressure information to a central location that is accessed by the patient's doctor.

Does controlling the pressure that causes the symptoms of heart failure work? The answer is yes. The FDA has just approved the first device that directly measures the pressures in the lung. It reduced heart failure hospitalizations by 30% at six-month follow-ups in 550 previously hospitalized patients. I got a lump in the throat reading the comment of noted Ohio State heart failure specialist Dr. William Abramson: "pulmonary artery pressure monitoring . . . represents our first meaningful improvement for the management of heart failure in nearly a decade . . . patients with chronic heart failure can reduce the need for costly and dangerous hospitalization while improving quality of life."

THE EVOLUTION OF the CCU now seemed complete. We had the capacity to monitor both disordered rhythm and the function of the heart following myocardial infarction, we had potent therapies, and we had the ability to assess the effectiveness of our treatment in each patient. Today, a destitute skid-row heart attack victim now receives far better care than the most powerful man in the world had received only a quarter century earlier. Three arrows: pacemakers, defibrillators, and methods of assessing cardiac function, aimed at different targets, had hit a bull's-eye in myocardial infarction. When I saw Willie the Phillie, the in-hospital mortality rate was 30%. With these three advances in the CCU, in the passage of less than a decade, we had reduced heart attack mortality rate by half.

And yet, if you stood at the bedside of a patient experiencing a heart attack, as I did so often in those years, you had to admit an awful truth. We were standing helpless watching the progressive death of heart muscle, waiting to treat its consequences. We had no strategy for preventing the death of heart muscle as the heart attack occurred. Today, we have that strategy. I am proud to say it began with one of our former cardiology fellows.

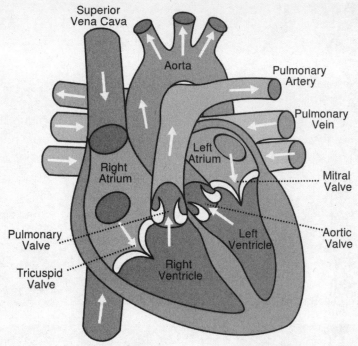

Superior
Vena Cava

Aorta

Pulmonary
Artery

Pulmonary
Vein

Left
Atrium

Mitral
Valve

Right
Atrium

Pulmonary
Valve

Left
Ventricle

Aortic
Valve

Tricuspid
Valve

Right
Ventricle

Inferior Vena Cava

Deoxygenated "blue" blood returns from the body, is collected in the right atrium, and then pumped by the right ventricle to the lungs, where oxygen is added. Oxygen rich "red" blood is collected in the left atrium and then pumped by the left ventricle into the aorta for distribution throughout the body.

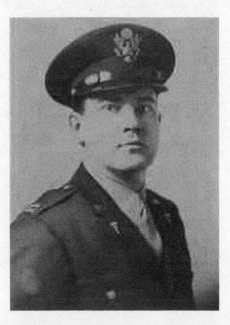

Square-jawed redhead Army officer Dwight Harken was an intriguing mix of a fiery-tempered surgeon and a charming raconteur.
Courtesy *Wilts and Gloucestershire Standard*

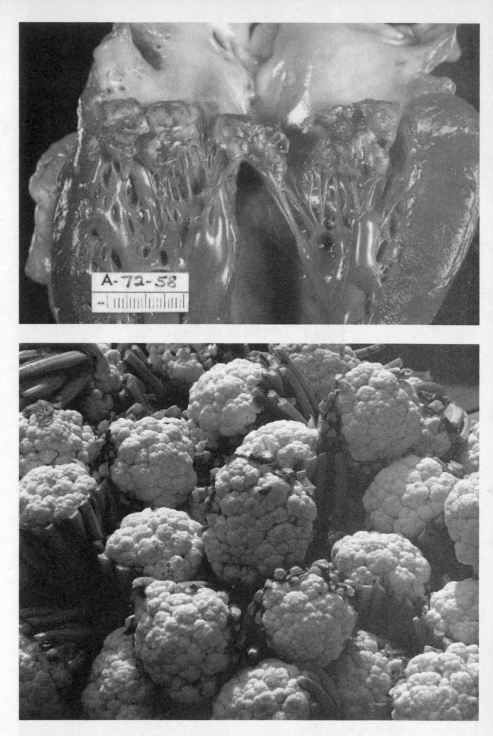

Early pathologists bequeathed a cuisine of terms to modern medicine, seeing "vegetations" growing on a heart valve (top) that resemble clumps of broccoli (bottom).

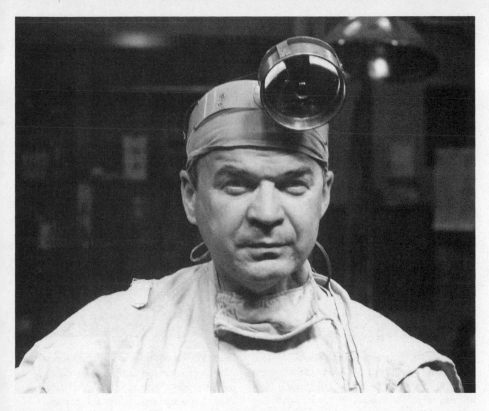

Walt Lillehei survived personal tragedy in his medical training to pursue a professional career that traced the most exhilarating heights and devastating lows of anyone in my experience.
Courtesy University of Minnesota Archives, University of Minnesota–Twin Cities

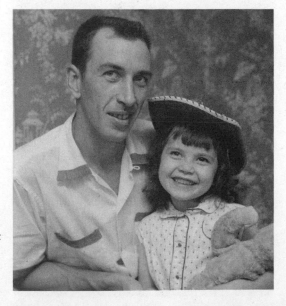

The "impossible surgery" on cute little "Annie," shown here with her father, astounded the world and won the heart of a nation. Innovative surgeon Walt Lillehei was not so fortunate. Courtesy University of Minnesota Archives, University of Minnesota–Twin Cities

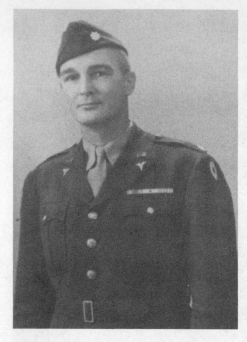

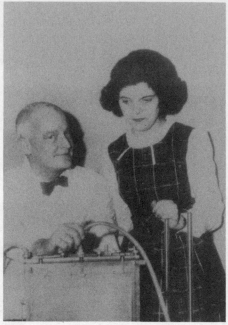

John Gibbon, the scion of generations of physicians, was the polar opposite of fellow Philadelphian Charles Bailey. His single-minded two-decade quest to create a heart-lung machine was interrupted by service in the Pacific theater. Courtesy of Thomas Jefferson University, Archives & Special Collections

John Gibbon with the world's first successful heart-lung machine patient, "Martha," a college student with an atrial septal defect. What happened next is arguably the most improbable event in our entire chronicle. Courtesy of Thomas Jefferson University, Archives & Special Collections

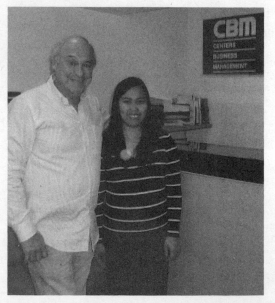

One of my most treasured experiences in cardiology is how Sam Bachner, the man of La Mancha, saved the life of a little girl named "Maria." So you can imagine my astonishment when I called him years later to learn what happened to that little girl. Courtesy Samuel Bachner

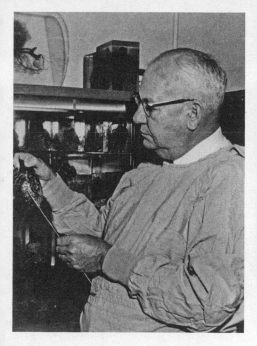

When Claude Beck was the first to realize a dream of mankind that stretches back to biblical times. Courtesy Dittrick Medical History Center

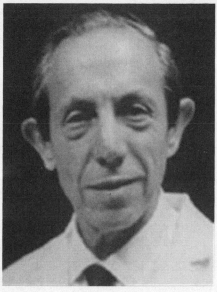

Boston intellectual Paul Zoll, the cardiologist who worked with Dwight Harken in London's wartime hospital, returned home to pioneer breakthroughs in treatment of disorders of the heart's electrical system. Courtesy Zoll Medical

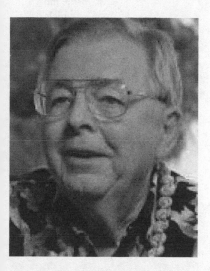

Earl Bakken, as I know him from many dinners together in Hawaii, catapulted from repairman to unimaginably successful entrepreneur when opportunity beckoned, a quintessential representative of The American Dream. Courtesy Earl Bakken

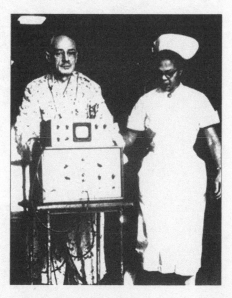

In the early years, the patient was tethered to his life-maintaining pacemaker. Courtesy of The Bakken Library and Museum and the Heart Rhythm Society

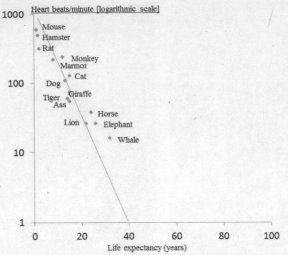

Modified from by author from Levine HJ. Rest heart rate and life expectancy. J Am Coll Cardiol. 1997 Oct;30(4):1104-6.

The relationship between the logarithm of heart rate and life expectancy is linear.

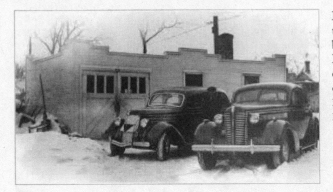

Medtronic, the pioneer of the medical device industry began as two guys in a 1950s Minneapolis garage and evolved to tens of thousands employees today. Courtesy of The Bakken Library and Museum and the Heart Rhythm Society

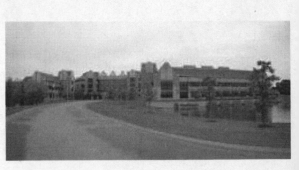

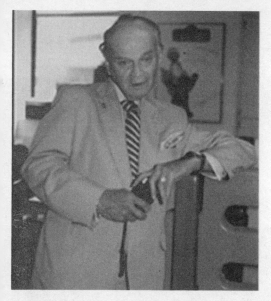

Brilliant, inventive, sensitive, funny Walt Lillehei lived a turbulent life according to his own rules. Courtesy William Hoffman

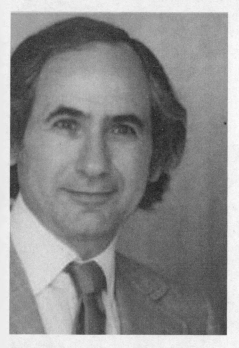

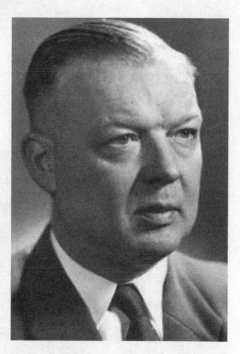

Albert Starr was only 32 years old when he and retired engineer Lowell Edwards overcame innumerable obstacles to create a mechanical valve to replace a diseased human valve. Their first valve was a ball-in-cage structure that bears no resemblance at all to its human counterpart. But it worked.

Werner Forssmann's story is one of the strangest in medicine.

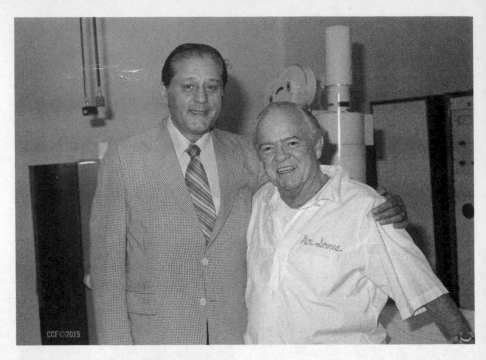

Profoundly principled Argentine surgeon Rene Favaloro and lovable rebel Mason Sones considered themselves brothers as Favaloro pioneered coronary artery bypass surgery. Courtesy Cleveland Clinic Historical Foundation

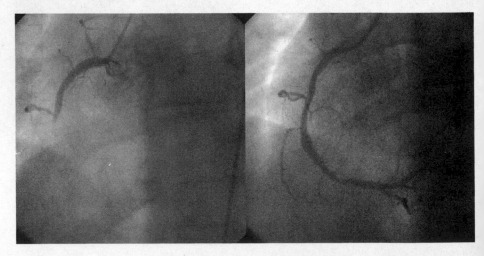

Injection of X-ray-dense solution into a vessel creates an angiogram. On the left is a right coronary artery obstructed by a blood clot on a ruptured plaque in a patient with acute myocardial infarction; on the right, blood flow has been restored by inflating a balloon at the site of plaque rupture.

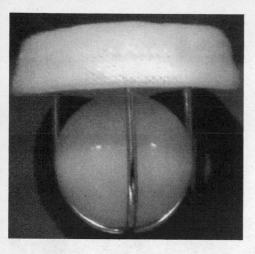

Retired engineer Lowell Edwards and youthful surgeon Albert Starr overcame innumerable technical obstacles in creating a mechanical valve to replace a diseased human valve. Their first valve was a ball-in-cage structure that bears no resemblance at all to its human counterpart. But it worked.
Courtesy Albert Starr MD and Edwards Laboratories

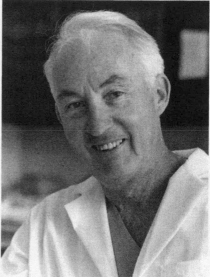

Cardiac transplantation was almost entirely the product of years of research in the laboratory of Norman Shumway. So how could public acclaim for his monumental accomplishment be snatched from him on a Sunday morning in South Africa?
Courtesy Stanford Medical History Center

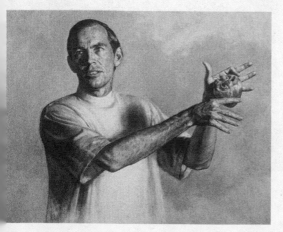

Handsome, charismatic Christiaan Barnard was a world celebrity, a favorite of the press, but not the medical establishment.

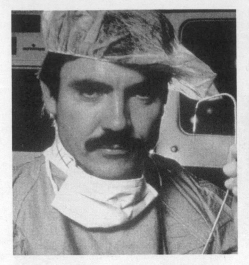

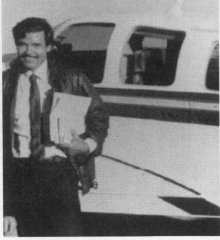

Every bit as charismatic and movie-star handsome as famed surgeon Christiaan Barnard, Andreas Gruentzig was described by one of his nurses as a cross between Clark Gable and Errol Flynn. Courtesy Emory University

Andreas Gruentzig, a lover of fast cars, was drawn to flying. After buying his own plane and earning certification as a solo pilot, he upgraded to instrument flying. Courtesy ptca.org

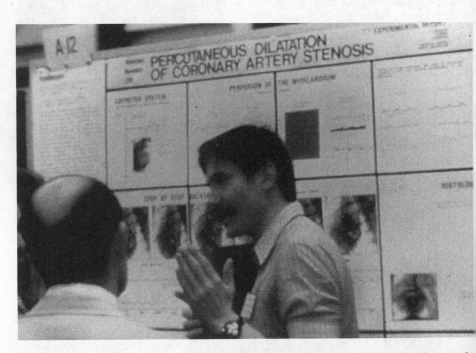

Andreas Gruentzig's appearance with a poster displaying angioplasty in an animal at the annual American Heart Association meeting encountered a very skeptical reception. For Gruentzig, however, failure was fuel. Courtesy ptca.org

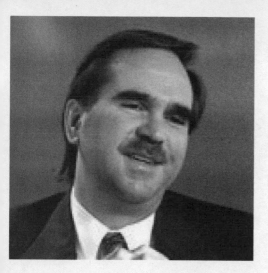

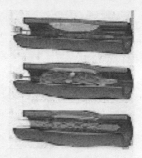

Geoff Hartzler, throughout his life a rebel, faced down both Gruentzig and the medical establishment. Courtesy ptca.org

Stenting an atheroma: at the top, a yellow atheroma partially obstructs a blood vessel above a balloon-tipped catheter with a crimped cylindrical stent. When the balloon is inflated (middle), the stent crushes the atheroma into the vessel wall. When the balloon is deflated and the catheter withdrawn (bottom), the stent holds the vessel open.

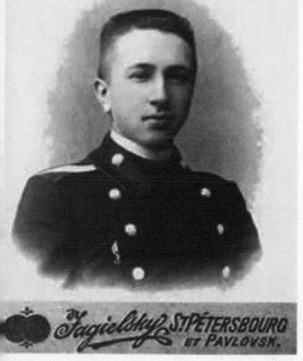

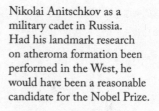

Nikolai Anitschkov as a military cadet in Russia. Had his landmark research on atheroma formation been performed in the West, he would have been a reasonable candidate for the Nobel Prize.

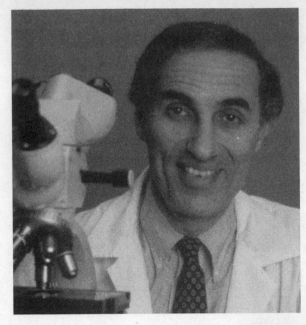

Russell Ross, a dentist by training, chose the path less followed, making basic science observations that led to our understanding of atheroma formation and rupture. Courtesy University of Washington Medicine Department of Pathology

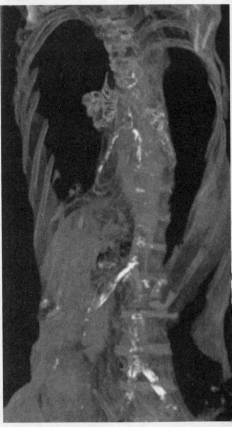

Meet the first person ever diagnosed with CAD: it is Princess Ahmose Meyret Amon, who lived during 1580–1550 BC, and died aged 40–45 years. This computerized tomographic image of her mummy shows bright white calcium in her left and right coronary arteries, as well as leg vessels. For more, see Allam AH, et al., "Atherosclerosis in Ancient Egyptian Mummies." *Journal of the American College of Cardiology*, Cardiovascular Imaging. 2011;4:315–327. Courtesy Dr. Gregory Thomas

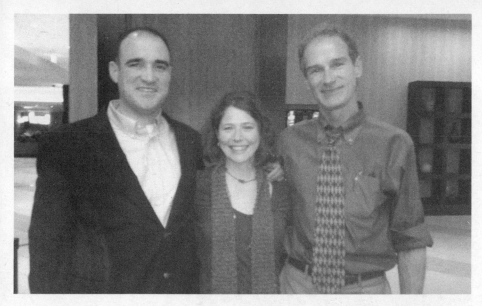

"Greta," "Tyler," and "Jon" when I interviewed them in San Francisco. Greta's story is the most remarkable that I have encountered in my years as a cardiologist. Courtesy Author

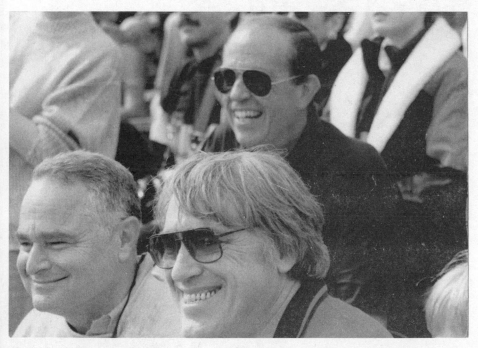

As three college buddies enter middle age, they stage an annual reunion. "Mort" on the left, "Don" in dark glasses (behind), and me at a football game could hardly imagine the events that soon would consume our lives. Courtesy Author

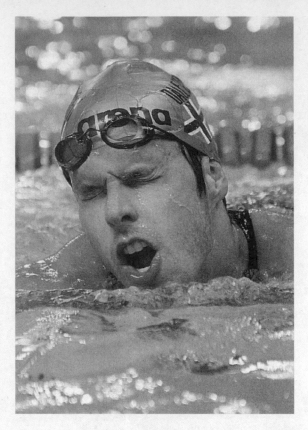

Like London Marathoner Claire Squires and English soccer player Fabrice Muamba, competitive world-class athletes are not immune to sudden death. Norwegian swimmer Alexander Dale Oen won gold at the European Championships. A year later he died suddenly at a pre-Olympic training facility. Autopsy revealed coronary artery disease.

Today's wireless pacemaker. Compare this device to the one used by Paul Zoll at the beginning of our story. Courtesy Dr. Eugenio Cingolani

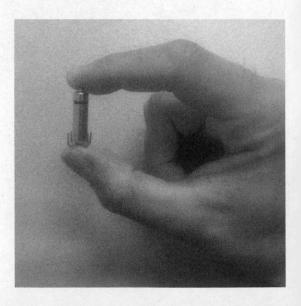

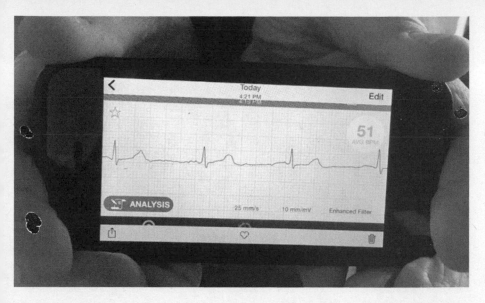

The ECG recorded on the iPhone of a cardiac patient with whom I currently consult. He suffers from episodes of a common heart rhythm disorder (atrial fibrillation). The ECG is recorded by grasping two electrodes attached to the back of his phone, and can be immediately sent to me anywhere in the world, from anywhere in the world. Courtesy Dr. Alexander Dubelman

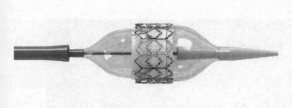

The transcatheter aortic valve. To allow insertion into an artery in the leg, the balloon is deflated and the valve is crimped onto the shaft. After the yellow tip facilitates valve positioning in the aorta, the balloon is inflated, forcing the valve into correct position. The balloon is deflated, and the catheter is withdrawn. Courtesy Edwards Laboratories

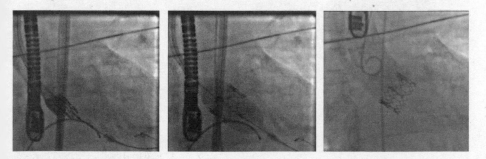

Enmeshed in the images of several monitoring devices, we see the catheter properly positioned (left), the balloon inflated to deploy the valve (middle), and the valve in place after the balloon is deflated and the catheter withdrawn. Valve placement takes about 10 seconds, the entire procedure 1–2 hours. Courtesy Author

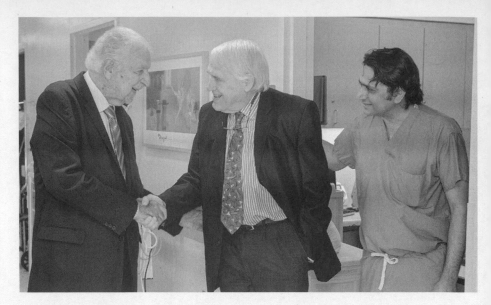

My mentee Raj Makkar and I congratulate 102-year-old Leon Saliba at his successful 2-year follow-up of Dr. Makkar's placement of a coronary artery stent and a prosthetic aortic valve.

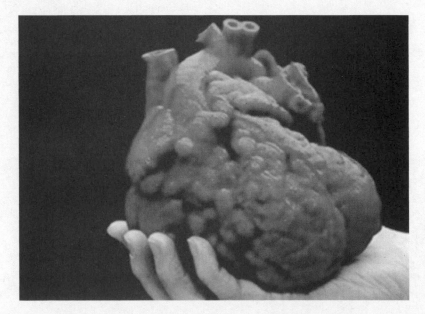

A precise scale model of a tiny infant's heart before surgery, created from multilayer images of the child's heart and a printer. The heart can be created in any size, and sectioned at different angles, allowing the surgeon to closely examine every defect, and plan his surgery for no unpleasant surprises. Courtesy Norton Healthcare

16

THE CLOT BUSTERS

I don't want to play 10 years and then die of a heart attack when I'm 40.

—Pete Maravich, All-American basketball player who died suddenly at age forty in a pickup game

THROUGHOUT THE 1970S I (and many others) focused on that era's central topic: managing the devastation caused by myocardial infarction (heart attack). At that time we all believed that myocardial infarction was a final exclamation point, the culmination of a relentless progressive stenosis (narrowing) of a coronary artery plaque. A moderate narrowing caused angina, which was Mother Nature's way of saying it's time for bypass surgery. Left unattended, the narrowing ultimately became so severe that the need for oxygen in a segment of the heart muscle exceeded the supply. That segment could no longer survive. Without a way to open the narrowing during a heart attack, we focused on reducing its need for oxygen, using drugs that slowed the heart rate and diminished its vigor of contraction.

We imagined that a solution might lie with emergency bypass surgery, but creating such a program posed a logistic nightmare. If a heart attack occurred during the day, the surgeons, operating rooms, and heart-lung machines were typically busy with other elective procedures, so waits of three to four hours were often unavoidable. If the heart attack occurred at night, rapid mobilization of the entire team of surgeons, nurses, and technicians was at least as frustrating, and then wreaked havoc with the next day's operating schedule.

In 1979 one of my former cardiology trainees, Dr. Marcus DeWood, came back to visit me. Marcus had recently settled into practice in Spokane, Washington, and sought me out for advice about the results of a small research project he had organized. He and his local cardiac surgery group had been able to establish a new program offering around-the-clock emergency bypass surgery for patients with acute myocardial infarction. At that time, no other hospital in the United States had yet succeeded in establishing a program like it. I was eager to see Marc's results, believing that emergency coronary bypass might well reverse the imbalance between oxygen supply and demand precipitated by a heart attack.

I had attended the autopsies of patients who died of acute myocardial infarction, so I knew that a blood clot, called a thrombus, was sometimes found in the coronary artery. We considered it an uncommon incidental finding of no great importance, agreeing with my friend Dr. William C. Roberts, chief of the cardiac pathology at the National Institutes of Health, who said, "Although it may play a major role in causing atherosclerosis, coronary thrombosis may well play a minor role, or none at all, in precipitating a fatal coronary event." Roberts, like the rest of us, believed that diminished blood flow led to death of the heart muscle, and blood clots then formed in the damaged arteries. As an international lecturer, I had pontificated innumerable times with professorial grandiosity on the imbalance between oxygen supply and demand, not blood clot, as the cause of myocardial infarction. But Roberts and I were wrong.

In his modest way, Marc almost apologetically unveiled his discovery, careful not to insult the ego of one of his mentors. He knew I was wrong, but he would let me discover it for myself. When his surgeons opened the culprit artery to attach a bypass graft, Marc was stunned to find that the vast majority of his still-living patients had a thrombus that completely obstructed their coronary artery. His mentors, among them me, had taught Marc that heart attack was the product of oxygen supply/demand imbalance, and that the thrombus came later. He showed me photo after photo of clots he had fished out of the vessels. There they were: evil, glistening, gelatinous red worms, now lying inert with a ruler lying next to them. They were about a half-inch to an inch long. Marc said nothing, looking at the photographs, as I shuffled through them a second time. As I sat back he raised his eyes and spoke softly.

"In almost every case," he said.

I am not sure how long it took me to absorb the full import of that sentence. I do know that during our meeting I felt like St. Paul on the road to Damascus . . . I had just experienced an astounding revelation. All my life, I had been wrong and now I saw the light. Like Paul, I underwent an instant conversion. "Marc," I finally said, "you have made an incredible discovery . . . it will completely change the treatment of acute myocardial infarction. You have got to publish this as soon as possible."

Less than a year later Marc formally announced to the world in *The New England Journal of Medicine* that a heart attack was not caused by our imagined progressive narrowing of a coronary artery. A heart attack was caused by the sudden occlusion of a coronary artery by an unseen blood clot, a coronary thrombus. His manuscript astounded the cardiologic world. It now stands as one of the most widely quoted manuscripts in the vast corpus of clinical cardiology research in all my years of cardiology. He reported that he had found thrombus in the coronary artery of 87% of patients operated on within four hours of the onset of symptoms. In one single powerful stroke Marcus DeWood's photographs collapsed the venerated citadel of oxygen supply/demand as the cause of heart attacks.

Before we chronicle the impact of Marc DeWood's revelation, let's look at it in the broad context of scientific discovery. He had begun with beliefs rooted in the past, yet he had illuminated the future. As Dr. Siddhartha Mukherjee observes of cancer research in *The Emperor of All Maladies*, "Scientists study the past as obsessively as historians because few professions depend so acutely on it. Every experiment is a conversation with a prior experiment." Like ancient city architects, in medical research we build upon the work of those who came before us. When we do well, we confirm and extend the knowledge that preceded us. When we succeed brilliantly, however, we destroy the existing structure. And thus every great new theory is a refutation of the old. DeWood's discovery of the unanticipated blood clot demolished conventional wisdom on the cause of heart attack.

DeWood's revelation left us with a baffling question: How could a generation of pathologists and cardiologists have missed all these clots at autopsy? I had stood at the autopsy table of many heart attack patients as the pathologist opened each coronary artery along its entire length. Like Bill Roberts I was quite sure, certain really, that there were no clots in most of those vessels. The pathologists and I had blundered. How? Put simply, we should never have believed our lyin' eyes. We assumed that what we saw in death represented what existed during life. We assumed that the autopsy gave us a chance to see in intimate detail what we had been unable to see hours before during life. Our assumption was founded on centuries of experience with every other disease in every other organ. But this time the autopsy was wrong. Dead wrong.

As a blood clot forms, the body's natural mechanism for dissolving the clot also swings into action. This process, called thrombolysis, can dissolve a small clot in a matter of hours, a large clot in a day or so. This mechanism makes biologic sense. Blood clots form to stop bleeding. But once the bleeding is controlled, we want to restore flow to the tissue beyond the clot. Both thrombosis and thrombolysis are a biologic necessity. In the case of the coronary artery, the sudden appearance of a clot in a coronary artery caused death of heart muscle. But in two-thirds of the cases of death from heart attack, by the time we opened the culprit vessel on the autopsy table the clot, like a snake in the grass, had slithered off after creating its devastation. DeWood sealed his proof that clots in coronary arteries disappear with time by analyzing patients who came in at twelve to twenty-four hours after symptom onset. By that time only 65% had a coronary thrombosis. We had not missed the clots at autopsy; they were not there. The nefarious clot had wreaked its damage and disappeared. As unwitting members of the flat-earth society we assumed that our single snapshot several days after the heart attack represented what existed at its moment of onset. Our logical error recalled my medical school's yearbook with a photo of a curmudgeonly professor with a humorless grin and the caption, "True, it's a small point, but you fail."

IN THE EARLY 1980s Eduardo Flores, a forty-two-year-old father of two and a chef at a popular Mexican restaurant in Southwest Los Angeles, had just returned to work from a three-day bout with the flu. Perfectly bilingual, Eduardo's face and brown skin limned his ancestry, more Peruvian Indian than Caucasian. His nose formed a continuous straight line with his forehead; his black hair had flecks of gray. Eduardo had always been a powerful man, with a hairy barrel chest and legs like tree trunks. Entering his fifth decade of life, you could still imagine the physique of the football tackle he had been in high school, although the recent years had not been particularly kind to his waistline.

Eduardo had returned to work with the perpetual good humor and openness that marked his life. Why not? For his first forty-two years he had never been seriously ill. Aside from childhood appendicitis, he had never been hospitalized. It was true he was a smoker since high school, but with a dedicated wife, the constant amusement of a toddling two-year-old son, and another on the way, he had vowed to eliminate cigarettes from his life.

Eduardo's indigestion began a few minutes past three in the afternoon after he gulped down a quick lunch. Looking back, although the pain was not initially severe, his mind retained the commonplace details at the moment the discomfort first entered his consciousness: baskets of chips on the counter near the kitchen's swinging door, the dishwasher stacking clean plates, his salad man chopping green peppers. Had his subconscious warned him at that instant that this pain was destined to be different from any other? He recalled wondering idly if a chef should ever admit to indigestion caused by his own menu. He popped a couple of Tums and continued preparing for the dinner crowd. Over each minute of the next half hour, however, the discomfort of indigestion ratcheted up, notch after notch, blossoming first into his chest and into his jaw. By now it dominated his every thought. He told his sous-chef to get help. A few minutes later, he was engulfed with a sudden unshakable feeling of impending doom. Just after 4 p.m. Eduardo Flores stood up from a chair someone had brought in, staggered forward a few steps, and collapsed to the floor. Without prior warning, once powerful Eduardo Flores had been struck down, brought to his knees by a stunningly swift, now excruciatingly painful, terrifying blow to the chest.

HAD EDUARDO FLORES collapsed when I entered college, he quite likely would not have survived to reach the hospital. But if he had, he would have been given a stool softener, some pain medication, and put to bed for three weeks with gradual progression from bed to sitting in a chair. Every doctor of that era recalls the great anxiety surrounding that bedside-to-chair moment. He would have had spent another three weeks at home at bed rest. That was all we had to offer.

The cardiology fellow who met Flores in the Emergency Department saw a characteristic change in his ECG. The familiar narrow spike of the normal ECG had become quite wide and almost rectangular. In the macabre humor of medicine, the upright rectangular shape of the ECG is called "the tombstone ECG," the signature of the highest risk type of myocardial infarction. This ECG pattern indicates a clot obstructing the left anterior descending coronary artery near its origin. Pathologists have called this vessel "the widow maker" with good reason. I had told the staff that I wanted to be notified when we had a patient for a new clot-dissolving treatment for myocardial infarction because I wanted to witness the breakthrough that I thought would revolutionize the management of heart attacks around the world. When the call came, I grabbed my tape recorder and raced up a flight of stairs to observe the treatment in the cath lab to record an oral history of the event.

MY EAGER ANTICIPATION was based on a research program in our Specialized Center of Research. DeWood's discovery created a new direction for therapy. We began the search for an agent that would very rapidly dissolve the clot in the coronary artery. Ironically a potent agent for dissolving blood clots had been identified some forty years earlier. Called streptokinase, it had even been tested in acute myocardial infarction in the late 1950s by Philadelphia hematologist Dr. Sol Sherry. His group reported that when streptokinase was given within four hours of symptom onset, hospital mortality was reduced, whereas if treatment was delayed beyond that time it had no beneficial effect. Yet we cardiologists had ignored Sherry's report. After all hematologists were members of a different guild, and we were blinded by our belief that coronary thrombus did not cause myocardial infarction.

Even if we could dissolve a clot in a patient's coronary artery, however, a new question arose. Would restoring blood flow through the obstructed vessel have any benefit? How long did it take heart muscle to die after it was deprived of blood flow? Would our treatment be too late? We had no answers to these simple questions. In San Diego, investigators in Dr. Eugene Braunwald's laboratory reported that if they released a tie around a coronary artery after half an hour, the heart showed evidence of partial recovery. Meanwhile in our animal laboratory Willie Ganz created a coronary thrombus in an anesthetized dog by inserting a copper coil. The heart muscle beyond the clot turned blue and stopped contracting within five or ten heartbeats.

Willie called me in to see what happened next. He infused streptokinase directly into the obstructed vessel. Standing beside him in the laboratory, I was dumbfounded by what I saw, an event as spectacular as anything I have ever seen in the research lab. Willie's infusion dissolved the clot, and it did not take long . . . sometimes it dissolved in as little as ten minutes. As the clot dissolved, I saw the blue noncontracting, apparently dead segment of heart muscle become pink, and it began to contract again. In that moment, I knew that I was a witness to what would become a worldwide breakthrough in the management of acute myocardial infarction.

A footnote to history that still amazes me today is that when Willie and I submitted his preliminary results in a modest grant request to the National Institutes of Health for financial support of what was to become landmark research in cardiology, his request was rejected because his anonymous reviewer turned wine into water, asserting that the clotting system of dogs was not necessarily similar to man. But when innovators battle the establishment, innovators usually win. Seriously miffed, I found other sources to support Willie's research, and years later I nominated Willie for the American College of Cardiology's annual Distinguished Scientist Award, which he received at the college's annual convocation ceremony to a standing ovation from many hundreds of cardiologists. I never learned who had so firmly planted his jackboot on the neck of progress. I only hope that his retribution requires that he pay full price for this book. Meanwhile in Russia, Germany, and our hospital a new cadre of pioneers began their first attempts to infuse streptokinase into the coronary arteries of patients with acute myocardial infarction.

* * *

WHEN OUR CARDIOLOGY fellow diagnosed acute myocardial infarction in chef Eduardo Flores he immediately activated the signal for a "Code White," which meant the cath lab was to be readied for immediate infusion of streptokinase directly through a catheter inserted into the coronary artery. When we first began giving streptokinase we feared that the drug might cause irreversible bleeding, perhaps from an unrecognized stomach ulcer or even within normal brain tissue. So to minimize the dose we infused it directly into the culprit coronary vessel, mimicking the way Willie Ganz had dissolved clots in the animal lab.

In treating acute myocardial infarction, you are on the clock. Every action by each team member is done in controlled haste. I watched our cath lab director Dr. Harold Marcus rapidly pass a catheter from the groin into the left coronary artery, then inject contrast material to outline the vessel. As I saw blood enter Eduardo's left coronary artery, then abruptly stop, my brain flashed momentarily on Marc DeWood's photo of the evil red worm lying inert on a towel. There it was in life; the clot abruptly cut off blood flow and Eduardo's heart muscle fibers beyond it were dying. In acute myocardial infarction, time is muscle: the faster the obstruction is cleared, the less heart muscle dies. Now Harold began the intracoronary streptokinase infusion, and we waited for the clot to dissolve. After about half an hour, Eduardo's ECG began to change. Like a snowman melting, the rectangular "tombstone ECG" began to disappear, returning toward its familiar normal spiked shape. Eduardo also reported that his chest pain was markedly less. These are two cardinal signs of restoration of blood flow in a coronary artery, which we call a "reperfusion." We knew we were witnessing signs that his artery had reopened.

Until that moment I knew that Eduardo stood poised on the edge of a chasm, the netherworld of misty benevolent light that accompanies death, according to many who have been resuscitated. In the years before thrombolytic therapy we had spent years trying to develop a prognostic index of death in our newly arrived patients, based on factors like age, blood pressure, heart rate, body temperature, etc. But we found that the best index we had was what we called the Nora Index. Nora was a crusty CCU nurse with many years of experience. In the crude language doctors sometimes employed to insulate themselves from our 30% mortality rate of that era, the Nora Index was "when Nora says they're gonna die, they're gonna die."

Thrombolytic therapy changed all that. Eduardo's Nora Index was off the charts when we began the infusion. He was undoubtedly sliding inexorably toward death until the clinging red worm was abruptly dissolved. When Eduardo's ECG began to change, we were ready to repeat the coronary angiogram. I held my breath as I watched Eduardo's coronary angiographic image appear on the TV monitor. In medicine we are trained not to jump, wave our arms, and cheer. But for me that instant felt, still feels today, like an explosive release of unanticipated pure joy, like the moment when injured Dodger Kirk Gibson hit his miracle home run in the 1988 World Series. Who says you cannot cheer at a transcendent moment like that? The red worm had disappeared! I had seen a miracle in my own lifetime. Blood flowed briskly down Eduardo's previously obstructed vessel. We had aborted Eduardo's acute myocardial infarction.

When he collapsed in his kitchen, Eduardo's risk of death had he been unable to get to a hospital was at least 50%. Now, lying on the table in that singular glorious moment he had about an 85% chance of walking out of the hospital, and returning to his life with his family and to his job. When he did I felt Eduardo probably had smoked his last cigarette. My experience is the patient who emerges intact from the emotional cataclysm of impending doom, as Eduardo had, undergoes a foxhole conversion. In the face of imminent death, he becomes a true believer . . . in Eduardo's case, in lifestyle change.

WE HAD OUR glorious, mind-bending answer: infusion of streptokinase into coronary arteries aborts a heart attack in progress. But wait: in medicine, great answers always raise new questions. If time is muscle, was not infusion directly into the coronary artery colossally inefficient? It took us at least an hour to mobilize the cath lab if a patient arrived in the middle of the night. Then each little step—scrub, drape, gown, anesthetize the groin—took more time before we finally directed a catheter into a patient's coronary artery to begin the infusion. And with each minute more heart muscle was dying. As our lab and others reported spectacular angiographic results, the question became inescapable. What about saving at least an hour, maybe more, by circumventing the cath lab? Could we start an intravenous infusion of streptokinase at the moment the patient burst through the emergency room door? It would quite clearly be a trade-off between an increased risk of bleeding due to a much higher dose of streptokinase and a decrease in the time required to restore coronary flow. By the mid-1980s we were ready for the first large-scale randomized trial of intravenous streptokinase. The landmark trial came from Italy, conducted by the Gruppo Italiano per lo Studio della Streptochinasi nell'Infarto Miocardico, nicknamed GISSI for obvious reasons. The group reported that intravenous streptokinase worked best when given early after the onset of symptoms. When GISSI reported that their survival advantage was maintained at one-year follow-up, intravenous thrombolytic therapy was anointed as the standard for treatment of a heart attack.

In the 1950s, when future president Lyndon Johnson sustained his first heart attack at age forty-six, we had no effective therapy at all. By the time of Johnson's final fatal massive heart attack on his ranch in the early 1970s we could have offered CCUs to control his arrhythmias and his heart failure, but we still had no effective therapy for his acute myocardial infarction. Now in the 1980s we had delivered another staggering blow to the ravages of CAD. We had discovered the cause of heart attack, and knowing its cause, we had devised spectacularly effective therapy. Average citizen Eduardo Flores had just received vastly more effectively therapy than that available to the president of the United States just a decade earlier.

Prior to clot-dissolving therapy I was forced to stand by watching as heart muscle died during a heart attack. Now we understood the cause of heart attack. We had a highly specific, effective therapy. CCUs had an immediate effect on mortality rate in patients hospitalized with myocardial infarction. By saving heart muscle during heart attack we had reduced the long-term risk of heart failure. In the prior decade, our early CCUs had almost halved the hospital mortality rate for acute myocardial infarction; now our newfound ability to dissolve clots in coronary arteries had reduced it by half again. In 2013 I reminisced about the treatment of heart attacks as we had helped it evolve with Dr. Eugene Braunwald, my generation's most recognized cardiologist. Pithy as always, Gene captured the essence of this story in a single sentence: "Jim, the coronary care unit is the most important advance in the treatment of acute myocardial infarction."

And now it is time for us to take a break from medicine to ask a deeper, more fundamental question. Why did these amazing advances, and the equally astonishing breakthroughs still on the horizon, occur in such a short period of time? Why did they occur when they did, where they did? The unrecognized answer to these two questions is central to both today's health care and more broadly, to the future of the U.S. economy.

17

THE BIRTH OF
BIOTECHNOLOGY

America demands invention and innovation to succeed.

—Kit Bond, former U.S. senator from Missouri

OPEN HEART SURGERY, coronary angiography, and the emergence
of the CCU set the stage for the modern cardiology's final assault on CAD.
But along the way our attack was joined by an additional warrior with
tremendous power and resources. Industry entered the battlefield, and
with it came what I call The Merger. It was the merger of industry with
academia.

From my perspective The Merger came about as an unintended consequence of two unrelated and little noticed events in the 1970s. The first
event was a then-confidential change in policy within the National Institutes of Health (NIH). Dr. Claude Lenfant was then director of the National Heart, Lung, and Blood Institute (NHLBI), one of the major
subunits of the NIH, and source of most heart disease research funding
in the United States. An urbane, nattily dressed, rather formal intellectual with a disarming French accent, Claude was both an accomplished
scientist and savvy politician. So when Claude spoke about Washington's
medical politics, I had learned to expect an indirect message, to focus on
his subtext. I was now director of one of the NHLBI's nine huge
multimillion-dollar flagship research programs, called Specialized Cen-

ters of Research (SCOR) in Ischemic Heart Disease. Every five years the nation's leading heart centers competed intensely for these nine grants, which were awarded only after on-site grilling by a group (usually about ten) of the nation's leading heart researchers. With many millions of dollars at stake, I spent months rehearsing each member of my team for their two-day visit. The SCOR programs were devoted predominantly to clinical patient-oriented research, and my program had competed very effectively by pioneering advances like the balloon catheter and clot lysis in acute myocardial infarction.

At the annual meeting of his nine SCOR directors Claude delivered an oblique confidential warning. A major NIH change in research funding policy was afoot. The NIH was planning to allocate a much greater percentage of its funds to the support of basic research, while encouraging industry to share the cost burden of clinical research, particularly trials of new drugs and devices. If industry funded clinical research, a far greater percentage of the NIH budget could be devoted to the tremendously promising research programs in cellular and molecular science. The NIH vision was that much more research would be accomplished at the same cost to the taxpayer. As the director of the only nonuniversity SCOR among the nine programs, I had little access to large basic science laboratories of medical schools like Harvard and Johns Hopkins. This was a potentially devastating blow to my patient-oriented, bench-to-bedside clinical research program, but I could not deny the logic of the NIH policy decision. Individual companies should pay for multimillion-dollar randomized trials of new devices and drugs since they stood to profit from those that we proved were effective.

All of us missed what now seems like an obvious corollary of this at first little noticed event . . . an unintended consequence. Until that change in policy we physician-investigators were the ones who conceived and designed clinical research. Our scientific peers judged the merit of our proposals. But with industry paying for the trials that determined whether their new drug or device was effective, the power to design trials and to select investigators to conduct the trials passed from scientists to corporate executives. The massive influx of corporate money accelerated drug and device development, and led to randomized trials that never would have been possible within the NIH budget. The principal negative aspect of the NIH policy decision—industry's control of the design and conduct of much of the important clinical research—was not recognized in these early years. But years later, critics would say that was the moment the fox strolled into the henhouse.

The second event that led to The Merger was a little noticed amendment to U.S. patent law in 1980, fathered by two leading senators of that era. Whereas the change in NIH funding policy for clinical trials affected predominantly the pharmaceutical industry, the patent amendment changed the device industry. At the time, the NIH controlled most medical research funding, and thus legitimately claimed patent rights on any invention developed with the use of their funds. The problem was that the federal government had no structure for developing a patented idea into a commercial product. Those of us involved in new device development saw our inventions being strangled by bureaucratic red tape. Birch Bayh (Democrat from Indiana) and Robert Dole (Republican from Kansas) forged a bipartisan solution. The Bayh-Dole amendment ceded the NIH patent rights to the involved academic institution. By eliminating government control, academia could patent an invention and then deal directly with industry to commercialize it. The rationale for the amendment was sound: American industry was losing out to international competitors who did not have to deal with the barriers presented by transfer of innovations from university laboratories to government and then to industry. Again, however, there was an unintended consequence. When industry became a source of grant money for academia, the once brittle hands-off relationship between academia and industry became intimate. Industry's leverage in dealing with academic institutions and research physicians had made another quantum leap. The biotechnology industry was about to be born.

The influx of money from industry to academia was monumental. For instance, the year that the Bayh-Dole amendment passed, industry was investing $26 million in academic university research. Fifteen years later, this investment had increased nearly 100 times to $2.3 billion. This single factor was to be the tipping point in the war on CAD. The federal government had shown great wisdom: first, to provide seed money for innovation, then again when it stepped aside to allow industry to bring these fantastic technological innovations in both drugs and devices to practical daily use. A nation that had led the century through investment, education, productivity, and innovation was about to do it again. The new era would be driven by a partnership between physician-researchers, basic scientists, and industry. Forays in technologic innovation that could not have been begun or completed without huge financial investment now became possible. The first new industry to emerge would be biotechnology.

AS WE GAINED experience with streptokinase infusion, we became aware that it was far from being a perfect drug. The basic science community now asked, "Can we make a better thrombolytic agent?" In Europe, using cells from human melanoma cancers, Belgian scientist Dr. Désiré Collen purified an agent that was more specific for thrombus and caused less allergic reactions than streptokinase. It came to be called tissue plasminogen activator or t-PA. A start-up company in Northern California initiated collaboration with Collen's group with the idea of producing commercial amounts of t-PA. Their plan was to use a new technology called genetic engineering.

Genentech had been founded in 1976 when young venture capitalist Robert Swanson called Stanford University scientist Dr. Herbert Boyer who, with his university colleague Dr. Stanley Cohen, was working in an emerging new field called recombinant DNA technology. Boyer agreed to a ten-minute meeting with Swanson. The meeting stretched into a three-hour lunch, and ultimately led to the formation of the first pharmaceutical biotechnology company. The company's mission was to create genetically engineered medicines using recombinant DNA technology. They chose Genentech's name, like Medtronic before it, by fusing the names of its principal disciplines: genetics, engineering, and technology.

Boyer joined Genentech, Cohen remained at Stanford. Boyer began by collaborating with scientists at the Beckman Research Institute. In 1977, as the United States launched its first space shuttle and John Travolta danced in *Saturday Night Fever*, they successfully inserted a human gene into a bacterial cell for the first time. Genes produce proteins, for instance enzymes that regulate the body's systems. Although this first step resulted in no commercial product the achievement was a crucial proof of principle. If a human gene could be inserted into a bacterium, then millions of bacteria could be induced to act as little factories for the protein that gene produced. The next year Genentech scientists announced a jaw-dropping achievement that had great commercial potential. Using their new technology they succeeded in mass producing one of the world's most familiar proteins: human insulin. On that day, the treatment of diabetes was forever changed. Heady with success, now they wanted another drug.

Collaborating with Collen they were able to successfully clone the gene responsible for expression of t-PA, using cells originally derived from a Chinese hamster ovary. Again they were able to manufacture industrial quantities, this time it was t-PA. At that time, a young medical resident was finishing his training at nearby University of California in San Francisco Hospital. Collen's manuscript describing use of t-PA in dogs was the subject of one of the residents' weekly journal club meetings, where interesting articles were selected for discussion. Dr. Eric Topol, later to become a thought leader in his generation of cardiologists, describes his reaction:

> I was struck by the idea that (t-PA) could be used for acute myocardial infarction. I inquired further and was told to contact a lady named Diane Pennica at Genentech. Busy with plans for starting cardiology fellowship at the Johns Hopkins Hospital, I forgot about (t-PA) until I was packing and found her name scribbled on a slip of paper. I called her and was introduced to the members of the Genentech team. Although I moved to Baltimore to start my fellowship, I was soon contacted by Bob Swift at Genentech, and began a collaborative effort to use t-PA for acute MI. In February, 1984, my colleagues and I successfully treated the first patient with recombinant t-PA at the Johns Hopkins Hospital, a 57-year-old woman with an acute occlusion of her left anterior descending artery (in lay language, a clot in the coronary artery we earlier nicknamed "the widow maker").

Topol subsequently became the principal investigator on a large randomized trial in myocardial infarction. The trial reported that t-PA more rapidly opened coronary arteries than streptokinase, with a modest reduction in mortality.

Now a fierce transatlantic debate erupted, because t-PA was about ten times more expensive than streptokinase. At the 1991 American College of Cardiology scientific sessions, American t-PA advocates presented their data in the convention center's packed massive main auditorium. When the British, sensitive to the cost of the new drug, wholeheartedly disagreed with the Americans, a scientific shouting match erupted. The debate was heated.

The real nastiness, however, came days later when the ABC-TV public affairs program *20/20* railed against the high cost of t-PA, then revealed a financial relationship between Genentech and Dr. Burton Sobel, the editor of *Circulation*, one of cardiology's most prestigious journals. I soon learned from personal conversations that a number of American cardiology's thought leaders had quietly been given shares in Genentech as consultants. Dr. Arnold Relman, editor of *The New England Journal of Medicine*, jumped into the combustible relationship between academic medicine and industry with both feet. Relman was infuriated by the incursion of industry into the formerly pristine practice of medicine: "Editors and their staffs should be totally free of conflicts of economic interest. They should have no economic connection at all with any health related company," he said. As the debate raged on, Eric Topol, who had led a much-quoted trial of t-PA, added, "Streptokinase is the gold standard drug. t-PA, while a very good thrombolytic agent, is not worth over $2,000 per dose." The program foreshadowed a new and terribly serious moral conundrum, which we thought leaders were about to confront, the relationship between academe and industry. This issue dominates the ethics of today's health care. At that time, however, Relman's and Topol's voices were drowned out by the feet of American cardiologists rushing to use the new agent. As they left the packed auditorium, Americans and Europeans lurched toward different corners of the ring. Today t-PA is the most widely used thrombolytic agent in the United States, whereas streptokinase is more frequently used in European countries with budgetary concerns.

Genentech became the father of an entire new American industry. Robert Swanson's initial investment in a couple of corn beef sandwiches had a value of $46.8 billion when the Swiss pharmaceutical conglomerate Hoffmann-La Roche purchased Genentech in March 2009. By then, Genentech employed more than 11,000 people. Today as you enter South

San Francisco you will encounter a road sign that proudly introduces the city as "The Birthplace of Biotechnology."

From my ringside seat at these events, I fervently believed that at last we had the final answer for treatment of heart attack: dissolve the clot that causes it. And once again I was completely wrong. Would I never learn that on this journey, great answers create even greater questions?

18

A BALLOON IN ZÜRICH

Nothing in the world can take the place of persistence.
Wishing will not; Talent will not; Genius will not;
Education will not; Persistence is like a Genie that creates
a magical force in your life.

—LUCAS REMMERSWAAL, NEW ZEALAND AUTHOR

MASON SONES'S IMAGES of coronary arteries, which turned a giant oculus on the cause of angina, heart attack, and sudden death, triggered human intuition in ways impossible with words alone. Those images precipitated the emergence of bypass surgery and coronary care units and thrombolysis. And thus we arrive at the greatest of all spin-offs, coronary balloon angioplasty—the opening of coronary arteries using a balloon mounted on the tip of a catheter.

Like a bursting balloon, coronary angioplasty exploded our thinking, sending ideas hurtling off in every direction. Before coronary angioplasty, the cath lab was our center for the X-ray diagnosis of cardiac disease. After angioplasty, the cath lab became our hub for the treatment. The impact of balloon angioplasty is almost incalculable, because what began as a treatment for CAD spun off a fantastic spectrum of treatments for every form of structural, electrical, and heart muscle disease, and an entire new subspecialty called interventional cardiology.

The origin of angioplasty (from the Greek *angeíon,* meaning vessel or urn, and *plastos,* meaning molded) begins with radiologist Charles Dotter.

We first met Dotter when he developed a method of visualizing human coronary arteries by injecting X-ray dye into the aorta, only to be trumped three months later when Mason Sones inadvertently put a catheter direct into a coronary artery. Dotter shared striking personality similarities with Walt Lillehei. He was a practical genius who skipped a grade and disassembled and rebuilt all kinds of machines in his youth. He also was an exceptional painter and photographer. He was charming, funny, flamboyant, and he cared nothing for society's conventions. He was an incurable risk-taker. He flew an airplane. His passion was mountaineering. He set himself the goal of climbing every one of the sixty-seven peaks over 14,000 feet in the continental United States, and he did it. Every one. Like Lillehei, he, too, had radiation therapy (for Hodgkin's disease) and ignored his disease's lethal implication, celebrating his survival by climbing the Matterhorn at age fifty without a guide.

And, well, like Bill Mustard swallowing goldfish, Charlie was a trifle crazy. Dotter's biographer Misty Payne tells of Charlie lecturing at an 8 a.m. department of medicine conference:

> He was talking about what you could realize if you could get a catheter in the heart and what the graphs would look like. Well, he brought in a rather large—standing about six feet tall—cathode oscillograph, which is, you know, like a TV screen with these graphs on it. And he said, "I've been standing here and talking to you for about twenty minutes, and all this time I have had a catheter in my heart," whereupon he rolled up his sleeve, and there was the end of the catheter. And he said, "Now I'll show you what a normal heart reading looks like." So he went and he plugged himself into the machine, and we were all kind of gasping, you know. There's a man standing there with a catheter in his heart— and he moved it among the chambers of the heart as he stood there, and he explained what the graphs represented. It was an absolutely horrifying example, but it was the kind of thing he did, to say it is perfectly safe.

Within the affectionate definition of misfit that characterizes so many we meet in this history, even today I have to rank Charlie Dotter near the top. Creativity, it seems, sometimes finds a soul mate in a charismatic, show-off, unconventional, risk-taking personality.

Dotter was appointed chairman of the department of radiology at the University of Oregon at age thirty-two, the youngest in the country, and held the position for an academe-eternity: thirty-two years. When Dotter was appointed, vascular obstructions were treated by open surgery. In 1963, while performing an X-ray examination of blood vessels, Dotter accidentally completely opened a partially obstructed artery as he advanced his catheter from his patient's leg into the aorta. With the same chance-favors-the-prepared-mind attitude as Mason Sones and Marcus DeWood, Dotter was open to discovery by serendipity. He and his fellowship trainee Melvin Judkins decided to test the idea that obstructed vessels could be opened with catheters. They developed a set of stiff catheters of progressively larger diameter. In cadavers, they started with the smallest diameter catheters then pushed one after another through the obstruction until the vessel was finally completely open. It seemed to work. They were ready to test their system in patients.

Laura Shaw was a gruff eighty-two-year-old diabetic with a nonhealing ulcer and gangrenous toes due to obstructions in the arteries in her legs. She adamantly refused to have her toes amputated by her surgeon Dr. William Krippaehne. As a last resort Krippaehne, who knew of the cadaver experiments, sent her to Dotter to see if he could reopen the obstructed leg vessel.

Dotter was lucky. Shaw's angiogram revealed the obstruction was short, in a large diameter vessel, and was easily reached through the skin. He pushed a wire across the obstruction. Then, starting with a stiff small diameter catheter, Dotter progressively dilated the diseased vessel segment by forcing larger and larger diameter catheters through it. The response was startling. Within minutes color had returned to Laura Shaw's foot and it was now warm. Within a week, her pain disappeared and the ulcer healed soon thereafter. Dotter performed an angiogram at three weeks and again at six months: the vessel remained open. Vinegary Laura Shaw died of congestive heart failure three years later at age eighty-five, as she never failed to remind her surgeon, "still walkin' on my own two feet."

As he treated patient after patient, surgeons were not enthusiastic about losing their patients to "Dottering," as the procedure became known.

So they called him "Crazy Charlie." He had an answer. Soon every Dotter lecture included a photo of a surgeon's written requisition for a diagnostic angiogram of the legs with the surgeon's handwritten notation "visualize but do not try to fix." Dotter's angiogram showed a major and a minor vascular obstruction in the leg. Dotter dilated the major obstruction, but "did not fix" the minor one, since it was not necessary. Dotter had complied with a strict literal interpretation of the surgeon's orders, and still saved the patient's leg. A showman to rival Lillehei, Dotter topped off his lectures with a film on his technique which included a photograph of him and this very patient standing on the summit of 11,000-foot Mount Hood a year after the procedure.

Although Dotter opened obstructed vessels, his procedure had important limitations. His large diameter catheter left a gaping hole at the point of entry into the artery, which often required surgical repair. His rigid catheters sent torn-off chunks of atheroma cascading downstream to completely reobstruct smaller vessels. So, while Charlie Dotter proved that obstructed vessels could be opened by a distending force from within, the toxic mixture of his brash style and the strong opposition from surgeons doomed his method in the United States.

Europeans were not so hidebound. After seeing Dotter's technique described at a radiology symposium Dr. Andreas Gruentzig, a completely unknown young radiologist in Zürich, Switzerland, was inspired to think outside the box. Gruentzig's vision was that he could improve Dotter's technique, and then apply it to CAD, that he could treat heart disease with a catheter instead of cracking open the chest. Gruentzig's story of persistence in the face of repeated failure and rejection is the most inspiring in our half-century chronicle of cardiology, and stands as a message for each of us regardless of our occupation or circumstance.

ANDREAS GRUENTZIG WAS born in Dresden, an East German city near the Polish border, in 1940, during the period between the Nazi invasion of Poland and the entry of the United States into World War II. Five years later, on the evening of February 13, 1945, Allied firebombs reduced the "Florence on the Elbe" to rubble, killing 135,000 people. It was the single most destructive bombing of the war, more so than Hiroshima or

Nagasaki. The firebombing of Dresden was particularly tragic because the city had no strategic value at a moment when the Germans were on the verge of surrender. Before the bombing, his parents had moved the family to Rochlitz, a small town about fifty miles west, only to have their new home commandeered by Allied forces as a headquarters. Andreas's father was later lost during the battle for Berlin. Fatherless and impoverished, Andreas had to fend for himself in the early postwar years. His deliverance from poverty came through the classroom. At age seventeen Andreas escaped from East Germany to be taken in by his older brother in Heidelberg. Poor but focused by ambition, the immigrant kid graduated from medical school seven years later, chose radiology, and was accepted for training in Zürich. When he saw the Dotter procedure, Andreas cajoled his boss to allow him to travel to Nuremberg, Germany, to learn the procedure.

When he returned from Nuremberg to Zürich in 1970 Gruentzig performed Dotter angioplasty on a modest number of patients. But his boss in radiology came to feel that Gruentzig's puttering was not only taking him from assigned work, but also creating complications when an occasional dislodged atheroma created a surgical emergency. It was a now-familiar story: where Gruentzig saw opportunity, his boss saw complications. But Gruentzig had an intuition. In his mind's eye Gruentzig imagined that a forcefully expanded balloon pressed against the narrowed segment might dilate it without snowplowing off the atheroma like Dotter's catheters. That single idea became his life's obsession. He thought of it, dreamed it, lived it every moment of the day. As he had so many times before in his life, Gruentzig found an escape route: he maneuvered a transfer into the department of cardiology. Now his target would be the coronary arteries.

His transfer was hardly like being let out of jail. As in radiology, his boss soon told him that his pursuit of his passion would be strictly on his own time, after work hours. So with his loyal assistant Maria Schumpf, her husband, and his wife, Michaela, Andreas set to work at night in his kitchen. Six months became a year. Imagine trying to keep three normal people interested in the task of putting a balloon on the end of a catheter. Night after night Gruentzig mixed boundless enthusiasm with bottles of wine to cajole the little group to play his game of catheters. He and his friends began by affixing small cylinders of latex or rubber to the end of a catheter with thread and epoxy glue. When the little group finally mastered a method for attaching a balloon to a catheter, Gruentzig tested their prototype in cadaver vessels. His balloons burst.

Gruentzig's friend and colleague Dr. Spencer King published Gruentzig's notes describing what happened next: "I spent the next two years contacting manufacturing plants in an attempt to solve this problem. It was at that time that I met a retired chemist, Dr. Hopf, a professor emeritus of chemistry of the junior high school of Zürich. He introduced me to polyvinyl chloride (PVC) compounds. . . . After hundreds of experiments, most of which were performed in my own kitchen, I was able to form a sausage-shaped distensible segment." What Gruentzig had needed from the start was a bladder, which could withstand great internal pressure, like an auto tire or an inflatable toy. Now he had a distensible PVC bladder, which looked like a miniature football, one that could retain its shape at high pressure without bursting. At the same time it could deliver tremendous force to the vessel wall.

But now a new problem emerged. To negotiate the catheter through the tortuous vessels of the heart, it needed to be passed over a previously placed guidewire. Gruentzig would need two lumens (channels), one for the wire, and a second to deliver air to inflate his balloon. He had no way to construct a double-lumen catheter, and he could find no catheter company that saw any reward from the cost of designing and fabricating such an unproven, untested device.

Working in complete obscurity, Andreas Gruentzig had now spent three years of his life moving from failure to failure. On the brink of defeat, a young friend came up with an ingenious solution. He created a longitudinal groove on the length of catheter's outer surface, then covered it with a long thin tubing. Voilà, a second lumen to deliver air to inflate the balloon.

He had finally succeeded in constructing a homemade, cockamamie balloon catheter that everyone agreed would never work. But at least he could try his contraption in the coronary arteries of dogs. It worked! Now, armed with X-ray images as proof, he was finally able to convince a local manufacturer to construct a real double-lumen catheter. Elated, Andreas packed his before-and-after images of obstructed coronary arteries in dogs, and headed to the 1976 annual American Heart Association meeting in Miami in the United States. He imagined that he would astound the world of cardiology with the results of his animal research through his poster presentation. Many thousands of cardiologists walked past his poster. Most ignored the enthusiastic bubbling German completely. The ones who stopped were courteously deeply skeptical. His presentation was just a goofy curiosity by a home hobbyist. His technique was irrelevant to humans. World-renowned catheterization specialist Dr. Spencer King told me that when he saw it, he walked away, telling a colleague, "It'll never work."

At the meeting, however, one cardiologist saw merit in Gruentzig's enthusiasm. San Francisco cardiologist Dr. Richard Myler invited him to come to St. Mary's Hospital in San Francisco to perform the procedure on a patient. Gruentzig and Myler performed the first successful human coronary angioplasty under anesthesia during coronary bypass surgery in May 1977. Although now convinced it would work, Myler lived in a different era than Dwight Harken. He realized that he could not risk his career by using it in the cath lab, cognizant of the condemnation from colleagues and the massive California lawsuit that would follow any complication. Years later Dick Myler described the episode to me as his most bittersweet experience: exhilaration with their technical success, belief that he had a breakthrough technology at his fingertips, yet frustrated by insurmountable barriers to its implementation.

Dusting himself off after being ignored in Miami and stymied in San Francisco, Gruentzig returned to Zürich determined to treat a patient in his laboratory. He struggled for months to find a suitable patient, one in whom he had a high probability of success. He wanted to dilate just one atheroma in a large coronary artery. After months of searching he found his potential candidate in mid-September 1977. Adolph Bachmann was a thirty-seven-year-old Swiss businessman with severe typical angina. A two-to-three-pack-a-day smoker, his angina had progressed to the point that he required up to twenty-five nitroglycerin tablets daily. "I ultimately couldn't do anything. With the slightest exertion came pain," Bachmann told later historians. Coronary angiography showed he had a severe stenosis in his left anterior descending coronary artery. He needed surgery. The vessel was large; it would easily accommodate the untried balloon catheter. Bernhard Meier, the resident at the time, notified Gruentzig.

Gruentzig went to see Bachmann. His personal charm, sincerity, and honesty carried the day. As Bachmann recalled, "Gruentzig wasn't at all overbearing . . . He made it clear that I would be the first man ever to receive this pioneering procedure . . . The severe choice between the scheduled bypass operation and the alternative dilatation probe left little doubt in my mind as to which path was preferable . . . I said 'What's the big deal? The difference can't be so great.'" When Gruentzig scheduled the procedure for the next day in the catheterization lab, however, he ignited a conflagration similar to that faced by surgeon Walt Lillehei a quarter of a century earlier. In a hastily called conference with his hospital leadership, both the hospital's chief of medicine and chief of cardiology were vehemently opposed to the procedure. Gruentzig watched his dream evaporate as the sacred Hippocratic Oath was added to practical arguments like unknown risk and negative public backlash. As the meeting neared closure, the hospital's most respected leader, internationally famed pioneering surgeon Dr. Ake Senning, rose to speak.

"Let the young man try it," Senning said.

When no one deigned to challenge Senning, Gruentzig, against all odds, had carried the day.

At 7 a.m. the following morning Adolph Bachmann, conscious but sedated, was wheeled into the cardiac cath lab. With a dozen doctors watching, the laboratory crackled with tension. "Only those who dare to fail greatly can ever achieve greatly," Bobby Kennedy had said a decade earlier. This was Andreas Gruentzig's moment. But he encountered difficulty from the start. Before inserting the catheter, he tested his balloon. It would not inflate. Frustrated, he discarded the defective catheter. He tore open a new sterile package for a second backup catheter. It, too, would not inflate. By now Gruentzig could visualize a story to be told and retold for years in Zürich with just the right amount of schadenfreude. He ripped open a third package, attached a syringe to the end of the catheter, and pressed on the barrel of his syringe. The third balloon inflated. That tiny piece of polyvinyl chloride encircling a catheter tip was his career's brass ring. Could he grasp it?

Gruentzig poked a needle into a quarter-sized patch of skin above the femoral artery in Bachmann's groin, to inject a local anesthetic. The first steps were routine: needle into the femoral artery, guidewire passed through the needle, push the wire back up the aorta to the orifice (opening) of the left coronary artery, slither his catheter over the wire. He took his first step into the unknown, the unexplored ominous domain of the atheroma, the land of sudden unexpected death, passing the guidewire into the left coronary artery, sliding silently past the lurking atheroma. He slid his catheter over the wire, puffs of X-ray dye illuminating the landscape beyond, catheter creeping forward, finding the perfect position where the uninflated balloon near the catheter tip completely straddled the obstruction in Bachmann's coronary artery. Tension in the room escalated, Gruentzig staring at the monitor, surgeons and anesthesiologists poised to rescue Bachmann from his plight with emergency bypass surgery.

Imagine yourself in Gruentzig's profoundly uncertain moment, not knowing if inflating the balloon would cause a heart attack, precipitate sudden death by ventricular fibrillation, or open the obstruction in Bachmann's coronary artery. Gruentzig tells what happened next: "The catheter wedged the stenosis so that there was no antegrade flow and the distal coronary pressure was very low" (his catheter completely obstructed the artery, so no blood could flow beyond it, causing pressure to drop). Gruentzig's catheter was obstructing the most important coronary artery of Adolph Bachmann's heart. "To the surprise of all of us, no ST elevation, ventricular fibrillation or even extrasystole occurred and the patient had no chest pain." He inflated the balloon. "After the first balloon deflation, the distal coronary pressure rose nicely [suggesting the vessel was no longer obstructed]. Encouraged by this positive response, I inflated the balloon a second time to relieve the residual gradient."

Bachmann seemed just fine . . . at least no harm done. But to what benefit? The proof would lie in a repeat coronary angiogram. As Gruentzig sent a new load of X-ray dye cascading down Bachmann's coronary artery, onlookers gasped, hands flying to mouths as if to stifle a shriek, silently trying to comprehend the incomprehensible, to believe the unbelievable. It seemed like a magician, scrub suit for cape and catheter for wand had, with a couple of thrusts on the plunger of a syringe made an atheroma vanish completely! But each observer knew that what they had witnessed was no illusion . . . it was a medical breakthrough. Years later, pathologists would prove that the force exerted by his inflated balloon crushes the atheroma back into the wall of the blood vessel, completely reopening it.

I rank this miraculous, magical, astonishing moment in the history of cardiology in the same pantheon as Claude Beck's defibrillation of the fourteen-year-old boy. Thirty-seven-year-old Adolph Bachmann was about to become the best-known patient in the history of cardiology. Gruentzig recalled, "Everyone was surprised about the ease of the procedure and I started to realize that my dreams had come true." A new legend in cardiology had been born. Andreas Gruentzig was poised to be the most famous cardiologist of our time.

After the procedure, Bachmann had no further angina. King recatheterized Bachmann on his tenth anniversary. The vessel continued to look perfect.

Gruentzig returned to the annual American Heart Association meeting in 1977 to describe his first four angioplasty procedures in human beings. But this time he spoke from the podium. His voice washed over the heads of a rapt audience as he showed all-too-familiar angiographic images of coronary arteries obstructed by atheroma. Then came his Big Reveal. After balloon angioplasty, the obstructions simply disappeared. Cardiologists are a visual species: for us, seeing is believing. As each new image flashed across the screen, murmurs rose from the audience as people turned to each other to say, "That's amazing" and "Did you see that?"

What happened next was a first in my experience of listening to thousands of scientific presentations over forty years. In his words, "I also showed the slide of the fourth patient with the incredible success of main stem dilatation and it was during this case that the audience started applauding in the midst of the lecture. I was so surprised that I almost could not proceed with my ten minute presentation." When he finished, his audience rose as one, and his ten-minute presentation concluded with a standing ovation.

No one could to fail to grasp that this was a transitional moment in medical history. Moments later, the torch was passed to a new generation. Mason Sones approached him after the lecture and asked to see more than snapshots. He wanted Sonesian proof: the movie films that

Gruentzig had recorded during his procedure. Gruentzig said, "I invited him to share with me the cineangiogram [coronary angiogram recorded on movie film] which I had in my suitcase. We went to the exhibition hall and reviewed the film of this patient together at the booth of one of the exhibitors."

Gruentzig reported his first five cases in a letter to the editor of the prestigious English medical journal *The Lancet* in 1978. In the three years following his first case in Zürich, he performed coronary angioplasties in 169 patients. Ten years later, nearly 90% of his patients were still alive.

I FIRST GOT to know Gruentzig during his Zürich years when the two of us and our wives had dinner as a foursome in Aspen, Colorado. What a couple! His wife, Michaela, a psychologist, was very bright and very pretty. Andreas was Michaela's equal in charm and grace. He told wonderful stories and listened with great interest to my banal ones. He spoke with passion about almost everything, was at once ebullient, down-to-earth, and larger than life. I recognized the charisma that I had seen earlier in Dwight Harken and my mentor, Jeremy Swan. I left dinner that night feeling that Andreas had opened my mind to a new world of limitless possibilities I had never before imagined. For the first time we could enter our patients' coronary arteries; we could touch and manipulate our tiny adversaries that lay within.

In science, failure occurs in isolation, success draws a crowd. Gruentzig's kitchen receded into distant memory as the world's cardiologists clamored to be taught his procedure. With thousands of cardiologists wanting to learn, he found a way. He wore a microphone in his cath lab and sent continuous X-ray images from the laboratory to monitors in the hospital's auditorium as he performed live procedures. Hundreds of cardiologists sat in reverence like parishioners at a Billy Graham sermon. Immediately after each procedure Gruentzig strode from his lab to the auditorium lab to talk about the just-witnessed case. His approach was revolutionary. As his biographers David Monagan and Dr. David Williams concluded, "Almost no modern surgeon back then would have dared televise in real time the unpleasant sights and sounds of his unpredictable trade. But Gruentzig was passionate about holding nothing back, believing that the sheer dint of his scientific honesty would be the key to gaining credibility in the world of skeptics."

His open and honest attitude dissolved any residual skepticism. Gruentzig was his procedure's most severe critic, predicting that it would only be applicable in 5% of patients with CAD. On this single point he was vastly mistaken, proving why there are far more medical historians than prognosticators. Today I see few coronary lesions during our weekly catheterization laboratory conference that are beyond the reach of interventional cardiologists.

Gruentzig held three courses in Zürich. At the end of each course he put on a spectacular informal party at an exotic location. He tried to meet each individual attendee. At his final Zürich course in August 1980, Andreas Gruentzig invited Crazy Charlie Dotter, Mason Sones, Melvin Judkins, and other pioneers that made his own success possible. He chose a mountain high above Zürich's lake. At the end of the dinner, Gruentzig passed torches to each attendee beginning with Sones, Dotter, and Judkins. Sones, tipsy as was his wont, disappeared into a ditch on the trek downhill. When he was missed and retrieved, he had his rescuers take him to the wrong hotel. But the moment of symbolism could not be missed, the cardiologic equivalent of John Kennedy's inaugural speech, "Let the word go forth from this time and place, to friend and foe alike, that the torch has been passed to a new generation . . . born in this century, tempered by war, disciplined by a hard and bitter peace." Gruentzig, the acknowledged champion, now was known by a single name, Andreas. Theirs was a movement whose members glowed with a sense of camaraderie and shared vision bequeathed by Andreas. They were marching forth to create a new worldwide subspecialty. They would call themselves interventional cardiologists. Perhaps Andreas imagined it even then, I know I did not: interventional cardiology now dominates the present and the future of cardiac therapy.

Meanwhile Gruentzig's bosses made themselves the poster boys for the classic three phases of the establishment's reaction to new ideas:

1) It can't be done.
2) It probably can be done, but it's not worth doing.
3) I knew it was a good idea all along.

By the time they arrived at stage three, however, the East German Andreas Gruentzig, low man on their totem pole, let the world know that he was thoroughly fed up. He felt that he was more respected throughout the world than he was at home. He felt he needed to realize his potential in a more open society. He wanted to resettle in the United States. I tried to lure him to Cedars-Sinai, and the Cleveland Clinic made their pitch. But we were too late. Dr. Spencer King, the consummate Southern gentleman, had charmed the Charmer. He enticed Gruentzig to visit him in Atlanta. Gruentzig joined the Emory University staff. For charismatic Andreas, leaving the confines of Zürich had an eerie similarity to Christiaan Barnard sallying forth from Cape Town fifteen years earlier. Would he succeed or would he encounter unanticipated consequences?

19

CONQUERING ATLANTA

Never regret thy fall, O Icarus of the fearless flight! For the
greatest tragedy of them all. Is never to feel the burning light.

—OSCAR WILDE, IRISH DRAMATIST

FOR ANDREAS GRUENTZIG his move to the United States was
like bursting from underwater to gulp a breath of fresh air. Professionally
shackled in Zürich, he arrived with instant celebrity in Atlanta. At Emory
soon after his arrival, swashbuckling Andreas decided to undergo coronary angiography. His coronary arteries, of course, were entirely normal.
With a typical Andreas flourish, despite the puncture in his femoral (leg)
artery, he went dancing in public that night. In Atlanta, Andreas's creativity and spellbinding teaching were expressions of a flamboyance that
bubbled through every aspect of his life. Being with Andreas was like being in a cyclone. He had equal passion for partying and for work. He
charmed people, particularly ladies, and he could light up a room with
his zest for life. He seemed gloriously happy with a glass of wine, playing
the piano, and singing. He was an elegant dancer, tall, graceful, athletic,
and so strikingly handsome. One of his nurses captured him perfectly: he
was an alchemist's version of Clark Gable, Errol Flynn, and Omar Sharif.
Yet Andreas made no social distinctions. Even with the acclaim that show-

ered upon him, he was as friendly to trainees and staff as he was to those in positions of power.

The passion for life so apparent in his social life shone through his patient care, teaching, and medical research. In a seminar setting, if there was a Magic Marker and a whiteboard handy, he became a consummate artist drawing the heart and blood vessels. His hand-eye coordination extended to the catheterization laboratory, where he was an artist with catheter manipulation.

With fame came a flood of angioplasty referrals to his partnership with Drs. Spencer King and John Douglas. With the referrals and catheter company contracts came sudden wealth. You said Andreas to any cardiologist anywhere in the world and he knew you referred to the acclaimed, elegant, handsome, smiling, multilingual center of Atlanta's medical and Emory hospital society. Andreas loved the attention, but his wife Michaela did not. She returned to Zürich with their daughter, Sonja. Andreas's wandering eye settled on a new companion much younger than him. Margaret Anne Thornton was a bright young medical student with the classic good looks and charm of a Southern belle. Andreas was smitten. They were married in 1983.

Andreas's life morphed into the antithesis of his former life in Zürich. He bought a mansion. He and Margaret Anne put on lavish parties there at the end of his angioplasty teaching courses. He bought a Porsche. As he had in Zürich, he drove recklessly. He bought a vacation home on Sea Island, about an hour's flight south of Atlanta. To travel to Sea Island, he bought a powerful private plane, a Beechcraft Baron, and became a pilot.

According to his biographers David Monagan and David Williams, in his transition from Zürich to Atlanta some felt that Andreas's values changed, whereas others saw a natural progression that accompanies sudden new wealth and a new young wife. Some of the wives who knew his first wife, Michaela, remained loyal to her, making the relationship with Margaret difficult. His detractors muttered that he was becoming a modern Icarus, flying too close to the sun for his own good, while his supporters countered that no one soars too high if he soars on his own wings.

Andreas began leaving work at 5 p.m., putting strain on his professional relationships. Soon we heard that he was looking at other opportunities, at the possibility of leaving Atlanta to join his friend Richard Myler in San Francisco.

On a Friday in late October 1985, Andreas performed an angioplasty on a vascular surgeon, then hurried to fly with Margaret and their two dogs for their weekend in Sea Island, anxious to beat a powerful incoming storm. On Saturday morning he received a call that the coronary artery he had treated was closing, and that his partners Spencer King and John Douglas were taking his patient back to the cath lab. By now Hurricane Juan began to unload on the Southeast. Juan would ultimately kill sixty-three people and cause $1.5 billion in property damage. From his Sea Island cottage, Andreas looked out at torrents of rain slamming into the sand, steps away from frothing waves churning an angry Atlantic Ocean. Margaret's instinct was to hunker down, but Andreas, who had five cases scheduled for Monday, felt he was obligated to get back to Atlanta. He argued that he had some experience flying in bad weather, and that his new Beechcraft Bonanza had sophisticated instruments. Andreas checked with meteorologists, who reported that Juan's force was already dissipating over Georgia. His plane was at St. Simons's McKinnon Airport, just five minutes away. The control tower informed him that his planned northwesterly route from the airport to Atlanta was not particularly violent, although visibility was poor.

Andreas made his decision. He and Margaret and their two Irish Setters, Gin and Tonic, would fly at 3 p.m. Just as they were leaving Margaret's mother called to say she had heard a very different forecast, that Georgia was still being deluged. She begged them to reconsider. Her entreaty was ignored. Andreas couldn't wait; his compulsion for action took over. He would fly. As he prepares to return to Atlanta, let's meet one of my friends who owed years of his life to Andreas's balloon.

I KNEW AARON Stein as a friend for many years before I knew him as a patient. Aaron was about ten years older than me when I first met him. He was a short, balding, slightly overweight man in his mid-fifties whose preferred attire was shorts, a Hawaiian shirt, and sandals. His unimpressive features camouflaged his strongly held opinions and his intolerance of fools. He liked to describe himself as a nice Jewish boy from Brooklyn. But he wasn't. Aaron's street-smart intelligence poked up its head in every conversation, often with a scathing and hilarious wit. He was a tough, motivated, highly successful entrepreneur in the import-export business. He prospered as most of his competitors fell by the wayside. His secret lay in combining impeccable taste, a network of contacts in Asia, a willingness to use money to make things work, and tough negotiating with those who supplied him services. He was not in business to make friends.

Aaron had a youthful joie de vivre that made it seem like he would outlive us all. I was a little surprised when he called to say, "Jim, I went in for a routine physical and now my family doc is trying to tell me I have diabetes. I don't have diabetes. I don't add sugar to my coffee, I don't eat sweets, I cut the fat off my steaks, and I walk on the beach a couple times a week. *Goyishe kopf.* I shouldda gone to Bernstein. Can you talk to him?"

I had learned long ago never to challenge a family doctor with a curbstone consult unless you have the all information he has. So I called Aaron's doctor. Aaron's blood tests spoke clearly. He had diabetes. Worse, the doctor's opthalmoscopic exam of his eyes, which provides a direct view of arteries as they traverse the retina, revealed that Aaron had advanced atherosclerotic disease in his blood vessels.

When I got back to Aaron, he was as feisty as ever. Pointing an accusing finger at me as if I had joined the doctor's conspiracy against him, he challenged, "You tell me why I have diabetes when I am not obese?"

"Aaron. How did your parents die?" I asked. His father and his grandfather had early heart attacks and his mother had a stroke.

"It's in your damn genes, Aaron," I said. "Blame your parents, rest their souls."

When a disease is chronic and progressive, the doctor-patient relationship can subtly evolve as the disease progresses. At this point in his illness, my role was to be unyielding, like a parent finding the delicate balance between affection and authority. First Aaron had to admit he had a problem, and then take responsibility. "Aaron, listen to me. Stop arguing. This is what you need to do." I demanded he alter his diet. He resisted. I asked about exercise. He shot back, "I already get enough exercise on the golf course. When my friends collapse, I run for the paramedics." That was quintessential Aaron. But like the good child, in the end he listened.

Soon after Aaron's diagnosis, however, he began to have typical angina. A fiftysomething man with diabetes, typical angina, and vascular changes has a very high likelihood of having obstructive atheromas in his coronaries. Drugs proved insufficient to relieve his symptoms. I referred Aaron to Steve, one of the most talented interventionalists on our staff. As we expected, Aaron's coronary angiogram revealed CAD. Faced with a choice between the scalpel and the balloon, Aaron chose the balloon. Balloon angioplasty completely relieved his angina. But was that sufficient to slow his disease?

ANDREAS TOOK OFF for Atlanta under the watchful eyes of air traffic controllers in Jacksonville, Florida. He took off east, turned north, and quickly rose to 11,000 feet. He would be handed off to Atlanta Approach Control, and given exact instructions for his descent into the congested skies of Atlanta. As he approached Macon, Georgia, there were patches of heavy rain and dense fog, with cloud cover beginning at 600 feet and visibility to three miles. The conditions were challenging, but not difficult for an experienced pilot. Below him on the ground the fog was so bad that as he drove toward Macon to visit his mother, Spencer King reversed his course and went back home to Atlanta.

About ten minutes into flight, Andreas received his instructions from Atlanta Approach Control to descend to 5,000 feet, and perform a 360-degree clockwise loop, which was designed to delay him for a few minutes so that he could get in line for final descent into the Atlanta corridor. Andreas acknowledged the instruction. It was the route he had flown innumerable times on his return home from Sea Island. But instead of turning northwest, Andreas inexplicably turned southeast. A few minutes later, he reported that he had a malfunction in his autopilot system. Clearly he believed that he had turned northwest and now did not believe his instruments telling him he was flying southeast. Andreas's quaking voice revealed he knew he was in terrible trouble. "I have to fly with my backup," he reported. "The autopilot and whole first system is gone." Three minutes later his Beechcraft Baron 583AM disappeared from Macon's radar.

In a pine forest near Bolingbroke, Georgia, about eight miles north-west of Macon, deer hunters were hidden in a tree stand peering into the fog when they heard a high-pitched shriek like a World War II dive bomber, followed by an earthquaking explosion. Soon thereafter police, alerted by a nearby resident, found the wreckage of a plane. Clothing dangled from the broken limbs of pine trees surrounding a thirty-eight-foot crater. The devastation at impact made it impossible to identify the occupants. They found a few pages of a cardiology manuscript, and an emerald ring. Protruding from the wreckage like a memorial tombstone was the Beechcraft Baron's tail with its painted identifying logo, 583AM, chosen by Andreas and Margaret to commemorate their marriage in the fifth month of 1983.

The screaming crash of the Beechcraft Baron in a rural Georgia field shook the world of cardiology to its roots. Our generation's supernova had been suddenly extinguished. But Andreas left a legacy. He had worked with the National Heart, Lung, and Blood Institute to establish a multi-center registry of treated patients whose response to angioplasty could be followed over time. The results of the registry suggested that angioplasty was comparable to surgery for relief of angina. We estimate that today, about 600,000 angioplasty procedures are performed each year in the United States.

Today we have no hard-and-fast rule for choosing bypass surgery or angioplasty for relief of stable angina that is not controlled by nitroglycerin. My thinking for an individual patient is based largely on the severity of disease we see on the angiogram. If all the vessels have CAD, or if there is significant heart failure, I may favor surgery. For the rest, I often favor angioplasty because the recovery period is so much shorter.

ANDREAS GRUENTZIG'S STORY has a bizarre epilogue. In September of 1985 Andreas put on his last teaching course at Emory. He gave special tribute to the three great "fathers" of interventional cardiology: Charles Dotter, Mason Sones, and Melvin Judkins. He pondered the strange irony that the three great pioneers had all passed away within months of each other that year. Andreas was to join them in just a few weeks. Andreas's early tragic death levitated him from the king of angioplasty to cardiologic sainthood. He was just forty-six-years old and yet was already, and remains, the most memorable cardiologist of our times.

Andreas Gruentzig had persisted through years of isolated frustration in his kitchen by using failure as fuel, advancing rather than retreating from errors. Years later a series of Apple advertisements reminded me of Andreas. A large photo of one of the century's brilliant innovators—Albert Einstein, Bob Dylan, Martin Luther King, John Lennon, Muhammad Ali, Mahatma Gandhi, or Pablo Picasso—was shown with a small Apple logo beneath and just two words: Think Different. The ad was brilliant in its simplicity. I thought if a cardiologist had been selected, Andreas would be the first, glancing up from a glass of red wine at his Zürich kitchen table. Andreas Thought Different.

ANDREAS GRUENTZIG HAD proven that it was possible to crush an obstruction in the coronary artery that caused angina and heart attacks, restoring the coronary angiographic image to normal. But as groundbreaking as his idea was, an even grander idea lay inherent in his breakthrough: heart disease does not require the doctor to crack open the chest, touch the offending organ under direct vision. We can treat congenital heart disease, valvular disease, and electrical disorders of the heart with devices inserted through the skin. As he basked in deserved glory, however, Andreas Gruentzig's ideas were about to be challenged by the most unlikely of any of the characters in our story.

20

PRICKING ANDREAS'S BALLOON

Every really new idea looks crazy at first.

—ALFRED NORTH WHITEHEAD
ENGLISH MATHEMATICIAN AND PHILOSOPHER

We know that the nature of genius is to provide idiots with ideas twenty years later.

—LOUIS ARAGON, FRENCH POET AND NOVELIST

DR. GEOFF HARTZLER was a quintessential American Midwesterner who dressed like he was the bass guitarist for redneck country singer Johnny Cash. The son of a Mennonite minister, in his rebellious youth Geoffrey Hartzler was consumed by rock 'n' roll and his bass guitar. His talented high school and college bands had blasted music throughout his home state of Indiana. When I met him as a cardiologist, his big smile framed by his droopy mustache and his cowboy boots suggested he was more ready to perform the Texas two-step than balloon angioplasty. Not that Geoff cared a whit about what I, or anyone else, felt about a doctor who dressed like a cowboy. Geoff's whole persona said maverick.

Hartzler had first encountered Andreas Gruentzig in Miami at his poster presentation on balloon angioplasty in dogs in 1976. After Gruentzig's dramatic human results in 1977, the Mayo Clinic catheterization laboratory team planned to test his method in the leg vessels of 100 patients before attempting the procedure in the coronary arteries. Hartzler, a younger member of the group, ignored the plan, performing angioplasty on a lesion similar to Bachmann's. His aggressive nature did not mesh well with the conservative philosophy of his colleagues, and he soon moved on to St. Luke's Hospital in Kansas City, Missouri, where he quickly became one of the country's leading practitioners of coronary angioplasty by performing fifty-five procedures in his first six months.

Geoff shared with Lillehei and Bailey that complete indifference to criticism from others that would have devastated most of us. If he did not fit society's norms, he did not care. The certainty in the righteousness of his cause spurred Geoff to pursue treatment options that his colleagues scorned. That perspective was essential because his decision to perform angioplasty on multiple atheromas in the same patient brought him into direct and heated conflict with Gruentzig, who feared Hartzler's complication rate would soar, besmirching the reputation of the method he had pioneered. In an intriguing reversal, iconoclastic Gruentzig assumed the role of conservative establishmentarian in his ballet with Hartzler, the rogue dissenter.

Fearing early adverse outcomes could kill his baby while still in the manger, Gruentzig insisted that angioplasty should be restricted to one simple lesion like that of Adolph Bachmann, in which the probability of success was high. With tongue-in-cheek logic, Hartzler replied that after he had successfully dilated one lesion, if he saw another he did that one, too, since he was only treating one lesion. Hartzler's insouciance outraged Gruentzig. He countered Hartzler's cavalier attitude by refusing to be in the same room with him. Most of us sided with the charismatic German who urged us to build our wall carefully, brick by brick. True, the mustachioed Midwesterner's magical skills in catheter manipulation matched his dexterity with the guitar, but still he was a cowboy, a guy playing it too fast and loose. So that's what we called him, Cowboy Geoff.

Hartzler went completely off the reservation in 1980. Like so many of cardiology's breakthroughs, it happened because of a wildly fortuitous convergence of person, place, circumstance, and time. Geoff had a stable angina patient in the hospital scheduled for angioplasty, when the laboratory called to say that the procedure had to be canceled because the man was having an acute myocardial infarction (a heart attack).

"That didn't seem logical to me. It seemed that an hour before he was a candidate for angioplasty," Geoff said. At that moment, what seemed illogical to everyone else made sense to Geoff. Like Walt Lillehei years earlier, conviction in the rightness of his cause was the only impetus he needed. Geoff Hartzler jumped into the abyss with both boots:

> We brought him down to the lab. The right coronary was blocked . . . we put a catheter in. It went through this occluded vessel right where the stenosis had been shown the day before. I expanded the balloon and it was the most amazing thing I had seen. The ST segments came down to normal (the electrocardiographic signs of heart attack disappeared), the pain went away totally, and he was normal . . . We had opened this totally blocked artery. It was unheard of at that time. It was amazing. It was fantastic. It changed my thinking.

On that day, Cowboy Geoff revolutionized the treatment of heart attack. He had opened a blood vessel that was obstructed with a blood clot, not with a drug but with a balloon catheter.

The patient was discharged home in a few days, rather than the usual two-week stay. From that moment on, Geoff began using angioplasty as his therapy for acute myocardial infarction. We already had the highly effective clot-dissolving therapy for myocardial infarction, but that made no difference to Geoff. Conventional wisdom, and Andreas Gruentzig, held that putting a balloon catheter into the coronary artery of a patient dying from acute myocardial infarction was unacceptable, even crazy, yet Hartzler was doing it anyway.

Soon after he began his angioplasty program in acute myocardial infarction, Geoff invited me to be a visiting professor in Kansas City, making hospital rounds and lecturing. In a packed auditorium, Geoff presented a case of a patient with shock accompanying acute myocardial infarction, and asked me to discuss patient management. After I discussed the patient's very poor prognosis based on his ECG, chest X-ray, and hemodynamics, Geoff asked me how I would treat the patient.

In medicine our opinions are slaves to our prior experience. Hailing from the home of thrombolytic therapy, I pontificated over the use of intravenous streptokinase to dissolve the clot, while warning the prognosis for such patients in shock was very poor. Geoff countered by showing a film of his dramatic opening of the obstructed culprit vessel by coronary angioplasty. In case anyone doubted what he had done, Geoff topped off his visual tour de force by adding that the patient had walked out of the hospital in good shape a week later.

Even though I had been played as Stump the Chump, I refused to concede to my younger colleague. "That's terrific, Geoff," I said. "But here in the USA, we say 'In God We Trust, all others must have data.' I have data, and all you have is a case." Geoff heard my admonition and by 1983, he published his data on angioplasty in forty-one heart attack patients who were treated within an hour of hospitalization. Only one patient, who arrived in shock, died. The paper concluded, "All remaining patients had prompt pain relief, subsequent stable clinical courses, and no clinical or late angiographic evidence of coronary reocclusion . . . At follow-up, 94% of patients remained free of angina."

Although Geoff's results proved both the feasibility and safety of angioplasty during a heart attack, I, along with other thought leaders, insisted on randomized trials to determine if it was really a better therapy than thrombolysis, as he claimed. Three years later, a slew of trials established that angioplasty outcomes indeed were superior to thrombolytic therapy, provided the procedure is performed within less than two hours from emergency room arrival. And with that, the stampede to angioplasty as a treatment of heart attack began.

So despite his laid-back persona, his droopy mustache, and high-heeled boots, the Cowboy was right. Twice right. He was correct when he argued with Gruentzig about multivessel angioplasty and right again on that day in Kansas City when he argued with me about angioplasty in acute myocardial infarction.

Over the years that followed, whenever Geoff and I met, he loved to needle me, saying: "Hey, Jim, tell me again about data and "In God We Trust." My lame repartee to my young friend also was always the same: "Aw, Geoff, medicine is a discipline in which the fool of this generation can go beyond the point reached by the genius of the last."

Today, immediate angioplasty is the preferred treatment of acute myocardial infarction. This approach has reduced the in-hospital mortality rate to about 5%. That's a fall from 30% since my encounter with Willie the Phillie. It's tempting to put that spectacular reduction alongside similar jaw-dropping reductions in mortality from congenital heart disease and valve disease and rest on our laurels. And yet, when I come to talk about the future, you will soon see that another wave of spectacular advances is on the near horizon.

Like Andreas Gruentzig, Geoff Hartzler was an interventional cardiology meteor. At age forty-nine, just fifteen years after he first flashed across angioplasty's sky, he stepped away from the catheterization laboratory table. His years of wearing heavy lead shielding had compressed his vertebrae, leading to five back surgeries. In retirement he built himself a professional music studio in Kansas City where he played his bass guitar in a band called, what else, Heart Rock. Geoff died prematurely of prostate cancer in early 2012.

AND SO WE return to my friend Aaron Stein, whom we met in the last chapter, as his angina was being relieved by balloon angioplasty. After a year or so his angina came back. His cardiologist decided to perform an office treadmill exercise stress test to assess the severity of his CAD. But the doctor made a serious mistake. A few minutes delayed in getting to the office, he told his stress lab technician to begin the test. The doctor did not examine Aaron's resting ECG before the test, and his technician missed an obvious, admittedly unusual finding. Although Aaron did not mention chest pain, his ECG showed unequivocal evidence of a beginning acute myocardial infarction.

A few minutes into the treadmill exercise, Aaron began to complain of severe substernal chest pain and light-headedness. The technician immediately terminated the test, and instructed Aaron to lie down. When the doctor arrived just a few minutes later, Aaron's pain had not relented with either rest or nitroglycerin. His ECG screamed the reason: heart attack. But this was a special kind: heart attack with a lawsuit waiting to happen.

Getting to a hospital quickly is the single most important factor in surviving a heart attack. Data from Sweden's national medical data base, collected over fifteen years, showed that 29% of 385,000 heart attack patients died before reaching a hospital. In comparison, the mortality rate among those who made it to the hospital was less than 10%. Today the vast majority of heart attack deaths, about 90%, occur outside the hospital. The message is clear: for a person with a heart attack, the care we are now able to provide in a hospital is lifesaving.

ABOUT AN HOUR and a half later, Aaron had been whisked by ambulance from his doctor's office, through our emergency room, and into our catheterization laboratory. Our mantra for treating heart attack is, "Time is muscle," three words that conveyed the message that in the first few hours after onset, the size of the segment of dead heart muscle expands like the ripples from a stone tossed into a quiet lake. In the first few hours, if the occluded coronary artery is opened, cell death stops. So every minute counts. This is the single most important message I can give you readers who have CAD. If you have substantial chest pain that persists after nitroglycerin, go immediately to the emergency room. Angina disappears very quickly. Heart attack pain does not. There are three compelling reasons to move swiftly. The greatest mortality from heart attack is in the first hour after onset, and occurs outside the hospital. You'll survive if you get to the hospital. Second, the amount of permanent heart muscle damage is markedly reduced by early opening of the coronary artery. Third, our diagnostic skills are now outstanding: if you are not having a heart attack, we will be able to tell you.

I have imagined myself as a patient being the object of the controlled bedlam created by recording vital signs, starting intravenous lines, drawing blood, and recording an ECG, all while getting a brief history and performing a physical examination. Our goal is to get our patient out of the emergency room and on his way to the catheterization laboratory in less than half an hour.. Even as a cardiologist, I would be terrified by the experience, which to any ordinary eyes says that everybody in this room thinks I am about to die. When I was chief of cardiology, I recall watching a young ER resident physician wedge herself sideways into the middle of the tumult. Her job was to obtain a brief medical history and to conduct a cursory physical exam before the patient left the ER. I was deeply gratified to hear her voice rise above the cacophony with a reassurance, "I know this is a confusing blur to you right now. But each of us is doing something to help you. We know how to take good care of you. Now that you are here, you can feel confident that everything is going to turn out right." With access to new technology that we never knew, the generation of young doctors still understood that compassion comes first.

As I left the ER, I stopped to introduce myself to the young ER resident. "The way you treated your patient made my day," I said. From her reaction, I think I made hers, too.

IN THE CATH lab Aaron Stein went into ventricular fibrillation as our multitalented interventional cardiologist Steve inserted his catheter. Steve defibrillated Aaron, and proceeded with angioplasty. He opened the culprit vessel with a balloon and placed a stent. Today angioplasty has so completely replaced thrombolysis as the primary treatment for acute myocardial infarction in major medical centers that our trainees may go for a year without seeing the use of clot-dissolving drugs in acute myocardial infarction.

Discharged from the hospital after his angioplasty, Aaron and I sat across a table to discuss what was next. Aaron had reached new levels of fury. He blamed his doctor for the stress test that precipitated his heart attack. He wanted to sue. I listened for a while, then leaned across the table, and gripped his fist.

"Aaron, look at me. Let's agree that you will win the lawsuit. But what do you gain? You certainly don't need the money. So you gain whatever joy there is in punishing the doctor. Balance that against your downside. First, let's be clear: the doctor is a good man who made a big mistake when he delegated his responsibility to someone who was unqualified. But he did not cause the heart attack. Your ECG tells us that your heart attack was already in progress; the stress test made it obvious. But most important to you is that to win, you'll endure a year or more of joyless, irritating conferences and depositions with lawyers. You'll have to relive all the events with your expert witnesses. After that is done, you'll have to participate in heated negotiations. If those break down, you'll have to testify in a confrontational trial. What price victory?"

When Aaron cooled down, even though he had a slam-dunk lawsuit, he opted for personal peace. He did not sue. Although Aaron was able to put his doctor's mistake behind him, I suspected that he was not done with either CAD or the complications of diabetes.

IN LESS THAN a decade after Gruentzig's first angioplasty in Zürich, randomized trials in over 5,000 patients had proven that angioplasty is an effective therapy for relief of angina (chest pain on exertion) and for reducing mortality in acute myocardial infarction (heart attack).

Industrial collaborators now competed to create better technology. Whereas the first angioplasty catheters were stiff, bulky, and difficult to manipulate, today an entire new set of slippery wires, flexible catheters, and low-profile balloons has led to catheters that can be steered into any location in the coronary tree. Whereas my generation had learned to insert our large-bore catheters through an artery deep in the leg, a new breed of interventional cardiologists frequently uses smaller diameter catheters inserted through a smaller diameter artery in the wrist, with less bleeding complications and shorter recovery times.

But as with the original cardiac surgeons, our success bred an unanticipated failure, which only became apparent as worldwide experience accumulated. Within six months of opening a vessel stenosed (partially obstructed) by an atheroma, about a third of the treated lesions narrowed right back to their original diameter, "re-stenosed," and their angina returned. With some dismay, we realized that in the third of patients who suffered restenosis, we had returned full circle to where we had begun. In medicine, it's always that way: where God has a temple, the devil has a chapel. If we were honest with ourselves, in a third of our patients, we had accomplished nothing.

Around the world, my laboratory and others set out to find the cause of restenosis. Detectives in search of clues, we went to the microscope. Initially we thought we would find reaccumulation of the cholesterol responsible for the original obstruction. Surprise! Instead of new cholesterol accumulation, we saw masses of scar tissue heaped up at the angioplasty site.

We reasoned that when we inflated the angioplasty balloon we caused microscopic injury to the coronary blood vessel that was too small to be seen by angiography. Restenosis seemed to be the body's normal wound healing response in overdrive. So we spent millions of research dollars to discover compounds that markedly inhibited scar tissue formation following injury to the blood vessels of animals. To our dismay, when we tested these drugs in humans, we did not reduce the restenosis rate. I was completely baffled . . . we had done science step by perfect logical step. We identified scarring as the cause of restenosis, defined the mechanism of scar formation, and then found drugs that inhibited scarring in animals. And yet we had failed to prevent restenosis in man. Like maniacal architects, we drew and redrew our study design. Impossible. We had identified the cause of restenosis and yet we couldn't prevent it. Where had we failed?

THE ANSWER TO our conundrum arose from a completely unanticipated source. A new technology called intravascular ultrasound allowed us to see the coronary artery vessel wall in cross section (angiography shows the lumen of the vessel, not its wall). The new technology was a new set of eyes looking at the same problem. At the Washington Hospital Center in Washington, D.C., Dr. Martin Leon and his team of investigators saw the vessel lumen expand following balloon angioplasty, then slowly recoil back over a few months. Restenosis following angioplasty, it turned out, had two causes, not one. Both elastic recoil and scarring occurred after angioplasty. Each process made about equal contribution to restenosis. We had no silver bullet that could kill this two-headed beast.

IN 1986, JUST nine years after Gruentzig's landmark first angioplasty, two cardiologists in France independently found the solution to elastic recoil. Drs. Ulrich Sigwart and Jacques Puel used a hollow metal cylinder to prevent elastic recoil. They called the device a coronary stent. To visualize a stent, imagine a cylinder made of chicken wire. Crimp the cylinder on a collapsed balloon around the tip of a catheter. Inside a blood vessel, wedge the tip of the catheter against atheroma. Inflate the balloon inside the cylinder, forcing it against the vessel wall. When the balloon is deflated, the stent remains, a permanent scaffold for holding open that segment of the blood vessel.

Why do we call it a "stent"? Charles Thomas Stent was a nineteenth-century dentist to the Royal Household who created a formula for dental impressions. The new compound was so effective that his sons formed a company to sell Stent's compound. Sixty years later during World War I, a Dutch plastic surgeon used Stent's compound to stretch and fix skin grafts on facial wounds. He made the grammatical error of describing it as "stents mold," without a capital letter. From a peccadillo came immortality. His method of stretching and fixation by "stenting" became widely employed even as Stent's compound disappeared. Later, surgeons and cardiologists made the logical transition of "stenting" to tubes that stretched and fixed tissue in the body. Not many men have their name immortalized as a verb.

In the next year following its first description, Argentinean interventional vascular radiologist Julio Palmaz collaborated with San Antonio interventional cardiologist Richard Schatz to create a balloon-expandable stent for deployment in coronary arteries. Seven years later, after trials showed that stents cut the rate of restenosis almost in half, to 15 to 20%, the FDA approved stents. But answers create questions. Could we do even better? We had discovered that stents, just like balloons, induced the scarring response to injury. In eliminating elastic recoil we had precipitated even more injury.

And so once again, failure became success. We reasoned that stents could be coated with our drugs that had inhibited the scarring response but failed to prevent restenosis. Now the restenosis rate fell again, by more than half. We had failed twice, first with wound healing alone, then with recoil alone. Now we stood failure on its head, and proved that two wrongs can make a right. We created "drug-eluting stents." Drugs coat the stent's surface, inhibiting the scarring response, as the cylinder prevents elastic recoil. That bring us to today, where the restenosis rate has fallen to 5%.

Stents propelled us into today's era of treatment of heart disease, with the catheterization laboratory as its centerpiece. As we will see in our final chapter, we have a fabulous array of devices. We can close holes in the heart, implant pacemakers, suck clots out of coronary arteries, replace and repair heart valves, and implant cells to restore cardiac function. It all began with Andreas Gruentzig in a Zürich kitchen, determined to find a way to open a coronary artery with a balloon.

ABOUT A YEAR after my friend Aaron Stein's heart attack during an exercise test, he woke with slurred speech and profound confusion. He had a stroke. Aaron recovered with only modest impairment. He had to use a cane. He retained his conversational ability, but his stroke left him with a strange, selective memory loss. He could recall past events without difficulty, and still tell amusing stories, but could not accurately place them in time. Yet Aaron saw himself as defeated. He slept a lot more, and he admitted to crying episodes. Aaron was depressed. He had abandoned hope.

With his family, we focused on helping Aaron find meaning in life, on finding what he could still do. We suggested he could emphasize a life of the mind and the soul. Aaron returned to dedicated study of his Jewish heritage, a part of his life, which he had ignored since his teenage years. Aaron joined a small devout local temple. He was a natural leader and a counselor to others. The experience awakened a new Aaron. He became less impatient, less combative. He listened to other points of view. He mellowed. Our medical conversations became far less factual, far more philosophical.

But diabetes had a trump card even after our advances in cardiology had fueled his recovery from angina, heart attack, and stroke. Aaron was hit with a second heart attack. The additional loss of heart muscle led to congestive heart failure, leaving him barely able to handle the chores of daily living. His prior stroke and other illnesses disqualified him for cardiac transplantation. Now nine years into Aaron's care, Steve tried different drugs, then different drug combinations. Now what? The new role for Steve and me was to help Aaron, for the first time in his life, confront his own mortality. He continued his religious pursuits and he entered trials of new experimental agents for heart failure. He would improve a little, then slip back, a pharmacologic Sisyphus. When we reached a point where there were no more new drugs, something remarkable happened. Aaron consoled us. It was, I imagine, not the first time a patient consoled a doctor.

One night at home, Aaron passed away silently in his sleep. In his case, however, the strangler in the backseat had become the old man's friend.

It is easy to imagine Aaron's final years as a downward spiral to death. But to do so would completely miss the humanity of his last decade. A Greek myth tells us of Pandora ("all giving"), the first woman on earth, being given a chest by Zeus, who tells her never to open it. Consumed by curiosity, Pandora opens the box, allowing all evil emotions to escape into the world of mankind. She quickly closes the box, but it is too late. Everything has escaped, except for one emotion. Only Hope remained.

Hope fueled Aaron's last years when little else remained. A group of us helped life's journey to death by never abandoning it. Not hope that Aaron could become physically stronger or younger, but hope that he could every day become a better person. Aaron won that battle. He used his physical adversity to help him rediscover love of his family, of his fellow man, of himself. As he said, "You gave me time to become a mensch." In turning an unending string of physical defeats into spiritual victory Aaron taught me that perseverance in the face of adversity brings special gifts. In living through denial, anger, and depression Aaron had come to acceptance.

At Aaron's burial, my urge was not to cry, but to celebrate a life well lived. In Aaron's faith, each mourner is invited to throw a symbolic shovelful of dirt onto the casket. As I did, I murmured to Aaron and myself, "Someday I want to write a book, and when I do I want to tell your story."

PART IV

HOW TO CONQUER CORONARY ARTERY DISEASE

21

WHY DO ATHEROMAS FORM IN BLOOD VESSELS?

He who loves practice without theory is like the sailor who boards ship without a rudder and compass, and never knows where he may cast.

—Leonardo da Vinci, Italian Renaissance polymath

WHEN WE SAW that bypass surgery and angioplasty relieved exercise-induced chest pain (angina) and X-ray pictures showed blood flowing through previously obstructed coronary vessels, most of us believed that we would soon see people living longer. But a few dissenting voices questioned this logic. Dr. Thomas Preston is a University of Washington cardiologist whom I have known since our years together at a small Quaker college in Swarthmore, Pennsylvania. I no longer recall if Tom is a Quaker, most of us were not, but he embodies all their virtues: serious, intellectual, gentle, and polite, and in the Quaker tradition unafraid of standing alone.

Tom argued that although their chest pain was relieved, there was no evidence that they lived longer. He insisted that "as it is now practiced, its net effect on the nation's health is probably negative. Fully half of the bypass operations performed in the United States are unnecessary."

Preston accused the entire cardiologic community of bias, claiming that we refused to do a clinical trial because we "knew" that our patients would die without the surgery. In simple language, he was saying, "prove it saves lives." Preston's comments on angioplasty were similar, and equally scathing.

Preston's critique of our two "revascularization" procedures infuriated its practitioners. Some refused to talk to him. How could he examine patients, observe their dramatic relief of pain, see X-ray pictures of blood pulsing through the heart's arteries, and then conclude that revascularization would not prolong life? By being rigidly illogical, he was raising unnecessary fears and questions in patients' minds. Let the rain fall on him up there in Seattle, he was not going to rain on our parade. My colleagues in Los Angeles privately labeled Preston "the Anti-Christ of Angioplasty."

A few years later came the stunning results of the first randomized trials of revascularization (bypass surgery and angioplasty) versus medical management. Although revascularization relieved angina, it turned out that neither had much effect on either the heart attack rate or the mortality rate in patients with stable angina. Mason Sones's X-ray images of the heart's arteries had become cardiology's Rorschach test. We had acquired an "occulo-stenotic reflex": if we saw narrowing in an artery our instant reflex response was to dilate it. Tom Preston had seen the elephant in the room; somehow it had escaped our notice.

Heart attacks were proceeding unabated in people even after bypass surgery and angioplasty, when our patients had been relieved of angina. How could it be that we were relieving chest pain, restoring the blood supply, but not prolonging life? It made no sense. We needed to return to first principles. We were missing something. And whatever it was, it was a crucial detail about CAD. As we will see, it is the one detail you must know to avoid a heart attack.

FOR A MEMBER of the high-IQ club Mensa, Jim Fixx did some dumb things as an early adult. His father had his heart attack at age thirty-five and died at age forty-three. As Jim turned thirty-five, he weighed 240 pounds and smoked two packs of cigarettes per day. Then at age thirty-five he got wisdom. He decided to get in better shape. He began running. At age forty-five, he had stopped smoking, and lost sixty pounds. He published a well-researched book about the health benefits of running. His book, *The Complete Book of Running*, made it to the *New York Times* bestseller list and stayed there for almost two years, selling over a million copies. Jim became a regular guest on TV talk shows. He was hailed as a pioneer in America's fitness revolution, promoting the health benefits of regular exercise in middle age.

But it was too late. On July 20, 1984, at age fifty-two Jim did his daily ten-mile run along on a rural Vermont road. He stopped at a grassy hill about forty yards from the door of his motel. Jim's knees buckled; he slumped to the ground. Jim Fixx died at that spot in his jogging suit. Autopsy showed atherosclerosis in all three coronary arteries. Atheroma had narrowed one coronary artery by 95%, a second by 85%, and the third by 70%.

Jim had played a vigorous singles tennis match the day before his death. He had never complained of cardiac symptoms. As his former wife, Alice Fixx, said, "He never had any warning."

Jim's death exposed gaping holes in our approach to CAD. First, since entering the period of life when CAD makes its first appearance he had spent seventeen consecutive years following a healthy diet, combined with regular vigorous exercise. When had his severe three-vessel CAD begun? We had no good idea. Second, half of CAD-related sudden deaths occur in people like Jim Fixx, who had no prior symptoms. We were performing hundreds of thousands of bypass surgeries and angioplasties each year on people with symptoms. Both procedures relieved chest pain (angina) in the vast majority of cases. If we had known the obstructions were present in Jim Fixx's arteries could we have prevented his heart attack by angioplasty or bypass surgery? To solve these conundrums we needed to determine when, why, and how obstructive atheromas (cholesterol plaques) form in coronary arteries. What we discovered is crucial knowledge for anyone with heart disease in their family, because it provides your foundation for preventing CAD.

IN SCIENCE, GREAT ideas spring from great contradictions. An inexplicable paradox had erupted like crabgrass in our perfectly manicured lawn. Seeing atheromas disappear after angioplasty, we had made science's critical error, the logical assumption. If CAD was a disease caused by a mass that obstructed blood flow, then surely it followed that eradicating the obstruction and restoring flow would cure the disease. And yet it did not. It defied logic that we were opening narrowed vessels and bypassing obstructions but not having an impact on the rate of heart attacks. From patients who had angiograms before and after their heart attack, we realized that the coronary angiogram failed to predict which atheroma would rupture, and consequently where or when a heart attack will occur. Think of it this way: the angiogram reliably identifies a block in the road but it does not tell us where the avalanche would occur. In admitting this paradox we exposed humbling lacunae in our knowledge. Angioplasty for prevention of heart attack teetered uneasily on its pedestal. We had to admit we had only a rudimentary understanding of our lethal adversary, the atheroma. The time had come to fling open the long-shuttered windows on atherogenesis—how atheromas form.

The quest to understand atherogenesis was not new. Early pathologists had begun by simply describing what they saw. When we slice open a normal coronary artery lengthwise, we see a lovely smooth glistening pink surface punctuated by the openings of branch vessels. The blood vessel surface is slick to our touch. Now let's place an atherosclerotic vessel next to it. Diseased vessels are pocked by irregular yellow bulges that make the surface bumpy. In some cases we see little red hemorrhages beside the bulges. Think of pizza. The pathologists do when they gaze on the irregular conflagration of yellows, oranges, and reds. When the yellow protrusions bulging into blood vessel surface are sliced open, they extrude a heavy slippery substance that reminded early pathologists of the gruel they had for breakfast. To bestow the aura of science on their work pathologists called their discovery an atheroma, from the Greek *athera* meaning gruel and *oma* meaning tumor. They also saw that calcium was added to the gruel-tumor over time, making the previously soft and flexible blood vessel stiff and inflexible. More erudition was necessary: they added *sclera* (Greek for rigid) and *osis* (Greek for condition). Atherosclerosis is the pseudo-erudite term for atheroma-induced hardening of the arteries. The word tells us what we see, but gives us no insight about cause.

Three competing theories of atheroma formation emerged. In the mid-1800s the century's most brilliant pathologist, German Rudolph Virchow, identified both cholesterol crystals and inflammatory cells in atheroma. Virchow thought inflammation was the trigger, proposing "inflammation hypothesis." Against him stood those who thought atheroma formation began with cholesterol accumulation, the "lipid hypothesis." Still others thought the process was more like wrinkles, simply a natural outcome of aging, the "senescence" hypothesis. The battle to understand the nature of our tiny adversary was joined. The three hypotheses framed a scientific battle that consumed much of the next century. Which hypothesis would be proven correct?

Just before World War I, Russian pathologist Nikolai Anitschkov succeeded in creating atheromas in rabbits by feeding them purified cholesterol, sixty-one egg yolks over seventy days in one protocol. Animals fed cholesterol-free sunflower oil remained free of atheromas. For the next thirty years, Anitschkov used his microscope to lay out the progression of atherosclerosis for the world to see. He found that young lesions were reversible, but older, more complex lesions were not. Although he toiled in isolation in St. Petersburg he published in both Europe and the United States. A searing irony is that the work of the man who clearly described atheroma formation was unappreciated in his lifetime because of a quirk of geography. Even today although historians know of his work, his name is largely unrecognized in the modern world of Western cardiology. He was ignored, at least in part because existing Western dogma favored the senescence hypothesis.

The rejection of Anitschkov, however, was also promoted by Mother Nature. When other investigators set out to validate his claims, they reached for their standard laboratory animal, the dog. The cholesterol-fed dog, however, does not develop atherosclerosis. In carnivores like the dog, unlike rabbits and man, blood cholesterol is rapidly transferred to bile and excreted. With no elevation of blood cholesterol, no atheromas develop. For Anitschkov's skeptics, the rabbit model was simply too remote from the human condition. His cholesterol-fed rabbits had blood cholesterol levels two to five times that of humans, and their atheromas developed over weeks or a few months, whereas human disease only appeared in middle age. To the medical establishment of his day, Anitschkov was a scientific Dostoyevsky, a long-winded Russian who had created too many complex questions and not enough easy answers.

At the end of World War II, the preponderance of erudite medical opinion rejected the "lipid hypothesis" that cholesterol was the cause of CAD. Cholesterol advocates were too much hypothesis and too little fact, all hat and no cattle. In the 1946 edition of *Quantitative Clinical Chemistry*, that era's biochemistry bible, John Peters and Donald Van Slyke concluded that "although there can be no doubt that deposits of lipids, especially cholesterol, are consistent and characteristic features (of atherosclerotic lesions) there is no indication that hypercholesterolemia plays more than a contributory role in their production." Instead, pathologists supported the "senescence hypothesis." Atherosclerosis, death, and taxes were inevitable, even though atherosclerosis and death didn't get worse each time Congress met.

Faced with the emerging epidemic of CAD and no understanding of its pathogenesis, in 1948 the National Heart Institute made a decision that reverberates through the halls of academia today, sixty-five years later. They set out to define the risk factors that predicted the appearance of CAD in apparently normal people. The concept was to identify a relatively small town, collect all the known potential risk-factor information in all its citizens, and then follow them until death. The Framingham Heart Study is named after the town that was chosen. Framingham, Massachusetts, was an ideal site for a long-term epidemiology study, a typical small American town, midway between Boston and Worcester, where people were begotten, born, and died. The Framingham study continues today with the progeny of the original participants. Each participant's age, sex, blood pressure, cholesterol, body mass, smoking history, family history, and diabetes were recorded (later the cholesterol subfractions, good and bad cholesterol, were added). Then investigators sat back and waited for subsequent development of CAD. When the ten-year follow-up results became available in the mid-1960s, it was used to create charts that estimated the ten-year risk for developing the symptoms of CAD. When I discuss risk and lifestyle modification with a patient, I refer to the Framingham results, which provides a sense of the risk of disease and the benefit of therapy, always adding Einstein's caveat that, "Not everything that can be counted counts, and not everything that counts can be counted." The Framingham model, for instance, does not include genetic history as a risk factor.

At about the same time, University of Minnesota nutritionist Ancel Keys began a study that approached atheroma formation from a different perspective. Keys hypothesized that since cholesterol is a form of fat, the amount of fat in diet might determine who gets CAD. He collected data on the type and amount of fat in seven different countries' diet, the average blood cholesterol, and the cardiac death rate. Not surprisingly, Japan with its emphasis on fish consumption had the lowest blood cholesterol level at 160 mg/dl. Finland, with very high dairy fat consumption, had the highest, 260 mg/dl. Then came the jaw-dropping result: the ten-year heart attack death rate was a paltry 5 out of 1,000 men in Japan but a whopping 70 out of 1,000 in Finland, a fourteenfold difference. The remaining five countries had intermediate cholesterol levels and death rates. The data for all countries almost fit a straight line, suggesting that risk of death was proportional to the level of blood cholesterol. Then Keys brandished a second graph that was to influence Western eating habits to this day: the blood cholesterol level was proportional to the amount of saturated fat in the diet. The difference in fat intake was as stunningly different as the death rate. In Finns, saturated fats constituted about 20% of daily calories, whereas in Japanese it was only 3%. Again, the values for the other countries fell roughly along a straight line.

Keys drew this logical, stunning conclusion: dietary saturated fat raises blood cholesterol and in turn, cholesterol increases the risk of a fatal heart attack. Keys's study breathed new life into Anitschkov's lipid hypothesis. In the mind's eye it was an easy leap from Anitschkov's atherosclerotic rabbit munching cholesterol chow to a fat Finn toppling over after devouring a plate of Gouda cheese.

The Framingham study and the Seven Countries Study precipitated the Cholesterol War. Every producer of fat, from farmers with cholesterol-laden egg yolks to ranchers with fat pigs, fought back. Their scientific surrogates howled that Keys had marched from preconceived notion to foregone conclusion. He had not conducted his study to find the truth; he had done it to prove a point. He was biased. Further, they insisted that an association between two measurements does not establish causality. Keys might just as well have shown that family telephone bills cause auto accidents. Sure, telephone bills and auto accidents correlate, they argued, but correlation is not cause. Teenagers increase both the phone bill and the accident rate. The difference between the Finns and Japanese could be due to obesity or to different smoking rates, or any other unrecognized factor. The study, they concluded, was hogwash.

Confronting his critics across this scientific chasm stood Ancel Keys. His trial was his baby, his progeny to be defended against all detractors. Keys understood his child's limitations. He countered that his correlations remained true after statistical correction for every one of the Framingham risk factors. Neither the press, nor the public nor most of cardiology, however, cared a whit about such statistical nuances. Ancel Keys's Seven Countries Study had forever linked diet and heart disease in the public mind. And so the Cholesterol War was joined.

Even Keys had to admit that he could not dismiss one obvious objection to his statistics: genetics. Perhaps the Finns were genetically predisposed to get atherosclerosis, and the Japanese were not. This possibility could hardly be rejected when it was so obvious in a glance that Japanese and Finns were vastly different in other genetically determined features. A counterargument that suggested Keys's findings were not due to genetics soon emerged from Hawaii. Investigators compared blood cholesterol levels and heart attack rates among ethnic Japanese living in Hawaii, San Francisco, and Honshu, Japan. First-generation Hawaiian Japanese had a higher blood cholesterol level, and with it came a parallel increase in heart attack rate. Both numbers were even higher in San Francisco. The obvious conclusion was that the difference between the Japanese in Honshu, Hawaii, and San Francisco was not genetics. It was diet. We now know that as the winds of Western lifestyle carry our diet east and south to less-developed countries, coronary disease follows like an unwanted lightning storm. The prevalence of atherosclerotic disease clearly increases as societies modernize in the twenty-first century, bringing us full circle back to the long-rejected hypothesis that the Industrial Revolution caused CAD. Machines don't cause CAD; it is diet. Historians had been right, but for the wrong reasons.

As opinion swung toward the lipid hypothesis, the anticholesterol gang raged against the dying of the light. A 1976 *British Heart Journal* editorial concluded, "The view that raised plasma cholesterol is per se a cause of coronary heart disease is untenable." Edinburgh's leading cardiologist Michael Oliver maintained that "It is probably of little value to reduce raised serum cholesterol concentrations in patients with CAD." Michael was one of my favorites—a cardiologic version of contemporary writers Christopher Hitchens and Sam Harris. He was erudite, analytical, and charming, a curmudgeonly critic of unproven theories. Others disagreed. A British newspaper dubbed Oliver the "Abominable No-man," and the *Journal of the American College of Cardiology* crowned him "The Cholesterol Pessimist."

Hoping to resolve the debate the NIH organized a randomized trial of cholestyramine, a drug that inhibits cholesterol uptake from the gut. After seven years, the trial announced a very modest difference of 1.6% in coronary death and myocardial infarction (7% vs. 8.6%), favoring the treatment group. When the NIH and the lipidology establishment ballyhooed the result as "statistically significant," Vanderbilt University's Dr. George Mann fumed, "They have manipulated the data to reach the wrong conclusion. The managers at NIH have used Madison Avenue hype to sell this failed trial in the way the media people sell an underarm deodorant." *Atlantic* magazine science writer Thomas J. Moore went further, calling the report an "extravaganza that resembles a medical version of the military-industrial complex," then named five lipidology leaders, darkly suggesting that "It is likely that one reason these physicians consented to [promote the results] is that their laboratories were heavily involved in research funded by Merck."

The NIH countered by issuing the groundbreaking declaration that blood cholesterol lowering was now a major national health goal. But there was a problem. Cholestyramine lowered cholesterol and in theory could save some lives, but only the most dedicated believer would willingly swallow the massive pill for any period of time after experiencing the indigestion, burping, and loss of appetite that accompanied its ingestion. The NIH had run afoul of Karl Marx's century-old critique of Hegel that "In theory, there's no difference between theory and practice, but in practice, there is." For management of high-risk asymptomatic patients our arsenal of cholesterol lowering drugs remained empty.

The Cholesterol War ended suddenly, on a single day, not with a whimper but a bang. On November 19, 1994, the first large randomized trial of a cholesterol lowering statin drug versus placebo was published in the prestigious British journal *The Lancet*. Over five years of follow-up, simvastatin had lowered bad LDL (low-density lipoprotein) cholesterol by 35% and the risk of coronary death by 42% compared to placebo-treated patients. The investigators concluded, "This study shows that long-term treatment with simvastatin is safe and improves survival in CHD patients." On that day, the Cholesterol War ended. The lipid hypothesis, it seemed, had won.

ATHEROMA FORMATION (DEPOSIT of fat in blood vessels), we now know, begins with cholesterol. So let's describe it. Cholesterol is used for the construction of cell membranes, for making hormones like progesterone, estrogen, and testosterone, and for synthesis of the bile that helps digest food in the intestine. So blood has to transport cholesterol to all parts of the body. To transport cholesterol, Mother Nature links it to one of several proteins. The resultant spitballs of fat (called lipid) and protein are called, logically enough, lipoproteins. The two lipoproteins cardiologists focus on are low-density lipoprotein cholesterol (LDL), nicknamed "bad cholesterol" because high blood levels are associated with CAD (coronary artery disease) and high-density lipoprotein cholesterol (HDL), which is associated with low rates of CAD.

Most of the components of blood, even cells, move in and out of the blood vessel wall. Cholesterol enters the blood vessel as part of the LDL (bad cholesterol) molecule. When it exits the vessel wall, it is transported out as part of HDL (good cholesterol). That is why LDL is bad and HDL is good. Cholesterol trapping in the vessel wall reflects the balance between transport in and transport out, between LDL and HDL. When the amount of cholesterol brought into the blood vessel wall exceeds the removal capacity, when all the garbage trucks are full, some of the cholesterol gets left behind. Now that spot in the vessel becomes New York City during a garbage workers' strike. The cholesterol left sitting in the blood vessel wall is like butter. It turns rancid. In scientific parlance, it is oxidized. Rancid LDL cholesterol is a potent stimulus for the body's inflammatory response. That's why pathologists see a mix of cholesterol and inflammatory cells in coronary obstructions.

The inflammatory response is activated when the cells of the blood vessel, finding themselves contaminated with unwanted oxidized cholesterol, send a chemical call into the blood for help. The chemical signal attracts white blood cells, the immune system's firemen, to the scene. These newly arrived inflammatory cells charge into the vessel to gobble up the offending oxidized LDL. Bloated to Falstaffian proportions with fat, these cells become trapped in the complex matrix of the vessel wall. Unable to leave, the trapped cells ultimately die there. The oily mixture of cholesterol and dead cells becomes the gruel, the *athera*, that pathologists see when they slice open an atheroma. Other cells, trying to wall off the mess, put a scar on top. Over months and years, this collection of fermenting gruel enlarges. The mass of gruel, covered with a fibrous cap, bulges into the flowing bloodstream, creating the tumor-like *oma* of atheroma. The bulging mass is what we see in our X-ray pictures (angiograms) of the coronary arteries.

Sometimes tissue adjacent to the atheroma breaks down and bleeds beneath the blood vessel surface. The vessel surface becomes the knobby mix of yellow, red, and white that reminds pathologists of pizza. As trapped cells die, the gruel becomes calcified. The calcified atheroma is what we look for when we do heart scans for calcium.

That's how an atheroma forms. To simplify, atheroma are caused by a local excess of oxidized fat (cholesterol) in the vessel. Over many years, it can grow larger until it partially obstructs coronary blood flow, causing angina.

We finally understood how atheromas form. But knowing how an atheroma forms and expands still leaves us with a giant unanswered question. How could Jim Fixx be such a great runner for many years with atheromas in his coronary arteries, then collapse without prior warning? He died when an atheroma in his coronary artery ruptured. We understood how an atheroma forms; now we needed to know why some plaques rupture, causing heart attack and sudden death.

22

PLAQUE RUPTURE, HEART ATTACK, AND SUDDEN DEATH

The greatest discoveries of science have always been those that forced us to rethink our beliefs about the universe and our place in it.

—Robert L. Park, American physicist

CLINICAL RESEARCH HAD created balloon angioplasty and bypass surgery. But to explain why neither prevents heart attack even while restoring blood flow, we needed basic research. Clinical research leads to reforms, basic research leads to revolutions.

After Russell Ross graduated from the Columbia University School of Dental Medicine in 1955 he migrated west to Seattle for seven years of PhD studies in experimental pathology. He joined the faculty in the department of pathology at the University of Washington and later became its chairman. Tall and willowy, Russell carried himself like the urbane, intellectually curious, elegant symphony buff that he was outside the world of medicine. Ross began by being curious about how a wound heals. The deeper he delved into the body's healing process, however, the more he became fascinated by a counterintuitive, revolutionary idea. Could Nature have created a yang to healing's yin? His beguiling thought was that the factors that drove healing could also create disease. His hunch ulti-mately led him to study the disease he came to believe was the quintes-sential example of how the healing process creates disease. It was our millennia-old adversary: the atheroma, the cholesterol plaque in the cor-onary artery.

Peering down through his microscope, Ross was astonished. The very cells that created the scar on healing skin also thronged like members of the congregation around a developing atheroma. But why? Ross made an intuitive leap that enthralls all who love science. He hypothesized that the same cells drove both formation of the atheroma and a scar on the skin. Ross proposed his response-to-injury hypothesis of atheroma formation in the prestigious journal *Science,* suggesting that the atheroma was the product of the body's normal healing response. He was partly right. Ross and others soon discovered that an even more fundamental biologic process than wound healing was afoot. Atheroma formation and rupture was actually driven by the body's most basic of all defenses, the inflam-matory response. In the case of the atheroma, it was the inflammatory response to cholesterol trapped in the blood vessel wall. Who could have imagined that the long-forgotten inflammation hypothesis would one day marry the lipid hypothesis? The progeny of this marriage is our modern understanding of atheroma formation and plaque rupture.

WHEN WE DISCOVERED that blood clots cause heart attacks, pa-thologists made a fascinating discovery. The red worm was clinging to a torn blood vessel surface, and beneath that ruptured surface lay . . . an ath-eroma (a plaque). Like a dormant Mauna Kea, the atheroma had suddenly erupted without warning, discharging its molten gruel into the flowing bloodstream. Any tear in the blood vessel surface instantly activates the blood clotting system. With that recognition, a new phrase entered our lexicon. "Plaque rupture" was the cause of heart attack.

The world of cardiac pathologists—England's Michael Davies, Den-mark's Erling Falk, Renu Virmani in Washington D.C., and our own hospital's Michael Fishbein all set out to define what made the ruptured plaque different from all the rest of the "stable plaques" in blood vessels. Michael Fishbein walked me through the violent world of plaque rupture under high magnification; he took me to the world of the atheroma, and showed me the enemy up close. What I saw was that each atheroma has its own personality. Most look like dullards, half asleep, doing nothing much. A few atheromas, however, appeared hot-tempered, ready to explode. What's the difference? Mike showed me: on average, ruptured plaques have four times more cholesterol, four times more inflammatory cells, and the cap over this mess is very, very thin. The cap is ready to rupture, and when it does, the heart attack begins seconds later.

What accounts for these three differences between a quiescent plaque and one that ruptures? It is the magnitude of inflammation in each plaque. Inflammatory cells release enzymes that digest everything around them, including the cap that walls off the atheroma from the flowing bloodstream. The three characteristics of ruptured plaques led pathologists to come up with a new term: the "vulnerable plaque," the plaque prior to its imminent rupture. The vulnerable plaque is a sinister form of atheroma, among all the cholesterol-filled egg yolks it is the one that splatters. Viewed by coronary angiography, a stable plaque and a vulnerable plaque look the same. The angiographic image does not tell us that one plaque is quiescent and the other is potentially lethal. So like all photos, the coronary angiogram is accurate but it does not tell the whole truth.

Vulnerable plaques, the ones poised to cause a heart attack, come in all sizes. A small vulnerable plaque can cause a heart attack, even though it was too small to have caused chest pain on exertion. That's what happened to Jim Fixx. He had no symptoms prior to his heart attack because the vulnerable plaque that ruptured was too small to obstruct blood flow. But when a clot that formed on its torn surface, it completely obstructed coronary blood flow, causing a heart attack. Vulnerable plaques are like Usain Bolt, prepared to explode from the starting blocks. Stable large atheromas cause angina, but vulnerable plaques of any size can cause a heart attack.

Think about the implication of this insight for treatment of CAD. It is why half of the Framingham heart attack victims had no symptoms prior to their heart attack. The ruptured plaque was too small to cause angina before it ruptured. And that leads to a second stunning insight: it is impossible to greatly reduce heart attacks if you only put a stent across a large atheroma. A swarm of smaller Judases still lurk in the artery, ready to betray their master and cause a heart attack.

Every society and every generation casts disease in its own image. Anthropologist Meira Weiss finds that cancer patients view the malignancy as a Pac-Man chomping everything it encounters, a beautiful fruit with worms inside, or an octopus with sticky tentacles. AIDS, affecting the whole body, is seen as diffuse, decaying, and polluting, as amorphous as an amoeba engulfing its prey, as fluid as Dali's melting clocks. Metaphors for heart disease are far less lyrical. Heart disease is a something that needs fixing, like a piston pumping in a misshapen cylinder, a rusted pipe. Interventional cardiologists call themselves plumbers. But we chose the wrong metaphor. Coronary arteries are not rusting pipes. Heart attack cannot be prevented by performing angioplasty on one atheroma among the many that dot the surface of the blood vessel. One of those atheromas is a quiescent volcano, ready to erupt without warning. So angioplasty and bypass surgery are highly effective for relief of angina, but not for preventing heart attacks. The essential insight for patients is that prevention of heart attack requires a different therapy.

Our new understanding of the birth, adolescence, and maturity of our tiny terrifying assailant bought a stunning irony. We had known our adversary intimately, because we had once stared him in the face. Literally. In our teen years, from time to time the tiny fat secreting units in our skin, called sebaceous follicles, become obstructed. Fat is trapped beneath our skin. The trapped fat is oxidized, inducing a violent inflammatory response. The skin becomes red and tender. Driven by inflammation, the fat erodes to the surface of the skin and pops out. When it ruptures, a tiny blood clot forms at the site. We call it a pimple.

The ruptured atheroma is the identical process, but it occurs in the coronary artery. Fat (in this case, cholesterol) gets trapped beneath the surface of the blood vessel. It is oxidized. The ensuing violent inflammatory response causes it to burrow its way relentlessly toward the vessel surface. Both the pimple and the atheroma erupt like a packed garbage bag tossed into a busy street, spewing its contents on its environment. And when the atheroma bursts, just like a pimple, a blood clot forms at the site of rupture.

An atheroma is as simple as a pimple on the blood vessel wall. Who could possibly have imagined that? All we can say is that sometimes our physiology is not only queerer than we imagine, but queerer than we can imagine. As one of my students asked after I explained atherogenesis, "Do you mean to say that this century's leading cause of death is acne?"

MY PASSAGE FROM callow young clinical investigator to cardilogic leadership had moments of exhilaration and despair. Many of my mentees returned to become leaders in cardiology. They invited me to their cities and homelands as a visiting professor. I was fascinated to see the vast differences in medical practice around the world, An unanticipated secondary benefit was that my wife and I always added a few extra days to travel through most of Asia, Europe, the Middle East, and South America. When I was home my trainees allowed me, like my dad before me, to never miss my three sons' baseball and soccer games.

My low point in those years came when my eighty-seven-year-old father called me from his home about thirty miles south of Albuquerque, New Mexico. He had awakened with severe substernal chest pain and shortness of breath in the middle of the night. It had disappeared after a half hour, then he had two more episodes in the ensuing hours. His medical history was unremarkable other than the diagnosis of mild Alzheimer's disease. He had no history of CAD, had never smoked, was not diabetic, and had never had high blood pressure. He was not sure what his cholesterol level was, but he was not taking any medications. But substernal chest pain with associated shortness of breath in an eighty-seven-year-old still says CAD.

I called my friends Drs. Michael Crawford and Jonathan Abrams, who were then the current and past chiefs of cardiology at the University of New Mexico. We arranged for an ambulance to take my father to the hospital. Mike called me at about midnight after examining Dad in the emergency room of Presbyterian Hospital and said, "Jim, he has no chest pain at the moment, but he does have ECG changes that indicate CAD, and his blood work indicates he has had some minimal muscle damage. So with the recent history of stuttering chest pain, I think we can be sure that your dad has a ruptured plaque causing unstable angina. What's your thinking about what to do next?"

I went blank as a segment of my mind told me I knew nothing at all about what to do, that I was unqualified to make such a decision. For a few moments I was the helpless student in Philadelphia, thrust back in the cruel world of medical uncertainty, where there are no clear-cut answers. Then I regained my balance. I knew how we approached decisions. Unstable angina is a condition midway between stable angina and heart attack. Patients with the symptoms of unstable angina have a vastly different prognosis depending on other factors. About a decade ago, Harvard's research team identified seven risk factors that predicted adverse outcomes during hospitalization for unstable angina. The more factors a patient has, the more likely the partially occlusive clot in the coronary artery is to become completely occlusive; the more likely an unstable angina patient is to have a full-blown heart attack. People with only one factor have about a 5% risk; those with six or seven factors have an eightfold greater risk of going on to a heart attack.

IN THE EMERGENCY room we can stratify our patients into low, intermediate, or high risk. As a rule of thumb we treat low-risk patients with drugs and observation, and send high-risk patients (who have more than four factors) promptly to the cath lab. The strategy is based on outcomes. In low-risk patients, medical therapy is at least as good as angioplasty, whereas in high-risk patients, angioplasty is clearly superior. Dad had three factors, so he had an intermediate risk. And so our first wrenching decision: should Dad have medical therapy or angiography?

Mike and I agreed that we could treat Dad with medical therapy under close observation and hope that he stabilized.

In the morning Dad continued to have episodes of pain despite drugs to inhibit clot formation and dilate his coronary arteries. Failure to respond to therapy catapults a patient into the high-risk category. Mike and I agreed that we had to send Dad to the cath lab to see his coronary arteries. Hours later I got a call from the cath lab. It was the worst of all possible news. Dad had an atheroma in his left main coronary artery. It was only about

50% obstructive, but it seemed to be the lesion that had ruptured to precipitate unstable angina. Dad had three options: angioplasty of the left main coronary artery, bypass surgery, or continued medical management. All three choices were unappealing. Let's look at each.

Many cardiologists at that time would not perform balloon angioplasty on the left main coronary artery because it carried about a 5% risk of immediate procedural mortality. But beyond the immediate risk is the problem created by putting a metal stent in the vessel. After stent placement the patient should probably take an anticlotting drug for a year. The risk of a blood clot forming on the exposed metal skyrockets if a patient stops the drug. So we avoid stents in people who cannot be relied upon to take the drug religiously, like drug addicts, psychiatric patients, and of course patients with Alzheimer's disease. For Dad, a clot that formed on a left main stent would almost certainly be fatal. The anticlot drugs also increase the risk of bleeding, and markedly so in an elderly patient. Elderly people fall a lot, and a fall with a broken hip while on anticlotting drugs can represent a big problem. So angioplasty was unappealing.

What about surgery? Mike and I both felt that Dad would survive the procedure. We can operate on eighty- and ninety-year-olds, and Dad was in good health except for his brain and now his heart. But the problem with surgery in this age group is that it carries as much as a 5% risk of stroke, and perhaps a 20% risk of measurable decline in brain function. In younger patients, the decline typically disappears in months. But Dad already had impaired mental function. Surgery could accelerate his descent into Alzheimer's, robbing him of the remaining meaningful time he still had left.

And medical therapy? Should we continue with just drugs and bed rest when the treatment had already failed to control his symptoms? Should we hope that the partially occlusive clot in his coronary artery would regress with time, rather than progress to complete occlusion, knowing that if it progressed to occlusion it would undoubtedly be fatal? The risk of progression to infarction was significant. In the days before angioplasty and bypass surgery, we had called unstable angina "preinfarction angina" because about 20% of our patients went on to have a full-blown heart attack. As an eighty-seven-year-old, his risk was probably even higher. If Dad was sixty-five years old with no Alzheimer's disease, medical therapy would have been my third choice. But he was eighty-seven years old with Alzheimer's disease. Which course of therapy would you choose for your father? I will let you struggle with the decision for a few minutes while we return to put the atheroma formation and plaque rupture in broader perspective.

BOTH STABLE PLAQUES and vulnerable (ready to rupture) plaques are accidents of evolution. Our primeval ancestors were plant eaters, herbivores with no atheromas in their blood vessel walls. To counter periodic famine, however, they needed an energy storage system. Our ancestors were selected for survival because of their ability to store life-sustaining energy in the form of fat. With the emergence of civilization, our diet changed. When we began consuming vast amounts of red meat and animal fat, we created what author Michael Pollan calls the Omnivore's Dilemma. When the level of fat in our bloodstream exceeded the capacity of its transport system, some of the fat that entered the blood vessel wall got left behind. The stable plaque, the cause of chest pain on exertion, is the bastard child of a mechanism originally designed for survival.

Two of Nature's other essential lifesaving processes create the vulnerable plaque. At the heart of plaque rupture lies inflammation. The inflammatory response was developed at least 500 million years ago, as the sole immune defense weapon of most primitive multicellular organisms. It is so important to survival that it has been conserved throughout evolution of every species all the way to man. Introduce into your body anything that the immune system identifies as foreign, and you precipitate what we call the foreign body response. You have seen this response in your own skin with bacteria (an infected hangnail), fat (the pimple), or even a wood splinter. Yet when the fury of inflammation persists in any tissue for long periods of time, it changes from becoming beneficial to potentially lethal. In blood vessels, the inflammatory response to oxidized fat is responsible for erosion through the blood vessel's inner surface until the plaque ruptures. The pimple bursts.

Clotting at sites of blood vessel damage has saved the life of each of us. The tiny atheroma, however, managed to turn both inflammation and blood clotting upside down, Humpty Dumpty, and by so doing, it became potentially lethal. Nature has decreed that three mechanisms, which made survival possible—energy storage, inflammation, and blood clotting—would return to complete the circle of human life as our leading cause of death. Sunrise and sundown.

By the millennium, cardiology had consumed a century bantering over competing hypotheses of atherosclerosis. Like the blind men examining the elephant, we had seen different manifestations of the same beast. Finally, however, cardiology found its Grand Unifying Theory. The lipid hypothesis explains atheroma formation, the inflammation hypothesis explains atheroma rupture, and the senescence hypothesis explains the atheroma's long lifetime. Everybody was right.

WHICH TREATMENT DID you choose for my dad? Balloon angioplasty with a 5% risk of death on the table, survivable surgery with a 20% likelihood of further mental deterioration, or drugs which had thus far been ineffective in a patient at 30% risk of going on to a heart attack? Mike and I chose the medical option for Dad. We felt that the immediate risk of death and the long-term risk of missed drug doses and bleeding ruled out angioplasty. We decided against surgery because we feared further devastating mental deterioration. Perhaps I also felt that if either of these interventions failed, we would bear responsibility, whereas if Dad passed away on medical therapy, it would be the disease, not our therapy that was responsible. But deep down I knew that as a cardiologist, from the first moment I joined in the decision-making, I was responsible for my dad's outcome.

We made the right decision. In the next two days, Dad's condition stabilized. He returned home. I visited him frequently, and called each week. As his Alzheimer's disease progressed, my weekly calls became the high point of his week. I flew to visit him frequently.

At age ninety-three he fell, breaking his hip. After surgery, his mental condition never recovered; he was only sporadically able to recognize me. Dad passed away about a month after surgery, when a large blood clot dislodged from his leg and lodged in his lungs. Mike Crawford had given my father and his only son six good years together, far more than I hoped for on the night Dad called about his crushing chest pain. A moment that began for me as desperate uncertainty now stands as a treasured memory.

THE GREATEST DISCOVERIES in medicine are those that force us to rethink our beliefs about disease and our role in managing it. Let's see how this applies to our new understanding of atherogenesis (plaque formation) and your own cardiac health. For those of us without symptoms, we want to reduce the amount of cholesterol entering the blood vessel wall and accelerate its egress. In people with CAD we need to keep stable plaques from becoming vulnerable plaques. For those with ruptured plaques, like my dad, we need to stabilize them. This understanding of atherogenesis allows us to develop a realistic strategy for preventing heart attack and sudden death in each of us, instead of reacting after it happens. Our journey has brought us to that pivotal stage in medicine, where understanding cause precedes cure, where CAD becomes a preventable disease.

Central to the prevention of CAD and its complications in my own life, and possibly yours, is the statin class of drugs. The story of statins, the most important in the history of cardiology, teaches us more about the incredible twists and turns of scientific research and discovery than any other in our half-century chronicle. At the end you will shake your head and say, "Is that really how it happened?"

23

A MOLDY GIFT

*Not all chemicals are bad. Without chemicals such as
hydrogen and oxygen, for example, there would be no way
to make water, a vital ingredient in beer.*

—Dave Barry, Pulitzer Prize–winning American
author and journalist

AS RUSSELL ROSS was beginning his research on formation of cholesterol plaques, halfway around the world Japanese biochemist Akira
Endo was beginning a search for a way to inhibit cholesterol synthesis.
About two-thirds of the cholesterol in our body is made in the liver, the
rest enters through our intestines after we eat. Endo's dream was that he
might discover a drug that would lower blood cholesterol, bringing both
profit and fame to his employer, Japan's Sankyo pharmaceutical company.

Endo was the son of a farming family from the snowy far north of
Japan's Honshu Island. As a child he had been taught about nature by his
grandfather. One plant that fascinated both of them was a fungus that
was poisonous to flies, but had no toxic effect on people. This inconsequential childhood experience would play a central role in the rest of Endo's
adult life.

Years later as a young chemist hired by the Sankyo, Endo first distinguished himself by discovering an enzyme that removed natural contam-
inants from wine and cider. Sankyo rewarded his commercially valuable
research with a year of sabbatical study in the United States at a place of

his choosing. Endo chose the lipid metabolism laboratory in New York's Albert Einstein Medical College, the home of renowned coronary bypass surgeon Robert Goetz. Endo arrived in New York City just as it became the hub of the new internal mammary artery bypass surgery for CAD. Seeing the juxtaposition of bypass surgery while working in a lab devoted to the study of blood cholesterol metabolism inspired him: he would find a drug that blocked cholesterol synthesis.

Recalling his childhood in Honshu, Endo had a hunch. Knowing that fungi produced substances that killed invaders, he hypothesized that they did so by inhibiting the manufacture of cholesterol, which is essential for the formation of cell membranes in most species on the evolutionary ladder from bacteria to humans. Although fungi had acquired a distinctly negative reputation in modern times, from destruction of vineyards, to poisonous mushrooms, to insistently infecting dark crannies of the human body, Endo believed that mankind's lowly pest might also carry a silver bullet, an inhibitor of cholesterol synthesis.

Endo planned his hunt. His project was stunning in its potential for both boredom and failure, calling for a commitment to dogged persistence that recalls John Gibbon and his heart-lung machine. He would make extracts of fungi, then measure the effect of each extract on the synthesis of cholesterol by rat liver cells. If the first fungal extract had no effect, he would test the next, continuing until he found one that worked. His strategy was neither new, nor proven by prior discovery. In the 1970s the National Cancer Institute had blindly thrown drug after drug at cultures of malignant cells, searching for a cure for cancer, with stunningly little success. Endo's blind-ended research project was a pharmaceutical misfit, yet each day Endo arrived in the Sankyo lab near a south Tokyo train station like Sisyphus to push his metaphorical rock back up the hill, "doing grunt work every day until we got sick of it."

At least he was efficient. He ramped up his testing regimen to a capacity of ten new fungal extracts each day. As negative results piled up day after day, many of us would have despaired. But to Endo each day's experiment was a new quest. After all, no man steps in the same river twice, since the river is not same and neither is the man. In the next two and a half years Endo tested 6,392 fungal extracts. Two years of his life had produced, well, two compounds that inhibited cholesterol synthesis.

Just two. Both lurked in a remote and unlikely landscape: a fungus that infected the Japanese Mikan orange. But unknown Akira Endo had made the century's critical breakthrough in CAD prevention. While searching for a needle in the haystack Akira Endo had discovered the farmer's daughter. He had discovered a member of the statin drug family, the wonder drug for treatment of CAD.

That the future savior of millions of CAD patient lives might be a pest that infected an orange is curious. Even curiouser was that the fungus that produced the two statins was a member of the penicillium genus. Yes that penicillium. Endo's statin was produced by a mold called penicillium citrium. The source of penicillin, the wonder drug antibiotic, was its cousin penicillium notatum. By quelling infection, penicillin had ended the reign of infection as mankind's leading cause of death, allowing CAD to become the new number one killer. Statins are penicillin for the heart, and will soon dislodge heart disease as the number one killer. Endo chose one of the compounds to pursue further. He called it mevastatin.

Endo's research style reflected his own postwar society. Quiet, patient, deliberate. He would cross the stream by feeling each rock in turn, each step determined by his experience with his prior step. His next step was to identify how mevastatin lowered cholesterol. He found that it worked by inhibiting the most critical step in the synthesis of cholesterol. In an era when political revolutions were occurring violently in public squares, a scientific revolution had begun quietly in a cubbyhole within a laboratory next to a train station.

Mevastatin was an elusive participant. To isolate a paltry 23 milligrams of the drug, he had to plow through 600 liters of fungus extract. But still those 23 milligrams might be cardiology's Holy Grail, the bookend to Russell Ross's cause, the way to prevent CAD.

His next step would be the proof. Endo could hardly control his excitement as he tried his drug in laboratory rats. Unknown at that time, blood cholesterol in rats exists predominantly in the form of HDL (good cholesterol). Statins are specific inhibitors of LDL (bad cholesterol) synthesis, with little effect on HDL. He was thunderstruck when the drug had little effect on the rat's total blood cholesterol.

Discouraged, Endo was baffled about where to turn. Just as everyone had predicted, he had invested his life in a project with a dead end.

It was time to visit the local bar. One night a fellow research scientist offered him some chickens he had used for research and was about to sacrifice. Endo could test his drug in another species. Who knows, maybe hens are different from rats. Endo took the offer, and mevastatin lived another day. The hens' cholesterol fell by 50%.

Back on track, he extended his studies to monkeys. Their blood cholesterol promptly fell by 20 to 35%. Endo was thrilled. Sankyo patented mevastatin in 1974 and Endo published his results in 1976. Endo presented his data the same year at the International Symposium on Drugs Affecting Lipid Metabolism in Philadelphia. His report drew little interest from attendees at the symposium. Sankyo executives, confirmed in their skeptical view of Endo's research, and convinced that a blood cholesterol lowering drug would have no important market, deemed Endo's discovery unworthy of further investment. In 1970s Japan, when a boss told an employee to stop, he stopped. No discussion was necessary. Told to quit and without funding, mevastatin and Endo teetered on pharmaceutical oblivion.

But Endo thought differently. Like Werner Forssmann and his catheter in 1929 Germany, Endo accepted his superiors' verdict and yet pursued his own instinct. At Osaka University, four hours' drive away, he knew that Dr. Akira Yamamoto had a cohort of patients with inherited elevated cholesterol level, a rare condition called familial hypercholesterolemia. Yamamoto, with no effective therapy for elevated cholesterol, was delighted to try Endo's compound. Endo got the drug to him. With no idea about what might be an appropriate or inappropriate dose in a human, Yamamoto gave the drug to an eighteen-year-old girl. She promptly developed the most common side effect of statins, muscle weakness. Yamamoto's superiors ordered him to discontinue drug testing. Endo had driven up another blind alley.

But here chance intervened. Yamamoto was as mavericky as Endo. He reduced the dose and secretly tried again in other patients. Yamamoto stared in astonishment as one blood chemistry slip after another piled up on his desk. He was looking at eighty-point drops in blood cholesterol in his patients, an average reduction of 22 to 35%. This astonishing outcome was the largest reduction in blood cholesterol ever recorded. Yamamoto excitedly told Endo that he had found a substance like none he had ever seen before. In today's regulated research environment we cringe at every step in this out-of-control scenario, which would unquestionably result in termination of both investigators and legal proceedings against the pharmaceutical company and clinic for lack of institutional control. Yet Endo had succeeded by listening to his own counsel.

Endo took Yamamoto's results to his bosses at Sankyo. How could they deny such promising results? Suppressing their outrage at Endo's insubordination, and anxious to save face, the bosses reversed course. They agreed to initiate a clinical trial. Endo had cleared his last hurdle. Patience and persistence. Patience had shown him the path to success; persistence had carried him there. If the clinical trial confirmed Yamamoto's results, and he of course believed it would, his dream would become a reality.

Shortly after beginning the trial, the bosses called him into the office. They would continue the trial but Endo did not fit the Sankyo mold. His career at Sankyo was finished. On a bleak December day in 1978, with his fellow workers forbidden to assist him, Akira Endo lugged boxes filled with the shards of his shattered dream to a waiting truck.

Endo had chosen the path less taken, only to discover, like many iconoclasts before him, that it led to a dead end. If Endo wanted to continue his research, it would have to be at Tokyo Noko Agricultural University. But his bosses had decreed that Endo's work on mevastatin would proceed no further; indeed his discovery would never be developed as a drug.

ENDO'S DISCOVERY OF statins and its subsequent abandonment bears a striking parallel to the fascinating story of its moldy cousin penicillin. On September 3, 1928, Scottish chemist Alexander Fleming returned to his laboratory at St. Mary's Hospital from a vacation at his country house. Always untidy, before leaving Fleming had stacked his discarded petri dishes with cultures of staphylococcus bacteria in a corner of the lab for cleaning on his return. As Fleming picked up the long-ignored cultures, he saw that some cultures had circular patches of dead bacteria, with a contaminating fungus in the center.

Fleming reveled in chance discovery. Six years earlier he had chanced upon a similar discovery when his nose inadvertently dripped onto the petri dish. The bacteria died, leading Fleming to discover lysozyme, a natural bacterial inhibitor in human tears and nasal fluid. The discovery proved that a substance capable of killing bacteria could be nontoxic in humans. In the ensuing six years, Fleming had set out to find a practical wonder drug that would have the same effect. He had not found one but now, recalling his prior experience, Fleming decided to investigate further.

Fleming grew the fungus in pure culture, and determined that it was a member of the penicillium genus. The mold turned out to be an airborne contaminant that wafted up from the lab of a mold expert conducting studies on the floor below him. Calling his extract "mold juice," Fleming conducted experiments on cultures of a number of bacteria known to cause infections in humans. He discovered that the juice killed the bacteria that caused scarlet fever, pneumonia, meningitis, and diphtheria. Like Endo, he had discovered a wonder drug. But like Endo, he suffered a similar fate. His publication the following year in the *British Journal of Experimental Pathology* generated little interest in the scientific community.

Fleming persisted, year after year. But he was poorly equipped to carry his discovery further. He had difficulty cultivating the mold, and had even more trouble extracting its antibiotic product. After ten years of searching without success for a collaborator who could isolate a clinically usable penicillin, he abandoned his quest, and moved on to different research. But Europe was now in the second year of World War II, and young men were dying across the battlefields of Europe from minor wounds that blossomed into blood-borne infection throughout the body. Desperate for a wartime antibiotic, the British and U.S. governments authorized funds for discovery of a wonder drug. At Oxford, Australian Howard Florey and his German-Jewish immigrant trainee Ernst Chain took a second look at Fleming's failed discovery. Within a year they had devised a method for purifying and concentrating penicillin by controlling the pH of the mold juice and then freeze-drying it.

But still, the extraction was colossally inefficient, requiring many gallons of juice to produce an amount of brown powder that barely covered a fingernail. That final critical step, an efficient method for extracting penicillin from mold juice, was designed by Florey's lowly graduate PhD student Norman Heatley. Mass production of penicillin began soon after the bombing of Pearl Harbor. Where Fleming's single laboratory could not succeed, the collaboration of thousands of people and thirty-five institutions including universities, government agencies, research foundations, and pharmaceutical companies did. By D-day in 1944 the Allies had sufficient supplies of penicillin to treat all wounded forces, saving countless lives.

Fleming was characteristically humble about his role in one of medicine's greatest discoveries, describing it as the "Fleming Myth." He never failed to laud Florey and Chain for transporting penicillin from his dream to mankind's reality. "I certainly didn't plan to revolutionize all medicine by discovering the world's first antibiotic . . . But I suppose that was exactly what I did," he mused. Fleming, Florey, and Chain received the Nobel Prize in Physiology and Medicine in 1945. But for me, the graduate student Norman Heatley stands as a metaphor for all my young physician-scientist mentees who are sometimes unrecognized contributors to the work of their mentor. As Sir Henry Harris, who succeeded Howard Florey as head of the Dunn School at Oxford, observed, "Without Fleming, no Chain; without Chain, no Florey; without Florey, no Heatley; without Heatley, no penicillin."

WHEN SANKYO ABANDONED him, only one person still believed Akira Endo had discovered an important drug. When Endo presented his research two years earlier at the lipid symposium in Philadelphia, physician scientist Roy Vagelos, a brilliant son of poor Greek immigrants, had just been installed as the new president of Merck pharmaceuticals. Vagelos had excelled everywhere, from college at the University of Pennsylvania, to medical school at Columbia, residency at Massachusetts General Hospital, and research at the National Institutes of Health before becoming chair of the department of biochemistry at Washington University in St. Louis. In his new job at Merck, Vagelos deeply wanted a signature blockbuster drug. CAD was the nation's number one killer. Vagelos knew each step in cholesterol synthesis and he saw that Endo might have found a way to block the most critical one.

After Endo's 1976 oral presentation in Philadelphia, later in Tokyo Merck and Sankyo signed a one-page disclosure agreement granting Merck access to Endo's methods and results. From Sankyo's perspective it was a trivial document. They were discontinuing their research on mevastatin, and if Merck somehow discovered a way to use the drug, Sankyo held the patent. The paper was as worthless as Endo's research.

But history suggests that perhaps there should have been a second page. The agreement failed to protect Sankyo's interest if Merck discovered a different member of the statin family using Endo's methodology. And that was precisely what Vagelos intended to do.

Two years later Merck had succeeded in creating a new system for testing thousands of soil extracts for the elusive cholesterol synthesis inhibitor. In November 1978 as Endo packed his boxes to leave Sankyo, Merck's statin program brought in the gusher. Prepared to test thousands of samples, Merck had discovered a cholesterol synthesis inhibitor in its very first week of testing. Merck called their drug lovastatin. They initiated testing in normal volunteers; lovastatin reduced blood cholesterol with few short-term side effects. But in 1980, Sankyo's animal lab reported that high-dose mevastatin induced intestinal lymphomas in dogs. When Merck learned that Sankyo had terminated their clinical trial because statins caused lymphomas in dogs, Vagelos felt he had to follow suit. He could hardly continue testing a drug in patients if it was known to cause cancer in animals. Cardiology's blockbuster drug was headed to the dustbin of history. Statins were twice dead.

Sometimes a man and an era, like Churchill and World War II, are made for each other. So it was with Vagelos and statins. Hardheaded Roy Vagelos had to see for himself. Vagelos and newly hired research director Edward Scolnick designed their own comprehensive animal laboratory toxicity studies. That decision changed the course of history. The lymphomas reported by Sankyo's investigators turned out to be scientific error. The "tumors" were due to massive doses of the statins. There were no tumors. None at all.

American leaders in lipidology had been searching for a drug that lowered cholesterol. Their first drug, cholestyramine, the source of so many academic insults, was not the answer. It had proven to be impotent and patient-unfriendly. With strong support of physician advocates, Merck was allowed to resume safety and efficacy testing in patients. In November 1986 Merck sent a van from Philadelphia to Washington, where it plopped 104 volumes at the feet of the FDA, to support their claim that their new statin was safe and effective for lowering blood cholesterol. Following a recommendation for approval by its advisory panel, the FDA approved the drug in August 1987, with what may rank as their all-time least-enthusiastic approval. The FDA allowed marketing with the caveat that Merck stipulate that although the drug lowered cholesterol, it had no proven clinical benefit. By now, eleven years had elapsed since Endo's landmark discovery.

Merck finally had its foot in the door. A second more potent cousin of lovastatin, called simvastatin (Zocor) was now ready for testing. Merck initiated a five-year clinical trial. In April 1994, a full eighteen years after Endo's discovery, investigators announced the results of the Scandinavian Simvastatin Survival Study using simvastatin in heart disease patients with elevated blood cholesterol. During five years of follow-up the treated patients had a 35% reduction in their cholesterol, and an astonishing 42% reduction in heart attacks compared to placebo.

For practical purposes, the San Andreas Fault of cardiology disappeared that day. No longer did bitter camps confront each other across the cholesterol divide. The argument was over. The following year, Merck sold over $1 billion of Zocor.

It was just a single number: 42%. But it precipitated a final great paradigm shift, a complete change in our worldview. It had popped up suddenly like the first mountain flower of spring on a desolate landscape. The new fantastic idea, both simple and profound, is: CAD is a preventable disease. The idea dominates today's thinking.

And the Rest of the Story? In 1994 Akira Endo went to see his doctor. Endo's blood total cholesterol was 240 mg/dl, and his LDL cholesterol was 155 mg/dl. "Don't worry, we have very good drugs to lower your cholesterol," his doctor assured him, not knowing that he spoke to the discoverer of statins.

Endo, however, was not forgotten by the scientific community. In 2008 he received the Lasker Award for his labors in a warren next to a south Tokyo train station. The Lasker Award is one of the world's most respected science awards, recognizing those who have made major advances in the understanding, diagnosis, and treatment of human disease. Eighty-three Lasker laureates have received the Nobel Prize, over thirty in the last twenty years. There is still time for Endo.

As Endo received the Lasker award it was too late for vindication of Russian Nicolai Anitschkov, the father of the lipid hypothesis. He had been brought down by the disease he defined, dying of a heart attack on Pearl Harbor Day in 1964. How renowned would he be today had he been born in a different place, in a different world environment? Author Daniel Steinberg muses, "If the full significance of his findings had been appreciated at the time, we might have saved more than 30 years in the long struggle to settle the cholesterol controversy and Anitschkov might have won a Nobel Prize."

In the ensuing chapters, we will begin to imagine strategies to save ourselves, our family members, and our patients with hearts too good to die. And yet, let's pause a moment to recall that but for a nonconformist Japanese and a bullheaded Greek, it seems likely that the word "statin" would never have entered our vocabulary.

24

YOSEMITE

Wake up, O sleeper, rise from the dead, and Christ will shine on you.

—Ephesians 5:14

LET'S SEE HOW everything we learned during those intervening years came to bear on Greta Adams's life. When Greta's heart fibrillated, Jon reacted instantly. "V fib" he shouted and at the same time, like a judge calling for order, slammed the gloved fist of his right hand down hard in the middle of Greta's sternum. Called "the chest thump," this is the first step in treatment of ventricular fibrillation because it induces a weak electric shock to the heart. Rarely the thump will restart a heart in ventricular fibrillation. But above Greta the monitor stayed silent. The electrocardiogram showed ventricular fibrillation and arterial blood pressure was zero, meaning no blood was being pumped to the rest of Greta's body. Jon initiated CPR. Four minutes without blood flow would mean irreversible brain damage and death. Jon was on the clock.

Cupping one hand behind the other and delivering the weight of his body through his shoulders, Jon began rhythmically depressing the middle of Greta's chest. Each thrust depressed her sternum about two inches. Greta's left ventricle was squashed against her vertebrae at a rate of once per second, causing ejection of sufficient blood into the aorta to maintain life. Behind him the lab erupted into controlled frenzy. Well-drilled for emergencies, each person in the lab took action: a terse "Code Blue, two" into a wall phone, a rolling crash cart, syringes filling, lubricating gel on paddles, a defibrillator "arming" to deliver 400 joules of energy. The defibrillator appeared at Jon's side. Jon grabbed its two paddles, pressed one high on Greta's right chest and the other on her left chest below the heart. "Clear!" he shouted, to be sure no one was in direct contact with Greta as the electric jolt went through her. Her body convulsed, then fell back. "Still v fib," Jon shouted. While a technician took over pumping on the chest Jon injected cardiac stimulants through the catheter in Greta's heart and repeated the shock. Still v fib.

An anesthesiologist crashed through the cath lab's double doors. Standing at the head of the cath table, he bent Greta's head back to straighten her trachea (windpipe). Holding open her mouth with his left hand, he inserted an illuminated blade called a laryngoscope into her mouth, then advanced it forward until he could see the vocal cords. He squinted through his narrow field of view, ignoring the bouncing created by the rhythmic pumping on Greta's chest.

"Hold a couple of beats," he said, and at the instant the bouncing stopped he pushed a flexible airway tube past the cords.

"OK to resume," he said after several seconds. He attached a compressible airway bag to the tube and began rhythmic expansion of Greta's lungs. The Code Blue team was now a surrogate for Greta's heart and lung function.

Another try at defibrillation, another failure. Jon grabbed a coronary stent, reasoning that perhaps Greta's left coronary artery obstruction had closed completely. If that was the cause of her sudden death, a stent inserted across the obstruction might open a floodgate of oxygenated blood to her heart. He had never placed a stent in a dead person with a nonbeating heart. It was an experience he hoped never to repeat. As the pumping on Greta's chest bounced her limp body on the table, Jon struggled to maneuver a collapsed stent into Greta's left anterior descending coronary artery until it straddled the obstruction. He inflated a balloon within the stent. The obstruction, crushed into the wall of the blood vessel, disappeared. Later when I reviewed the angiographic images with Jon, I was awed by his technical skill, and the transient eerie image of his technician's hands pressing rhythmically on Greta's chest wall, above her lifeless nonbeating, fibrillating heart.

Jon repeated the cardiac drugs and repeated the defibrillation shock. No effect. Medical cardiology was out of options. For Greta Adams the words of Pope Paul VI now seemed prophetic, "Whatever you want to do, do it now. There are only so many tomorrows." At that moment, it seemed there were no more tomorrows.

Jon had one last arrow in his quiver. Jon reached back to where modern cardiovascular medicine first took root. He called a cardiac surgeon.

"Can you put her on heart-lung bypass?"

"Jon, drop her body temp with a cooling blanket, to diminish her brain's need for oxygen. I'll see you in the OR. But even on the machine, there's only a tiny chance we can get her heart to restart when you can't" was the reply.

Greta's expert team performed consummately coordinated CPR (cardiopulmonary resuscitation). One cath lab technician pumped on her chest sixty times a minute while the anesthesiologist forced air into her lungs, and Jon and his crew lifted Greta's inert body off the cath table, onto a gurney, out of the lab, and raced down the hall to the surgical suite. As soon as they entered, the surgery team focused on connecting a complex system of tubes to Greta's arteries and veins as Jon's crew continued CPR. Greta was being connected to a modern version of John Gibbon's heart-lung machine.

By the time the cardiac surgeon stripped off his mask, Jon and his crew had been manually pumping on Greta's chest for two hours. Neither Jon nor I have ever seen a patient survive without brain damage from this duration of cardiopulmonary resuscitation. In fact, because the chances of recovery are vanishingly small, manual cardiopulmonary resuscitation is rarely continued for two hours.

Jon, emotionally drained, could barely face his next task. He called the hospital chaplain and went to discuss the grim news with Tyler Adams. He could only wait until tomorrow, hoping for a miraculous recovery of heartbeat. Yet even if Greta's heartbeat returned, no one could say whether her brain had survived the cardiac arrest and the brief interruptions of pumping when the tube was inserted into her airway, the stent was placed in her left coronary artery, and she was moved to the surgical suite. Recalling the success of body cooling for preserving brain function in the early days of cardiac surgery, he could only hope that cooling might also be part of Greta's salvation. As she exited the surgical suite, Greta was neither clearly dead, nor clearly alive. She was suspended in cardiac purgatory.

Attached to the machine, Greta was transferred to the surgical recovery room. Tyler, deeply religious, later tearfully recalled for me how he spent the hours of the bleak night and early morning desperately praying, imploring, promising, begging God for Greta's return.

The nursing staff kept the vigil overnight, but no heartbeat returned. In the morning, still with no heartbeat, medical science had run through all its options. What began as a chest thump had progressed through defibrillation, cardiac drugs, tracheal intubation, a stent, hypothermia, and the heart-lung machine. All had failed to restore life.

As science sank exhausted, faith emerged. In the morning Tyler knelt over Greta and begged her to open her eyes. Was that a flicker of movement? It was, so by some otherworldly definition perhaps she was alive. The heart-lung machine had staved off certain death in the limited sense that oxygenated blood was circulating through her body but her brain and heart were ensconced in a metaphorical netherworld, no longer loving yet still much loved.

At her bedside Jon faced a crushing new dilemma. Greta's brain function was undetermined, but quite possibly irretrievably damaged or gone. Had Tyler received an otherworldly message to continue or had Greta entered the realm of futile therapy? On a Friday afternoon, Greta Adams, in the prime of her young life, had been visited by life's most terrifying demon: sudden death. For health-care providers who witness it, it is never forgotten. For the parent, spouse, and children left behind, it is devastating beyond description. But when Saturday morning came, an evanescent response to Tyler's plea could be taken as a sign that Greta might still arise from the ashes of the past eighteen hours.

A doctor's responsibility is to extend life, but it is not to prolong dying. The eighteen-hour battle to maintain Greta's life had sapped Jon's options, his staff, even hope itself. The unpromising choices had become increasingly stark: procrastinate by moving Greta and her machines to the CCU for extended observation or admit defeat and turn them off. If Greta's brain was still intact, but her heart was gone, Jon forlornly argued, perhaps she could have a heart transplant. With little hope but unwilling to give up in the first twenty-four hours of care, Jon sent Greta to the CCU, the modern home of resurrection.

Had Greta reached the Mother of All Uncertainties in which no one could even say if she was alive or dead? An elephant was now in Greta's private CCU cubicle. When was it time to turn off life support? In the euphemism of medicine, should they "see how she does off the machine"? If not now, when?

For millennia, and indeed when I entered medicine, no one needed an expert to say when someone was dead—cessation of heartbeat and breathing meant death. But during my early years in cardiology, science trumped nature. When we became able to maintain these two functions artificially and indefinitely, death demanded redefinition. Death of the brain, as the third organ critical for sentient existence, became the obvious candidate. Assessment of brain death, simple in concept, has proven to be controversial beyond imagination. According to the American College of Neurology, the diagnosis of brain death is made twenty-five to thirty times a year in every major medical center. How do we do it, and wherein lies the rub? The diagnosis of brain death requires the presence of three cardinal criteria: absence of response to painful stimuli (like firm pressure on the nail beds), absence of reflexes (like pupils constricting in bright light) which are mediated by the lowest level of the brain, called the "brain stem," and absence of spontaneous respiration. If a patient is on a respirator, it is turned off to allow observation for spontaneous respiration. All potential causes of temporary and reversible causes of brain suppression, like drug overdose, hypothermia, and confounding conditions such as severe electrolyte and endocrine disturbances must be excluded. When a question remains after clinical assessment, neurologists can use supplemental tests including the recording of brain waves, brain imaging by magnetic resonance imaging or X-ray, and measurement of blood flow into the brain.

The reason that the diagnosis of brain death can become explosively controversial is that a brain-dead person may have spontaneous movements of limbs, or open eyes, or what seems like a facial expression and yet be completely and permanently unaware of their environment. An inexperienced individual, typically a family member, can misunderstand such movement as purposeful, and infer the possibility of recovery. Medical

centers try to prevent these tragedies through a small standing committee of specialists, which provides an independent review and opinion in
such cases.

When disputes over a loved one's state of consciousness burst outside
medical control, the results are often tragic. On an early morning in February 1990 in St. Petersburg, Florida, Terri Schiavo, a pretty raven-haired
thirty-six-year-old, concerned about her weight, but otherwise healthy,
walked down the hallway of the apartment she shared with her husband,
Michael. She had been faithfully pursuing a liquid diet, which included
about ten to fifteen glasses of iced tea daily in an effort to reclaim the figure of her youth. Suddenly she collapsed to the floor, unresponsive. Michael's frantic 911 call brought paramedics who encountered a woman
lying prone in the hallway with no respiration and no pulse. They attempted resuscitation and rushed her to Humana Northside Hospital
where she was intubated (a breathing tube was inserted into her windpipe).
But it was far too late. Lack of oxygen during her cardiac arrest had led to
massive brain damage. On hospital admission her serum potassium level
was noted to be extremely low (2.0 mEq/L, about half the normal
level), probably due to her excessive fluid intake. Very low serum potassium level is a cause of sudden death due to ventricular fibrillation. Terri's
sudden death was one of a brief rash of cardiac arrests in young women
trying the fad liquid diet that quickly disappeared after its risks were recognized.

After ten weeks in a coma, Terri was given the diagnosis of persistent
vegetative state. Her husband, Michael, however, refused to give up. He
flew her to California for an implantation of an experimental electrical
stimulator in her brain. The device induced no benefit. He arranged other
therapies that he hoped might support her return to consciousness; these
too failed. Terri's always-supportive parents, Robert and Mary Schindler,
put Michael up in their home for some months, and gallantly encouraged
him to "get on with his life." Michael even introduced some of his dates
to Terri's parents. But after seven years of completely unsuccessful therapies aimed at restoring her brain function, Michael finally conceded the
irreversibility of Terri's condition. When he discussed removing her feeding tube, however, the Schindlers vigorously opposed him, arguing that
she responded to her environment. In such tense situations, hospitals are

reluctant to act. Michael petitioned the Pinellas County Circuit Court to remove her feeding tube.

Since Terri had no living will, a trial was conducted to assess Terri's own wishes concerning her life support. Neurologists, other physicians, and court-appointed experts testified that Terri had no brain function and that there was no possibility of improvement in her condition. The Schindlers countered that "Terri was a devout Roman Catholic who would not wish to violate the Church's teachings on euthanasia by refusing nutrition and hydration." Based on all the evidence, the court determined that Terri had made reliable oral declarations that she would not wish to continue life support and ordered Terri's feeding tube to be disconnected. Two days after it was disconnected, however, her parents obtained an injunction from a second court, and the tube was reconnected.

Terri's case wandered through a seven-year maze of hearings, petitions, and trials. Among the most compelling pieces of evidence on both sides were images. One court ordered six hours of videotape of Terri with her parents and neurologist. Both the neurologist and the judge after watching all six hours of tape concluded that it provided no evidence of interaction between Terri and her mother. The parents, however, made six still images from the video, which implied consciousness.

The MRI of Terri's brain showed massive loss of tissue. An EEG showed no measurable brain activity. After an October 2003 hearing, her feeding tube was again removed. The parents turned to politicians. Within a week Florida State Representative Frank Attkisson convinced his legislature to pass "Terri's Law," which gave Governor Jeb Bush the authority to order the feeding tube reinserted. Bush ordered reinsertion of the tube. The liberal American Civil Liberties Union represented Terri's husband, Michael, and the conservative American Center for Law and Justice spoke for Terri's parents. Her case finally reached the Florida Supreme Court, which struck down Terri's Law as unconstitutional. When the feeding tube was ordered removed again in 2005, Republicans in the Senate and House of Representatives passed bill S.686, which transferred jurisdiction of Terri's case to the federal courts. President George W. Bush, on vacation in Texas, flew back to Washington to sign the bill.

Soon thereafter, "the Schiavo memo," written by the legal counsel to Florida Republican senator Mel Martinez, created a political uproar. The memo suggested the Schiavo case offered "a great political issue" against Florida Democratic Senator William Nelson, who had refused to co-sponsor the bill. Although Terri's dilemma had attracted powerful sup-port from the religious right, the broader electorate was unconvinced, and Nelson easily won reelection in 2006. Ultimately, the U.S. Supreme Court declined to hear the case, ending the legal saga. Once again the feeding tube was disconnected, and thirteen days later Terri Schiavo's fifteen-year ordeal ended as she finally passed away peacefully on March 31, 2005.

Terri Schiavo's autopsy the following day revealed extensive brain damage. Her brain weighed only 615 grams, barely half that of the brain of a thirty-six-year-old woman of her height and weight. Disarray of the remaining brain cells was apparent under the microscope. There was no possible medical doubt that Terri had lost all cognitive brain function. The MRI, brain wave, and cerebral blood flow analysis years earlier, of course, had already established that there never had been a reasonable medical doubt. Viewing the autopsy evidence, the chief medical examiner stated that the damage was "irreversible, and no amount of therapy or treatment would have regenerated the massive loss of neurons [neurons are brain cells]."

The debate over Terri's consciousness, fueled by well-meaning people not qualified to make such a judgment, was a fiasco that consumed hours of court time and millions of health-care dollars. The Florida courts had heard fourteen appeals. The federal courts had litigated five lawsuits. Both the Florida legislature and the U.S. Congress had passed laws about Terri, and had seen their laws struck down. The U.S. Supreme Court had to re-fuse to consider her case four different times. After all this expenditure of time and treasure, the outcome was the original thoughtful decision made by a deeply concerned husband with his physician consultants. Two polls conducted during the height of the controversy suggest that a large ma-jority of Americans understood the central issue, feeling that the life sup-port decision should rest with Terri's husband, Michael, and that legislative intervention was inappropriate.

GRETA'S CONDITION CARRIED the possibility of evolving in a similar direction. She still responded to painful stimuli, and the pupils of her eyes still reacted to light, so clearly she was not brain-dead. Still, if Greta continued with neither heartbeat nor respiration, the cost of continuing on would be incalculable. Further, even if she recovered cardiac and respiratory function she could emerge, like Terri, in a permanent vegetative state. The best medical judgment, however, said continue on, for one compelling reason: the four-minute rule for brain death. Properly performed CPR provides enough blood flow to the brain to maintain its viability. Greta's CPR had begun immediately after her loss of consciousness, whereas Terri's interval was much longer. And now with the heart-lung machine, she had a reliable source pumping oxygenated blood throughout her body. Jon's strategy and Tyler's prayers rested on the uncertain hope that during the period from her cardiac arrest to turning on the heart-lung machine, Greta's brain had remained intact.

Sometime during that day, no one knows precisely when, Greta's heart contracted once. Then again. Every person in the room stood immobilized like statues, silently staring at the ECG monitor, astonished, transfixed, struggling to focus, denying, disbelieving, believing. There it was. Greta's heart was beating, not powerfully, not regularly, not rapidly, but it was beating. As if awaking from a deep sleep, Greta's heart rubbed its metaphorical eyes and began to wake up. The next day, a small cadre of doctors stood wordless at her bedside, watching the ECG monitor for a full minute. Finally one broke the awed, reverent silence of the congregation.

"Normal sinus rhythm," he said. Greta, still unconscious, had a normal heartbeat and a normal blood pressure. Her heart was suggesting it was ready to return from purgatory. Over the ensuing hours, Greta's heartbeat and blood pressure remained in the normal range, much as we see when a patient comes off the heart-lung after cardiac surgery. Tyler stood at her bedside, engulfed in the tears, hugs, and prayers of family members. Today he chokes up as he recalls those hours when Greta's heart regained its footing while her brain remained silent. Uncertainty, fear, hope, helpless desperation . . . he could only wait and pray.

During the next few days, Greta's brain function returned like a person recovering from a prolonged surgical procedure under anesthesia. As Greta recalls it today, she woke up and looked at her surroundings with a furrowed brow. "What happened? What's going on?" she asked. When Tyler came into the room, she recognized him immediately. In about a week, Greta got out of her bed, and the next day she was able to walk to the bathroom. Greta Adams was back; Mommy would be coming home. But was her marathon now complete, or had she only passed through purgatory to return to her starting line, the catheterization laboratory?

Should she go home to give her some breathing room? Should she return to the scene of her cardiac arrest for coronary angioplasty? Greta's experience was so rare, so unheard of that there was no publication, no textbook to provide advice.

Jon reasoned that he did not know which of the obstructions he saw on her coronary angiogram just before her ventricular fibrillation was responsible for Greta's angina or her ventricular fibrillation. She already had a stent in the left main coronary artery, but she still had an untreated severe stenosis in her right coronary artery. So she was still at risk for sudden death.

Jon concluded that the risk of going home exceeded any potential benefit. Greta would return to the site where her tumultuous journey began, but this time she would undergo right coronary balloon angioplasty. The stent he had placed during her cardiac arrest looked perfect. After a second stent was placed across the plaque in Greta's right coronary artery, she returned home to her family.

With the use of a defibrillator, heart-lung machine, hypothermia, stents, and visits to the operating room and the CCU, Greta had nearly emptied cardiology's metaphorical medicine cabinet. But not quite. With CAD at age thirty-five, the most important step in Greta's care was now about to begin. Analysis of Greta's blood revealed the likely cause of her early development of CAD. Greta had marked elevation of her LDL cholesterol. Greta needed a strategy designed to prevent the development of any new lesions in her coronary arteries and to prevent rupture of any existing plaques for the next fifty years. Before hospital discharge she started on a moderately high dose of a potent statin designed to lower her blood cholesterol into the low normal range. She was told that she would be expected to take the pill for the rest of her life.

About two months after Greta's discharge, Jon called Greta at home to see how she was doing. There was no answer, so he left a message. When she did not return the call in a day or two, he called again, now concerned. Still no answer. So he got out her chart to find her emergency contact, which was Tyler's cell phone. Again he called. No answer. His concern mounting, he left a message.

The next day Greta returned the call. She apologized for missing his call, she said. She and Tyler and Ben were camping, and doing a little hiking, in Yosemite.

THREE YEARS AFTER her hospitalization, Greta, Tyler, Jon, and I got together during a national cardiology conference. I described the book to Greta, Tyler, and Jon, and then asked Tyler to recount the details of Greta's hospitalization as he experienced them. The three of us listened deeply moved in awed silence as deeply religious Tyler recalled every detail of the awful hours following Greta's cardiac arrest. As he spoke Tyler seemed to be watching a long video replay. As image after image passed before him in his mind's eye, he tearfully reexperienced his abject despair, his entreaties to God, his glimmers of hope, and finally his exaltation. It was so moving that at one point I noticed that all four of us had tears in our eyes. In that moment, I marveled how astonishing intellectual breakthroughs in cardiovascular medicine become truly profound when expressed in the life of a single patient. For me, the indelible image of Greta and Tyler, each smiling through their tears, personifies that profound insight.

25

CONQUERING CAD IN OUR LIFETIME

The past informs the present. Memory makes the map we carry, no matter how hard we try to erase it.

—CARA BLACK, AMERICAN MYSTERY NOVELIST

WHEN WE BEGAN our journey at the end of World War II, we encountered disorders of the heart's muscle, valves, electrical system, and arteries. Today, congenital heart disease is repaired early in life, mortality for valve surgery is a few percent, and rhythm disorders are managed with implantable defibrillator-pacemakers and ablation of abnormal electrical circuits in the cath lab. Since my days in Philadelphia, it is fair to say that we have delivered devastating blows to congenital heart disease, valvular heart disease, and disorders of the electrical system. In today's world, that leaves the heart's coronary arteries as our overriding concern. This year's American Heart Association statistics suggest that the lifetime risk for developing atherosclerotic disease at age forty is 2 in 3 for men and 1 in 2 for women. CAD accounts for about a third of our annual mortality, and more than 2,200 Americans die of cardiovascular disease each day. So why do I claim that we are poised to subdue it?

The profound idea that CAD and its devastating complications are preventable is cardiology's new mantra. Let me be explicit: if you have CAD, I now believe that you can arrest its progression, stop it in its tracks.

If you don't have CAD, you can prevent yourself from falling victim. But we know that in medicine, what sounds like an answer immediately raises new questions. Great scientific answers are not endpoints; they are new beginnings. So even as trials show us that CAD and its complications are preventable, to prevent CAD in yourself and your family, we need the answers to three new questions: at what age do atheromas begin to form, can we identify high-risk people before the atheroma begins to form, and can we reverse atheroma formation early in its course?

The answer to our first question, when do atheromas begin to form, has begun to emerge in just the past few years. At the Cleveland Clinic cardiologist Dr. Steven Nissen and his associates used a catheter with a miniaturized ultrasound probe to examine the wall of the coronary artery. In one study they have examined the coronary arteries of 262 donor hearts at the time of cardiac transplantation.

The investigators determined the percentage of donors who had coronary atheromas as a function of their age. It is 15% in fifteen-year-olds, and increases to 60% in thirty- to thirty-nine-year-olds. These shockingly high numbers parallel long-forgotten age-stratified autopsy studies of young soldiers killed in the Korean and in the Vietnam Wars. The conclusion is stunning and undeniable: although coronary atheromas cause symptoms in middle and older age, they actually begin to form in youth.

But can we identify the youth that are at high risk of developing atheroma? In Bogalusa, Louisiana, in the 1970s Dr. Gerald Berenson began a long-term follow-up of children in whom he recorded the risk factors for CAD. When the children were followed into middle age, he found that risk factors present in childhood tracked right into adulthood. So high-risk adults were identifiable as high-risk children. In a subgroup of Bogalusa middle-school children who died in their late teens and early twenties, autopsy showed that those who had more than two risk factors had eight times more atherosclerosis in their aorta than those with no risk factors. In a bizarre mimicry of ourselves, atheromas go through their own adolescence and early adulthood with us before blossoming to full adulthood in middle age. And thus the inescapable conclusion: we can identify people who are at high risk of a heart attack in middle age many years earlier, even as children and young adults.

The insight that CAD begins in youth and that risk can be identified at an early age raises the critical practical question for our times: can we halt and reverse atheroma formation years before symptoms? Our clinical trials show we can prevent the complications created by atheroma rupture, like heart attack and sudden death. But can we prevent atheromas from forming?

An experiment conducted by Mother Nature provides an insight into the potential impact of early prevention. The Atherosclerosis Risk in Communities study collects risk-factor information in four U.S. communities— Forsyth County, North Carolina; Jackson, Mississippi; suburbs of Minneapolis, Minnesota; and Washington County, Maryland. Approximately 3% of this population has a genetic mutation that confers a potentially beneficial 20% lower LDL cholesterol (bad cholesterol). Do these people, with modestly lower LDL cholesterol for a lifetime, do better? Yes, and how! Individuals with this mutation have had a 62% lower rate of cardiac events during the first fifteen years of the population study. An obvious inference is that a low LDL over a lifetime would have a similar impact in young high-risk individuals.

Our most recent statin drug trial confirms this idea. It was conducted in healthy people at high risk of CAD but with no known disease. Possibly someone like you, certainly like someone you know. Monitors stopped the planned five-year trial because they felt it was unethical to continue. After just two years the group randomized to rosuvastatin (Crestor) had a 44% reduction in cardiac events compared to the untreated group, and the gap between the groups appeared to widen each month.

What would you do if you knew the cause of a devastating disease, knew how to identify apparently healthy people at risk before it develops, and possessed the means to prevent the catastrophic illness before it developed? You would take action.

And that is why in November 2011 the Department of Health and Human Services, in partnership with many other organizations including the American Heart Association, announced the Million Hearts initiative. Our immediate stated goal is to prevent 1 million heart attacks and strokes over the next five years. I have not a single doubt that this goal is achievable, because in my personal odyssey I came to learn that CAD is a preventable disease. Last year heart disease ceased to be the leading cause of death in Canada. With Million Hearts, it will no longer be the U.S.'s number one killer. How does the initiative merge the past with the present and the future?

The logic of the Million Hearts initiative is compelling: in the Framingham study, half of the people who experienced a catastrophic heart attack or sudden death had no cardiac symptoms prior to their catastrophe. To overcome the scourge of CAD, therefore, we will have to prevent heart attack and sudden death in patients with no known disease. Our two-pronged approach is disarmingly simple: lifestyle modification and pharmacologic intervention when necessary. Lifestyle modification focuses on diet, exercise, stopping smoking, and controlling high blood pressure. The primary pharmacologic intervention will be medications that reduce the level of bad cholesterol in the blood.

How well have we done over the past twenty-five years, and how well might we do in the future? A 2013 analysis of the National Health and Nutrition Examination Surveys (NHANES) puts numbers on speculation. High blood pressure doubles the risk of CAD. Treatment reduces the risk of heart attack risk by about 25%. The national control of blood pressure has increased sixfold in the past twenty-five years. The control of LDL-cholesterol has improved by a similar magnitude. That's why the mortality rate from CAD has fallen so precipitously. As effective as we have been, however, 70% of individuals who have both high blood pressure and high cholesterol still don't have both risk factors controlled, and the majority is entirely untreated. So there is a huge opportunity for further improvement in this high-risk group. With the Affordable Care Act many of this untreated group will enter the healthcare system, and with the Million Hearts initiative, many more patients will be controlled through either lifestyle modification or drugs. Let's use another of my patient-friends to illustrate what you need to do for yourself and your family.

THE THREE OF us had hilarious times as college fraternity brothers, and the friendships lasted a lifetime. Mort was the college politician and the head cheerleader. He became a university professor and served in the president's cabinet as an adviser on Russia. Donald was the literary and

artistic intellectual who later gained national notoriety as the lead prose-
cutor in one of the great criminal trials of our era. I was the varsity athlete and sportswriter. After graduation, through marriage, children, and
changing jobs, we Three Musketeers held a reunion once or twice a year
where we endlessly retold glorious tales of yesteryear. When we were in
our early fifties, the reunion was a Texas-UCLA football weekend in Los
Angeles. Both friends flew in from Houston.

Donald is a big man, about six foot two inches. In the thirty years
since college, he had put on about forty pounds. He was a partner in one
of Houston's high-stress corporate law firms that bore his name. He lived
life with joie de vivre; a cultured connoisseur of wine and art, he always
had a big toothy smile, and another witty story to tell. In our college years,
one of our friends toured the dorms a couple times a week handing out
free packs of Winston cigarettes, four to a pack. That's how we started
smoking. I stopped, Donald didn't. He now had a three pack-a-day habit.

Late Sunday night, as we waited outside a restaurant for a taxi to take
my friends and their wives back to the airport, Donald pulled me aside,
and casually, as if he were describing one of the abstract paintings that
hang on his living room wall, said, "Jim, I felt some discomfort in my chest
when I walked up the Rose Bowl steps yesterday at halftime. I've been
fine since. I figure it was the chopped onions I put on those two hot dogs."
He postscripted an apology, "Nothing to worry about, I know, but you
being a doctor, I thought I might as well mention it to you."

Donald might as well have dangled from the nearby overpass and casually said, "Hey, look." Really? Nobody, least of all a lifelong friend, gets
a free pass after casually informing a cardiologist that he's just started having chest pain with exercise. I yanked Donald out of earshot of the others
and launched an inquisition. His discomfort had first come on a couple of
weeks earlier walking up a hill after lunch to a rental car in San Francisco. He had experienced several episodes since that time. Each episode
had its onset with either physical or emotional stress. Sometimes the discomfort went from behind his breastbone into his left arm. It was relieved
in about a minute by rest. He had not mentioned the symptoms to anyone
before me. An overweight fiftysomething smoking man in a high-stress
occupation had just described typical angina, defined by its location,

precipitation, and relief. I was momentarily dumbfounded. How could an intelligent person have such alarming symptoms, act as if he felt fine, and withhold such information until the last critical moment?

"Donald, do you know what you have? It's what we call new onset typical angina." I explained the three characteristics of angina, and what it implied. "In a fifty-year-old man who smokes, this means you have a 95% probability of having coronary heart disease. People with recent onset angina are at significant risk of a heart attack."

"Maybe I'm overreacting," I said. Willie the Phillie's face flashed before me. "But with recent onset angina you never know what will happen next. Donald, I want you to come in to my hospital . . . as in now."

Donald's jaw fell like Facebook's opening stock price. Yet he emphatically shook his head and looked away, unwilling to make the transition from reunion reveler to invalid in a matter of seconds. "You're right, you're overreacting."

The taxi pulled up and the other three passengers clambered in, urging Donald to quit dawdling on the curb. And so, in a few seconds, I faced a quandary. Over outraged protests I could demand everyone get out, send the taxi away, and involve Donald's wife, Mort, and Mort's wife in the decision. Confronting uncertainty, I waffled. I chose the route less challenging.

"OK, Donald, if you're going to disagree and fly home," I hissed, "I am calling my cardiologist friend Sanjay in Houston. I am going to ask him to see you first thing tomorrow morning, and I want you there in his office. And one other thing. Not one cigarette between now and then."

Donald, looking pale, grim, and shaken, nodded. He squeezed into the taxi. As the taxi's taillights disappeared. I felt a wave of guilt. I knew the safest course, and in the pressure and uncertainty of that transient moment, I had acquiesced in what I believed was a second-best solution. Now I stood silently asking myself what if the unlikely happens between now and tomorrow morning? Was Donald on the cusp of becoming a statistic?

Sanjay saw Donald on Monday. Donald had smoked nervously on the way to Sanjay's office, and then had another episode of angina while Sanjay was examining him. He moved quickly to record Donald's ECG during the pain. It was profoundly abnormal. Sanjay called me to say that he recommended that Donald have an immediate coronary angiogram.

The bad news came quickly. The angiogram revealed that Donald had multiple atheromas in all three major vessels of the heart. For relief of his angina Sanjay and I agreed that Donald needed bypass surgery. I knew the city's leading bypass surgeon quite well from working on national committees together over the years, so I called him. More bad news. He was on his way out of town for the next two weeks, so the best younger member of his team would operate. I did not know the surgeon, but after talking with him, I felt he was the best alternative since I felt Donald needed urgent surgery.

I spoke to Donald that night. Dread whistled through the fiber-optic lines.

"You'll be fine," I reassured him. I thought he would be.

Immediately after surgery I spoke with the surgeon, who was pleased with his surgical result. A week later Donald had come through surgery without difficulty and was ready for hospital discharge. I had a feeling of deep satisfaction that my medical training had helped Donald emerge from his personal fog of war.

Then disaster struck. Donald returned to his high-stress legal practice. Soon thereafter he called to relate what he said was the most frightening moment of his life. He had walked uphill to a rental car in another city. As he opened the door he felt the onset of crushing chest pain. Unable to breathe, he collapsed onto the car seat, thinking that he was about to die. After a few minutes, however, the pain gradually abated. My first thought was that one of Donald's vein bypass grafts had closed. The saphenous vein bypass graft closure rate was about 15% in the first year at that time; internal mammary artery (IMA) grafts almost never closed. Donald had had both types of grafts, since he needed multiple bypasses, more than is possible with the IMAs only. In such situations we attach the IMA to the left anterior descending (LAD), because as "the widow maker" it is the most important heart vessel. I called Sanjay and we quickly agreed we needed to see Donald's blood vessels again. He needed repeat angiography. The angiogram showed that I had been only partly right; I was in the right church but the wrong pew. Donald had the misfortune to suffer a complication I have only seen once, thank God.

Unrecognized by the young surgeon at the time of the procedure, he had twisted the IMA almost 180 degrees when he attached it to the LAD. With restricted blood flow, the twisted graft had finally closed off. I called my surgeon friend. He was deeply apologetic. "We are all terribly distressed about the technical mistake that occurred in my OR," he said. "I have to tell you that with that graft closed, we have no surgical options. We think that the amount of disease he has in his coronaries makes his prognosis pretty poor." Donald was not a candidate for angioplasty and his surgical option had blown up in our faces.

In the short time that he had returned to work, Donald had not lost weight. He was not going to slow down. With the surgery option eliminated, our only option was prevention. Donald's survival was going to be dependent on changing his diet, starting an exercise program, losing weight, stopping smoking, and medication to drastically reduce his bad LDL. It seemed that Donald had not taken good health practices seriously over his first fifty years. With Donald's history, Sanjay and I were not optimistic that we would be able to prevent a future heart attack.

As Donald's medical brain trust gloomily viewed his future, we did not realize that when he had the edifying experience of impending doom in his rental car Donald had undergone a foxhole conversion. He stopped smoking. He changed to a healthy diet. He lost thirty pounds in weight and maintained it. And, he initiated a daily exercise program.

WE STARTED WITH diet. But how in the world are you to sort out useful facts from the often-conflicting cacophony of advice on diet? The good news is that in 2002, someone did the work for us. At the Harvard School of Public Health scientists Drs. Frank Hu and Walter Willett analyzed data from 147 studies of the influence of diet on heart disease. Their conclusions are unequivocal: "Compelling evidence from metabolic studies and clinical trials in the past several decades indicates that at least three dietary strategies are effective in preventing coronary heart disease: substitute non-hydrogenated unsaturated fats for saturated and trans fats; increase consumption of omega-3 fatty acids from fish, fish oil supplements, or plant sources; and consume a diet high in fruits, vegetables, nuts, and whole grains and low in refined grain products."

But they also tell us what is not known: "simply lowering the percentage of energy from total fat in the diet is unlikely to improve lipid profile or reduce CHD incidence." In simple terms, the long-revered low fat diet is not going to do much to your cholesterol or reduce your risk for CAD. And finally they tell us what remains controversial: "Many issues remain unsettled, including the optimal amounts of monounsaturated and poly-unsaturated fats, the optimal balance between omega-3 and omega-6 polyunsaturated fats, the amount and sources of protein, and the effects of individual phytochemicals, antioxidant vitamins, and minerals." In case you feel yourself fading back into confusion, they offer this broad conclu-sion: "Substantial evidence indicates that diets using non-hydrogenated unsaturated fats as the predominant form of dietary fat, whole grains as the main form of carbohydrates, an abundance of fruits and vegetables, and adequate omega-3 fatty acids can offer significant protection against CHD. Such diets, together with regular physical activity, avoidance of smoking, and maintenance of a healthy body weight, may prevent the ma-jority of cardiovascular disease in Western populations."

How much does poor diet influence the appearance of CAD? In 2012, a twenty-two-year follow-up study of 42,000 men analyzed one compo-nent of diet, soda consumption. The impact is startling. As Dr. Frank Hu of the Harvard School of Public Health summarized, "Even a moderate amount of sugary beverage consumption—we are talking about one can of soda every day—is associated with a significant 20% increased risk of heart disease." According to a July 2012 Gallup poll, however, nearly half of U.S. adults, 48%, report drinking at least one glass of soda per day, with soda drinkers averaging 2.6 glasses daily. So independent of your opinion of New York mayor Michael Bloomberg's quixotic ban on sale of soft drinks greater than sixteen ounces in retail food establishments, his heart and his thinking are in the right place, if preventing early death from CAD is a societal goal.

But really, how important is diet? A landmark 2012 study that analyzed data from forty countries suggests it is very important. In patients with known CAD a heart-healthy diet—rich in fruits, vegetables, nuts, whole grains, and fish—was associated with a reduced risk of cardiovascular death by 35%, second heart attack by 14%, stroke by 19%, and congestive heart failure by 28%, compared with those eating the poorest diet. While the study surely will not end the diet debates, it will have an impact on cardiologists' practice. Dr. Robert Eckel of the University of Colorado, who was not involved in the study, commented: "This is the kind of evidence we need; it's incredibly encouraging. I've been in the clinic today and I can't tell you how many times I've emphasized a heart-healthy diet to patients."

Why are these diet elements good or bad in relationship to what we know about atheroma formation and plaque rupture? Fish, fruits, nuts, and tea are good, most likely because they are high in antioxidants like omega-3s and a long list of other less well-known potent antioxidants. Antioxidants are important because they are anti-inflammatory. Inflammation plays a role in plaque formation and is the predominant force in plaque rupture. I agree with my friend Dr. David Agus, author of the bestseller *The End of Illness*, that individual diet supplements have not been shown to decrease CAD. The fiber in leafy vegetables is good, most likely because it accelerates intestinal transport and decreases intestinal absorption of unhealthy foods. The bad elements are trans fats, which are fats that are solid at room temperature, like lard, butter, and margarine. Milk fat and animal fat is bad. These dietary components are bad predominantly because they elevate blood cholesterol, increase its oxidation, and increase the expression of inflammatory substances. Simple carbohydrates like glucose (sugar) and fructose (sugar derived from corn) are bad because they predispose to increased fat storage, and ultimately to diabetes. Since bakery goods are high in trans fats, and soft drinks are high in sugar, these foods are particularly poor dietary choices.

Finally, in 2013 came a randomized trial that may end the debate about what diet is best, at least among cardiologists. The five-year trial compared the Mediterranean diet (fish, vegetables, fruit, nuts, extra virgin olive oil, red wine in moderation) compared to a low fat diet, conducted in people who had no known cardiovascular disease but were at high CV risk. The Mediterranean diet had a 30% lower rate of heart attack, stroke, and cardiovascular death even though they were not required to reduce their caloric intake. If you are not on this diet, consider it. It is precisely my own diet. I drink red wine because it is high in potent antioxidants. Red wine, however, has a U-shaped curve relative to risk. Excessive wine raises blood pressure and adds abdominal fat. Sixty years after Minnesota nutritionist Ancel Keys's studies initiated the low fat craze for preventing heart disease, this diet itself may have breathed its last. I was pleased to see Donald order grilled salmon, a salad, and red wine at our most recent dinner a few months ago, although I secretly wished he had left a little more of the Cabernet for me.

THE SECOND STEP in Donald's lifestyle modification is exercise. It should be yours as well, if you want to prevent CAD. Exercise improves the level of both good and bad cholesterol, lowers blood pressure, diminishes inflammation, and promotes weight loss. In diabetics, it favorably affects insulin utilization. In addition, exercise improves oxygen utilization by muscles, allowing individuals with compromised cardiac function to perform a wider range of daily activities. In contrast sedentary lifestyle is one of the American Heart Association's five risk factors for CAD, along with abnormal lipids, hypertension, obesity, and smoking. Physical inactivity is a worldwide problem. In a 2012 Harvard Medical School investigators found that global mortality attributable to physical inactivity is similar to cigarette smoking (more than 5.3 million deaths per year vs. 5 million deaths per year). Worldwide, a sedentary lifestyle was associated with a 16% increase in the risk of CAD and a 20% increased risk of diabetes mortality, along with increased risk of breast and colon cancer death. In the United States, 250,000 deaths annually are attributed to sedentary lifestyle.

Donald, of course, wanted to know the minimum of amount of exercise necessary to maintain good health. So here it is from the Surgeon General: "Every American should participate in thirty minutes or more of moderate intensity activity on most, and preferably all, days of the week." This level of activity is any exercise equivalent to brisk walking (three to four miles per hour), cycling, yard work, or swimming. This amount of activity is equivalent to 600 to 1,200 calories per week. Less than this amount is considered sedentary. A modicum of good news: you do not have to do your thirty minutes of penance all at once, you just have to do it. Donald agreed to hit the minimum target. The Surgeon General also notes that "Less than one third of adults meet the minimal recommendation for exercise. The combination of excess caloric intake and decreased exercise is responsible for the worldwide obesity epidemic."

If you are willing to run, that's good. But there are some facts you probably do not know about running that you should. Running is a special case of exercise. The greatest reduction in CAD mortality occurs when an individual moves from sedentary to becoming moderately active. Less is gained in moving from moderately active to very active. A recent report from the Aerobics Center Longitudinal Study, which includes 52,000 men and women with no known CAD, reveals a stunningly unanticipated outcome. A quarter of the group used running as a form of exercise. During fifteen years of follow-up 2,984 participants died. Runners had a 19% lower mortality rate than nonrunners. No surprise there. The fascinating and unexpected outcome was that people who ran ten to fifteen miles weekly had a whopping 27% reduction in death rate whereas running more than twenty-five miles per week had only a 5% reduction. Similar differences were found between people who ran six to seven miles compared to eight or more miles per hour, and running two to five days per week vs. six to seven days per week. So the benefits of running are best achieved with moderate levels rather than at greater distances, running speed, and frequency. At high levels of running, the relationship between mortality and running trends back toward less benefit. Running, like red wine, has a U-shaped curve relative to risk. As investigator Dr. Carl Lavie wryly observed, "The fact that it reached its plateau at such a low level is surprising, as is the fact that it didn't level off but actually went the other way. We never had a point where runners did worse than non-runners, but really, if you put it in almost a joking way, it showed that if you ran enough you got yourself back to the level of a couch potato. You lost the survival advantage."

ARGUABLY THE MOST strenuous of all athletic competitions is marathon running. In 490 BC, Persian King Darius sent his powerful army to attack the Greeks at Marathon. Pheidippides was a forty-year-old Greek courier who ran to Sparta to ask for support. Over two days he ran 150 miles. Arriving at the Marathon battlefield from Sparta he was amazed to learn that the Greeks had defeated the Persians. He ran the 26.2 miles back to Athens, extended his arms in exaltation, and proclaimed, "Joy to you, we've won." Pheidippides then collapsed and died. In 1879 Robert Browning's poem "Pheidippides" inspired founders of the modern Olympic Games to invent the 26.2 mile marathon. Pheidippides's death is the first report of sudden cardiac death in a long-distance runner.

The London Marathon is a public spectacle. I love the camaraderie that envelops the entire city, the sweaty runners, the pubs' cold beer, and the sin of deep-fried fish and chips. Loosening up at the starting line of the London Marathon on a crisp April 2012 Greenwich morning was thirty-year-old Claire Squires. With her hair pulled back in a ponytail to reveal fine facial features and a gorgeous smile, Claire was slim and fit, looking forward to a soggy embrace with Simon Van Herrewege, her boyfriend of three years, who waited at the end of a serpentine 26-mile-385-yard course. In the meantime she would have a glorious tour of London past hundreds of thousands that lined the streets, before ending her run in St. James mall near Buckingham Palace.

Claire was one of 37,000 people taking part that year. Claire was a fitness buff, having both climbed Africa's highest mountain, Tanzania's Mount Kilimanjaro, and run in the London Marathon the previous year. This year was special. She was running for the Samaritan Charity to honor her brother Grant, who had died of drug overdose at age twenty-five, and for her mother Cilla's twenty-four years of Samaritan volunteer work. From Greenwich, Claire headed east toward the halfway point at Tower Bridge, continued along the Thames River into Canary Wharf, then wended west into the final leg of the race, past the Tower of London. Nearing the finish she glimpsed London's iconic Big Ben and Westminster Abbey as she prepared to turn onto Birdcage Walk for the final 385 yards of her run. Soon after turning, Claire stumbled and fell. She lay motionless on the ground. First responders attempted cardiac resuscitation. An ambulance transported her to the hospital but to no avail. Her death was the tenth in the London Marathon since it began in 1981, and the first since a twenty-two-year-old fitness instructor died in 2007. Autopsies revealed that at least five of the prior fatalities were attributable to undiagnosed heart disease, of which four were CAD. The next day Claire's lovely smile graced every English tabloid. The tragic loss of such a young vital life deeply moved Londoners. Donations to Claire's charity rose from 500 pounds to 1 million pounds in the days that followed, as Claire was buried next to her brother.

* * *

CLAIRE'S DEATH RAISES the question of how often sudden death occurs in athletics and how it might be prevented. Italian studies suggest the sudden death rate in strenuous competitive sports is about 1 in 50,000 athletes. Similar numbers have been compiled in the United States by the National Collegiate Athletic Association. The incidence of sudden cardiac death in college-aged athletes is 1:43,000. The risk varies widely with both ethnicity and sport. At higher risk are male athletes (1:33,000), black male athletes (1:13,000), and male basketball players (1:7,000). The basis of these wide disparities is as yet unexplained. Intense physical exertion in athletic participation does increase the risk of sudden death. An Italian study reported a 2.5 greater risk for youth participating in sports compared with age-matched noncompeting population. But striking as these numbers may seem, they are arguably misleading. If we look at risk during the period of exercise, it is much higher. Swedish investigators studied risk in 926,000 competitive cross-country skiers over ninety years. Although the absolute risk was similar to runners, during the period of skiing itself the risk of sudden death was a hundredfold higher.

We now have a database to assess the rate of sudden death among marathon runners. In *The New England Journal of Medicine,* researchers from the Massachusetts General Hospital reported that 2 million people run in marathons and half marathons each year. The number has more than doubled since the turn of the century. The investigators used the Race Associated Cardiac Arrest Event Registry (RACER) database to determine the incidence of sudden death during or within one hour of completing the race in the United States between January 1, 2000, and May 31, 2010. Among 10.9 million marathon runners 59 experienced cardiac arrest. Their average age was 42; 86% were men. The rate was 1 in every 184,000 runners. Cardiac arrest was higher in full-marathon than half marathon participants, and higher in men than women. Senior investigator Dr. Aaron Baggish saw the results this way, "You're much less likely to have a cardiac arrest as a middle-aged marathon runner than you are as a college athlete, as somebody who's doing triathlons, or even as somebody who's out doing casual recreational jogging." From the Italian and American databases, roughly one in 50,000 to 150,000 marathon runners will experience a cardiac arrest. The New York Marathon now has almost 50,000 participants yearly, so we should not be surprised when an event occurs.

How should we screen an athlete for his/her risk of sudden death? For nonprofessional athletes, we have no agreement among recognized authorities. At one end of the spectrum is Italy, where athletes are not permitted to participate in minor sports without having had a medical history, physical examination, and ECG. Data from the Venice region of Italy, where athletes at all levels are banned from competition based on potentially hazardous conditions, clarifies these issues. The program slashed the number of sudden cardiac deaths in athletes by 90%—from 3.6 per 100,000 person-years in 1979/1980 to 0.4 per 100,000 person-years in 2003/2004. To achieve this result, the program disqualified 2% of all athletes. We can calculate that for every death prevented, about 1,000 athletes are needlessly banned from competing.

Whereas Italy has focused on preventing sudden death, North America has emphasized the limitations of cost and access, and the fact that false positives would send an unknown number of healthy kids to the sidelines. A study in the November 27, 2012, issue of the *Journal of the American College of Cardiology* calculated the Medicare reimbursement rate for the cost of pre-participation physical exam and ECG screening to be $263 per athlete. Projected for 8.5 million U.S. athletes the authors estimated that this program would cost more than $10 million per life saved, and that if followed for twenty years, it would cost $50 billion to save 4,800 lives. The numbers were disputed by an editorial written by Dr. Antonio Pelliccia of the Institute of Sport Medicine and Science in Rome. Pelliccia says ECG screening in Italy's mandatory screening program costs $60 per athlete, which most athletes can afford, and that it is reimbursed for those unable to pay. The American Heart Association and the American College of Cardiology and the Canadian Heart and Stroke Foundations do not recommend the use of ECGs for cardiovascular screening of athletes, whereas the European Society of Cardiology and the International Olympic Committee do.

Squires's death in London reignited the controversy over a universal screening approach for the 10,000 athletes in the upcoming 2012 Olympic Games. London cardiologist Sanjay Sharma, who heads the only sports cardiology clinic in the UK, screened the entire cadre of 1,000 potential English Olympians on thirty-two different squads, with the aim of identifying conditions that could potentially cause sudden cardiac death. Sharma's team identified 2 athletes with an abnormal extra electrical conduction pathway called Wolff-Parkinson-White syndrome, a known cause of sudden death. The athletes were told they would be required to have a catheter treatment to destroy the extra pathway before competing in the Olympics. At the same time the International Olympic Committee recommended that all countries conduct ECG screening, and if it was questionable, additional tests be considered. Most commonly the logical additional test would be an echocardiogram.

Dr. Sharma makes two arguments for this more extensive screening: "Our own experience of screening high-level athletes is that about one in one hundred has a condition that is congenital and could potentially cause problems later in midlife—such as heart failure or the heart becoming hypertrophied. And one in 300 harbors a condition that could potentially kill instantly. . . . Sadly, only 20% of athletes with these conditions manifest any symptoms whatsoever. Sudden death is often the first presentation." Furthermore, he argues, "we spend millions and millions on octogenarians to get back two or three years, and nothing on the youngsters to get back seventy years of life."

Among elite athletes in professional sports, those competing in basketball, football, soccer, and swimming are at increased risk. For this reason, professional athletes in European and American soccer and in the National Basketball Association, National Football League, National Hockey League, and Major League Baseball now all have screening ECGs. For the London Olympics Sharma positioned at least one automated external defibrillator for every mile of the marathon, and added bicycle responders in between carrying defibrillators. As Sharma says, "We need to get to that individual within two minutes if they are in ventricular fibrillation. With the system now in place, I believe the same protocol should now be done in the London Marathon." Think of it this way. With roughly 40,000 runners, we should expect a cardiac arrest every two to four years. I agree with Sharma that when defibrillation is applied very rapidly in a heart too good to die, the victim has a very good chance of full recovery. The 2012 Olympic Games had no cardiac arrests among the world's athletes.

And so we come to the critical personal question. Assuming that you or a loved one competes in athletics, do you deserve the same consideration as the Olympic and the professional athletes, particularly since your risk may be higher than a conditioned athlete's? As public policy an ECG and echocardiogram for every athlete would destroy our health-care budget. On the other hand, I do feel that if you are competing in a strenuous sport and are willing to pay for the tests, an ECG and possibly an echocardiogram is not an unreasonable investment. The risk is quite low, but of course the return may be quite high.

How bad is living at the other end of the spectrum, a sedentary life? In 2014 a study in the *Journal of the American Heart Association* funded by the Spanish government reported the outcomes of 13,000 healthy young university graduates, average age thirty-seven, followed over eight years. During that period 97 deaths occurred, less than the expected number of the Spanish population of the same sex and age. The striking finding was that watching television for more than three hours a day was associated with a twofold increased risk of premature death, compared to less than an hour per day. Dr. Miguel Ángel Martínez-González of Pamplona's University of Navarra concludes, "Our findings suggest that 1 or even 2 hours of television viewing is OK, but spending more than 3 hours watching television is probably not a good idea." How relevant are these data to our daily lives? Other studies have shown a correlation between hours of TV viewing and the development of diabetes, the risk of CAD, and mortality. Perhaps it depends on what you do when you sit: the investigators found no association between either time spent in front of a computer or driving time and mortality. Dr. Martínez-González speculates that, "Because television viewing is likely to be associated with snacking and consumption of sugar-sweetened beverages, a possible explanation could be a difference in energy intake."

I CAN SPECULATE what would have happened if my friend Donald had not changed his lifestyle. When diet and exercise are ignored, we run the risk of obesity. In early 2012 the Institute of Medicine, a nonpartisan organization of medicine's leaders, drew the depressing conclusion that obesity "constitutes a startling setback to major improvements achieved in other areas of health during the past century." Two-thirds of adults and one-third of American children are now overweight. In the United States in the mid-1980s the prevalence of obesity in every state was less than 20%; today it is greater than 20% in every state. In Mississippi, the fattest state, 32.5% of adults are obese. The twentieth-century was the smoking century, the twenty-first is now the obesity century. The annual cost of illness related to obesity in the United States approaches $200 billion.

We are now for the first time seeing adolescents with type 2 diabetes, essentially diabetes caused by obesity, a disease that previously only occurred in adults. In May 2012 the Centers for Disease Control and Prevention published a survey of 3,000 youths ages twelve to nineteen. An astonishing 21% of the adolescents had already had diabetes or pre-diabetes, and fully half of overweight teens had abnormal levels of blood pressure, blood cholesterol, or blood sugar. How did this happen? More than 90% of diabetic adolescents eat more than the daily recommendations of saturated fat and one-third watch TV for more than two hours a day. These are the risk factors for a heart attack. We know that kids at risk become adults at risk. Earlier I said that I was certain that the Million Hearts initiative is achievable; I did not say I was certain it would be. Our kids and their permissive parents are doing us in. If you have a significantly overweight child, take care of him/her. It's what parents do.

The handmaiden of obesity is diabetes. Most diabetics die of cardiovascular disease. How does diabetes lead to CAD? After we eat, our blood level of fat and glucose (sugar) increases, triggering the release of insulin. Insulin is the body's deliveryman, responsible for clearing fat and glucose from the blood into the cells. When caloric intake exceeds energy expenditure, however, glucose and fat do not get cleared completely from the blood. The persistent elevation of glucose and fat triggers continued insulin secretion. The body's cells compensate for persistently increased blood level of insulin by becoming resistant to it, aggravating conventional risk factors like high blood pressure. Good HDL cholesterol falls and bad LDL rises. High levels of bad cholesterol lead to it being trapped in the blood vessel wall as the low levels of good cholesterol reduce cholesterol egress. After years in this condition, the pancreatic cells, which synthesize insulin, become exhausted. As this happens full-blown diabetes emerges.

Diabetes is the perfect storm for CAD, raising blood lipids and blood pressure, oxidizing LDL cholesterol, and creating chronic inflammation that affects every blood vessel in the body. The worst-looking coronary angiograms I have ever seen, with every millimeter of every vessel covered with atherosclerosis, belong to diabetics. And that is why, on the brink of victory over CAD, we must also admit the possibility of defeat, not at the hands of the enemy, but ourselves.

AFTER HIS LIFESTYLE conversion, Donald's LDL cholesterol was still in the 150 mg/dl range. We needed to bring it into the normal range. Yet here is the deepest irony of cardiology: we do not know the normal range of LDL cholesterol. Among people without signs or symptoms of CAD in the United States, the value for bad LDL cholesterol is now about 120 mg/dl, but we know from Framingham that half the people who had a heart attack or sudden death had no symptoms prior to their cardiac catastrophe. In other words, on the day before their catastrophe they would have been members of the "clinically normal" population.

But Mother Nature is giving us some advice about the normal level of blood cholesterol if we will only listen. Humans are the only species that spontaneously develop CAD. No wild animal in the entire animal kingdom develops atherosclerosis. So intrepid epidemiologists have measured blood cholesterol in wild animals like the elephant, bear, wild pig, and rhinoceros. The average LDL in wild animals is approximately 60 mg/dl (recall the average U.S. adult has twice this value). The entire wild animal kingdom is also pursuing a healthy lifestyle without atheroma or heart attacks. (The Angus steer that donated the steak you had last night, however, is not of this group because it was specially prepared for you by the cattle industry to have delicious "marbling.") Let's look at humans with the animal kingdom in mind. We are born with an LDL level in the same range as animals. It gradually increases as we get older. A few adult human populations, however, do not exhibit this progressive increase in LDL with age. The world's remaining hunter-gatherer societies, diverse in geographic location and ethnicity, but arguably living the way humanity did 10,000 years ago, have LDL levels in the range of the rest of the animal kingdom. In modern societies, rural Chinese blood levels often fall within this range. And here is the most important trivia you've never heard. Among this diverse group of humans, CAD is rare. The consistency of these diverse human data sources, taken together with the

mammalian species data, supports the idea that the normal range of LDL
in adult humans is approximately 40 to 70 mg/dl.

Does lowering LDL into this range translate into measurable beneficial clinical outcomes? The most recent trial of this idea showed that
reduction of LDL cholesterol from 108 mg/dl to 55 mg/dl in high-risk
patients without known CAD resulted in a 44% reduction in actual cardiac events over a two-year period. The results were considered sufficiently
powerful that an independent safety monitoring board called for the trial
to be stopped, believing that it was unethical to withhold treatment from
the placebo group. In patients whose LDL level reached values less than
50mg/dl, an even greater reduction in adverse events occurred. Sanjay and
I chose to reduce Donald's LDL to 70 mg/dl using statin therapy, and we
were successful.

My message for you is that lower is better. In my view, if you have
CAD or diabetes, you should be taking a statin and your LDL cholesterol should be in the 70s or lower. If you do not have CAD, still aim for
the same level. It's the same disease, whether or not we have symptoms.

Not everyone, of course, needs a statin. Can you assess your risk of
having CAD if you have no symptoms? Yes, but it can cost you as much
as $200. We cannot spend that amount of money on every adult because
it would destroy our health-care budget. None of our tests are perfect, but
two stand out as superior to all others. These are the two I would ask you
to focus on. The first is the risk score used in our national guidelines, which
includes age, smoking, diabetes, blood pressure, and blood lipids. The score
provides your ten-year risk of a cardiac event. The blood lipid test runs
about $75, and is covered by all insurance plans. You should have the test
every five years after age 20. Our guidelines urge that you begin statin
therapy if you have a greater than 7.5% risk of a heart event in the next
ten years. Your doctor can calculate your risk.

Setting the guideline at 7.5% risk for ten years is a wise suggestion,
but quite honestly, it is insufficient for you and me. We know that among
those classified as low risk by the risk score, more than a third already
have CAD. How do we detect these people, who also clearly need statin
therapy?

The second test, calcium scanning, is more specific. If you have calcium in your coronary arteries, you have CAD. Period. The amount of

calcium in your coronary arteries also is given a score, and it also predicts your ten-year risk. If there is no calcium (your calcium score is zero) your chances of a heart event in the next decade are vanishingly small. So if your LDL is low and you have no calcium in your coronary arteries, why take a statin?

If you want to prevent that cardiac catastrophe and you can afford to spend a couple hundred bucks, do these two tests. Your doctor can then design a risk modification program for you. What about me? Twenty-five years ago I had an LDL of 160 and just a wisp of calcium in my coronary arteries. I started on a statin. Today I have an LDL of 70 and no increase in the calcium in my coronary arteries. And that's the way it will be when I hit age ninety.

How much does a statin cost? The prices for a generic statin vary widely. On the Internet I found pricing for $19 per month, but some chains like Walmart have plans for as little as $4 per month. If you were taught to pinch pennies (I was), be like me: get yourself a pill splitter for less than ten dollars, ask your doctor to double the dose of your statin pill, and then cut your pill, and bill, in half.

Given the cost of treating the complications of angina and heart attack, health-care economists have begun to wonder about applying a similar strategy in the entire population. The irony is that the cheapest strategy is to put everyone on a generic statin. Crazy? Maybe not. Two of my boys, both athletes, had an elevated LDL in their thirties, did not bother with the calcium scan, both take a statin, and their bad cholesterol is in the 70s. They experience no side effects from the drug. Many cardiologists might disagree, but my opinion is that, like me, they are better off than they were with an LDL in the 160s.

Among all the drugs I prescribe, generic statins are low risk and inexpensive. If you have an elevated LDL, talk to your doctor about a statin. For many of us it's a very worthwhile inexpensive investment, provided you can take the pill with no side effects.

WE STARTED WITH statistics so let's end with them. In December 2012 pathologist Bryant Webber compared autopsy results from 3,832 service members who died in Afghanistan and Iraq to similar studies performed in the Korean and Vietnam wars. In the Korean War, at the outset of our chronicle, 77% of the soldiers autopsied had evidence of coronary atherosclerosis. Twenty years later during the Vietnam War the prevalence of coronary atherosclerosis had fallen to 45%. Now, forty years after Vietnam, the prevalence of coronary atherosclerosis in soldiers dying in Afghanistan has fallen to a jaw-dropping 9%. We can reasonably attribute this change to lifestyle modification in our soldiers: more healthy diet, insistence on weight control, better exercise programs, and less smoking. We also know that over the last decade, the incidence of cardiac events in the general population has fallen by 36%. Over the last thirty-five years in the United States, mortality from heart disease has fallen five times as fast as the mortality rate for cancer.

That's the past, but what about the future? In 2013, biostatistician Dr. Mark Huffman of Northwestern projected the number of CAD deaths in 2020, given recent trends in the six principal risk factors for CAD (total cholesterol, systolic blood pressure, physical inactivity, smoking, diabetes mellitus, and obesity). Even if we do not improve on our current trends, he projects a further 30% decrease in CAD mortality reflecting improvements in total cholesterol, systolic blood pressure, smoking, and physical activity (about 167,000 fewer deaths), offset by increases in diabetes mellitus and body mass index (about 24,000 more deaths). If these projections are correct, the annual mortality from CAD in the United States will fall from approximately 800,000 to 465,000. If we succeed in stemming the epidemic of obesity and diabetes, this mortality rate will be even less. The optimist sees the donut and the pessimist sees the hole . . . we are succeeding but even more is possible. We know what's necessary to win the battle, but we cannot declare victory until the public takes responsibility for its own health. The opera won't be over until the fat lady slims.

AND WHAT ABOUT Donald, whose surgeon predicted his imminent demise? As he embarked on his new lifestyle and LDL cholesterol reduction, he had a few episodes of angina, but within a year, his chest pain on exertion disappeared. Two years ago Sanjay retired after taking care of Donald for twenty years. Donald's surgeon retired. Donald and I still get together once or twice a year. Last month he had a stress test, which was normal. Donald likes to say that I saved his life. It's not true. Donald's foxhole conversion did. He made the decision to stop further progression of his CAD. From his normal stress test, I infer that some of his atheromas have regressed in size. From his two decades of absence of symptoms I infer that we have fended off the rupture of existing plaques. Every one of the steps Donald took was essential. I believe smoking cessation and exercise reduced chronic inflammation, proper diet and weight loss had multiple beneficial effects on his blood chemistry, and lowering his cholesterol stopped atheroma formation, induced regression, and cleared out inflammatory cells around the atheromas. I imagine that the atheromas are still there, smaller than they used to be, and in a deep sleep. And that's the way they will stay. We have defeated a tiny monster as insatiable as the guillotine.

For both Donald and me, the time had come to step down, to let go of the titles, and, well for me at least, to write a book. Combining mentoring with being on the cutting edge of the advances in clinical cardiology has been exhilarating. Although I loved my years on this larger world stage, even today I remain ambivalent, recalling my dreams as a little boy under my dad's living room table. What would life have been if, like my father's friends, instead of mentoring and consulting, I had spent my years seeing twenty patients a day? Daily hands-on patient care is deeply rewarding. Paradise Lost or Paradise Gained? Looking back, it seems to me I had both—the best of both worlds. So today I find myself more often asking young doctors questions rather then giving answers, suggesting they carry forward the legacy of a generation that never lost touch with compassion as they challenged conventional wisdom.

26

THE PRESENT CREATES THE FUTURE

The positive thinker sees the invisible and achieves the impossible.

—NISHAN PANWAR, CONTEMPORARY INDIAN WRITER

IF WE GAZE only on the past and the present, we will surely miss the future. So let's imagine the future management of diseases of the heart's four components: its muscle, its electrical system, its valves, and its arteries. I envision a new landscape with awe-inspiring achievements by a next generation that matches those of my own.

HEART FAILURE: CREATING NEW HEART MUSCLE

LET'S START WITH damaged heart muscle. We estimate that 5.7 million people in the United States have heart failure, the natural outcome of heart muscle damage, most commonly during a heart attack. Currently, half of our patients with heart failure die within five years of diagnosis. The economic burden of heart failure is the largest in all of health care, costing $35 billion per year in the United States. So heart failure is one of medicine's greatest problems. We currently rely on drugs, lifestyle measures, and cardiac transplantation for management of heart failure.

Here's the great irony of heart failure: even though normal heart muscle cells are naturally replaced each year by its own stem cells, damaged cells are not. In other words, although we humans clearly possess the intrinsic capacity to regenerate heart muscle cells after a heart attack, it does not happen. But there's more. Some animals like the zebrafish, newts, and mutant mice regenerate heart muscle as easily as a starfish regrows a limb. Somewhere along evolution's wandering trail, we lost the capacity for regenerating heart muscle. The good news is we can get it back.

FOR SIXTY-SIX-YEAR-OLD commodity broker Edward Sukyas his solitary one-hour walk along Third Street in Beverly Hills is his source of vitality, a metaphor for so much that is good about being alive: each unique smell emanating from competing restaurants and coffeehouses, the gabble of different languages, the hubbub of bustling humanity. After all, it mirrors his own ebullient life, one fully lived. His daily walk had begun more than a decade earlier soon after his father had died of a heart attack, and now it is an essential part of his day. With two children of his own, he looks forward to a grandchild already on its way.

Edward was educated at the Lycée Stendhal in Milan, Italy. He is fluent in seven languages. He has traveled the world. A Canadian citizen, he has lived in nine countries. Edward has been intimate with the back streets of Tangiers where he owned a carpet factory and he has lived the hectic nightlife of Cabo San Lucas as the owner of a French-Italian haute cuisine restaurant. And on this day his walk embodied the duality of his healthy-unhealthy lifestyle: adherence to both morning goat cheese omelets ("loosely rolled instead of folded, the French way, of course") contrasted with a very good exercise regimen. The south side of Third Street, wafting aromas of garlic and oregano through the doors of Locanda Veneta, was a metaphor for the gourmet side of life. At the moment the chest pain began he could hardly imagine that on the north side of the street stood a new metaphor, Cedars-Sinai Medical Center. A plaque was poised to rupture in one of Edward Sukyas's coronary arteries. He was about to have a heart attack. It was August 17, 2009.

THE FUTURE OF heart muscle disease is regeneration through stem cells. The potential impact of unlocking stem cell therapy for regenerating heart muscle is so tantalizing that about eight years ago, my former fellow Dr. Raj Makkar (he calls me Papa Jim) and I initiated studies of bone marrow stem cell therapy in animals with acute myocardial infarction. Other labs had some impressive results suggesting successful regeneration of heart muscle following delivery of stem cells.

To test the effectiveness of stem cell strategy in already existing heart failure, we delayed the injection of the stem cells until one month after inducing a myocardial infarction (heart attack) in a pig. The heart's function stabilized compared to untreated animals.

We used these results to convince the National Institutes of Health to allow us to initiate the first study of stem cell therapy in patients with a heart attack in the United States. We proved the safety of infusing bone marrow cells in patients with heart attack, but the number of patients was too small to prove effectiveness. Soon thereafter our Medical Center succeeded in recruiting Dr. Eduardo Marbán, one of the world leaders in cardiac stem cell therapy as director of our Heart Institute.

Dr. Marbán has advanced the field by developing a method for extracting stem cells from the heart itself, then multiplying them in culture, and delivering them back to the injured heart. From animal studies he concluded that these cardiac stem cells reduce scarring after myocardial infarction, increase the mass of living heart muscle, and boost cardiac function. Now amply funded by the California Institute for Regenerative Medicine, the next step was to use a biopsy of our patients' own heart muscle to grow many millions of cardiac stem cells in culture dishes, and then reinject the cells back into each patient's own arteries. So as the plaque in Edward Sukyas's coronary artery ruptured, our staff was preparing to open a new chapter in the treatment of heart attack.

* * *

EDWARD PAUSED ON his walk, staggered by the sudden onset of pain in his chest and back. He phoned his wife Kathy for help. When she arrived minutes later, Edward already knew. "I think I'm having a heart attack," he gasped. He was right. But for Edward there was an element of astounding good fortune in the midst of tragedy. Within an hour of the onset of pain, he had been whisked through the Cedars-Sinai emergency department to our sixth-floor cath lab where cath lab director Dr. Raj Makkar stood ready. With consummate skill and speed, Dr. Makkar placed three stents in Edward's obstructed coronary arteries. As Edward says in our hospital journal, "It was over in half an hour." But having arrived at this point in our chronicle, you and I realize nothing is further from the truth. Edward's life had been saved, but he had sustained extensive death of heart muscle, and now faced the risk of heart failure.

THE FIRST RANDOMIZED study to test the safety of Dr. Marbán's cardiac stem cells in patients with heart failure following heart attack was now in progress. Edward was twice lucky. Only one more patient remained to be entered in the trial. Our staff described both the uncertainty and the promise of cardiac stem cell therapy. For a former carpet maker, restaurateur, and commodity broker, it was an easy decision: "You have to accept a certain dose of risk in life," Edward said, and he became the study's last recruit. A few weeks after his heart attack he returned to the cath lab where Raj Makkar infused millions of Edward's own cardiac stem cells into his coronary artery.

Edward resumed his walks six weeks after his heart attack, and then returned for a battery of tests over the next year. His test of lung function (called oxygen consumption) improved from 1.9 liters before treatment to 2.5 liters at six months and 3.2 liters at one year. "I almost didn't need those results to know how I was doing," Edward recalls. "Before my heart attack, I had shortness of breath when I was under effort, such as exercising or climbing stairs . . . I don't experience that anymore."

Dr. Makkar published the results of our Heart Institute's trial in 2013. Edward's results fit with the other treated patients. He has a smaller heart muscle scar, and the heart muscle in the area of his heart attack functions better, compared to the patients who were randomized to receive standard care. Dr. Marbán calculates that the stem cell recipients grew the equivalent of 600 million new heart cells, or about 60% of the billion cells lost in a typical heart attack. As Marbán likes to say, "We are recruiting nature's own healing process and just amplifying it."

Since the study was very small, Dr. Makkar does not claim his patients' clinical outcomes are different with cardiac stem cell therapy. Consequently, we cannot say we have yet achieved what we set out to do with stem cell therapy, which is to reverse heart failure. That will require larger trials with longer follow-up. Once again we have glimpsed an incandescent light behind a partially open door. Regenerative medicine is that light. When we finally succeed, we will have achieved a breakthrough as important as any in this chronicle.

WHEN EDWARD SPEAKS of his experience today, he captures the ineffable spiritual bond, the shared exhilaration between patient and doctor I have so often experienced in risk-taking, ground-breaking clinical research. "These doctors are at the frontier of something big, a major advance in medicine . . . In my own infinitesimal way, it's like I planted a flag."

And the Rest of the Story? Edward's French cheese omelets, chocolate éclairs, and sauce Béarnaise have receded into poignant memory. "When you come from the Mediterranean, food isn't just food," he laments. "It's what ties you to your social environment." Today he gets by with gourmet ways to prepare salmon and chicken and sea bass. And well, no one's perfect: a slice of roast beef every two weeks. Edward's brisk walks continue, but nowadays a new metaphor looms when he pauses on the south side of Third Street to inhale those delicious Italian aromas of Locanda Veneta. It's his metaphor of survival, regeneration, and longevity. And it's on the north side of the street.

THE HEART'S ELECTRICAL SYSTEM: LIVING IN A WIRELESS WORLD

TREATMENT OF DISORDERS of the heart's electrical system is also poised to undergo a revolution. Paraphrasing my friend Dr. Michael Gold, director of cardiology at the University of South Carolina and an expert in such disorders, "The future is wireless." Here's why. Today, pacemaker hardware consists of a battery and computer algorithms that control delivery of electrical impulses to the heart. This hardware, about the size of a matchbook, is placed in a surgically created pocket under the skin in the chest wall. The pacing impulse is then connected to wires that we thread through blood vessels back into the heart. And therein lies the rub. The wires, being flexed sixty times a minute by the heartbeat, can be a problem. Some get infected; others break. Broken wires, often locked in place by layers of scar tissue, can be very difficult and even dangerous to remove when they become nonfunctional.

We are now beginning to test clever ways of eliminating the wires. Imagine an electrode the size of a grain of rice, which we can implant directly in the heart muscle. It is a passive receiver whose power comes from an ultrasonic generator inserted in a small skin pocket in the chest wall. The receiver converts the generator's acoustic energy into an electric pulse. Voilà. No more wires. The first generation of such new devices has been implanted in over one hundred European patients. In the near future we will have wireless systems capable of both pacing and defibrillating the heart.

An alternate version of a wireless pacemaker is a device a tenth of the size of conventional pacemakers, which are about the size of a triple A battery. It is implanted directly in the heart, having been inserted through a leg vein in the catheterization laboratory. In a European study thirty-two patients are now being followed to establish the pacemaker's longevity, and ease of replacement. And this is just the beginning. The small company that developed the device was recently bought by the giant medical device company St. Jude.

When perfected, these devices will alter the lives of millions of people: around the world 4 million people currently have implanted devices, and 700,000 new devices are implanted each year.

WORRIED ABOUT THAT disturbing feeling in your chest? How about recording and displaying your ECG on your cell phone, and instantly sending it to your doctor? I have one attached to my iPhone, and

I read the ECG myself. My iPhone app stores any duration of the ECG recording on my phone, and operates for 100 hours on a 3.0V coin cell battery.

Right now we are seeing a mad scramble among innovators to create the most user-friendly and medically useful device. The one that currently draws gasps, even from cardiologists, has a casing with two electrodes that inconspicuously attaches to your cell phone. Grip the two electrodes with your two thumbs, and in seconds, your ECG appears on the face of phone. Send it to me from the ninth hole after that hole in one, and continue on with your friends. I will text you back if it looks like more than indigestion. Oh, yes, and with different sensors you can send me your blood glucose if you are a diabetic. In the future, most of the measurements we make in cardiology will be transmittable from a remote location by a patient with a cell phone. Yes, the digital and wireless revolutions have arrived in cardiology.

HEART VALVES: REPLACING VALVES WITHOUT SURGERY

THE MOST STUNNING advances in cardiology, however, are now occurring in the treatment of valve disease. Let's look at two of them.

Mitral valve dysfunction, where cardiac surgery all began, is now being treated in the catheterization lab. In Western countries, following the conquering of rheumatic heart disease by antibiotic therapy, the only patients I see with mitral stenosis are immigrants from third world countries. On the other hand I see many patients with mitral valve insufficiency: when the left ventricle contracts, the two leaflets of the one-way mitral valve, which separates the left ventricle from the atrium, fail to come fully together. Blood jets backward from ventricle to atrium, then into the lungs, causing congestion and shortness of breath.

About a decade ago California cardiologist Dr. Frederick St. Goar devised a clip that could be passed into the heart in the catheterization lab. The clip grasps the two leaflets of the mitral valve and brings them together, creating a narrower, double-barrel valve opening.

My mentee Dr. Saibal Kar now has the nation's largest experience with this device. Compared to surgery, patients have strikingly improved heart function and quality of life at one year. Positive outcomes are somewhat greater with surgery; safety outcomes favor the clip. The role of the clip will become more clearly defined as long-term follow-up becomes available. Even now, however, for frail and elderly patients who are poor candidates for surgery the mitral clip represents a lifesaving advance.

IN THE COMING decade many heart valves will be replaced without surgery. When I see my mentee Dr. Raj Makkar perform the procedure, I feel it is the single most jaw-dropping, mind-boggling event in my career in cardiology. I can only marvel, how in the world did that doctor put that valve inside that patient's heart without opening the chest?

LEON SALIBA IS the son of immigrants, born in the hills of Beirut, Lebanon, who came to the United States in the early 1900s. Leon was born in tiny Campbell, Missouri, in 1911, but grew up in Los Angeles. Leon is now 102 years old. As the son of a poor dry goods merchant, Leon realized early in life that he would have to make his own way. He would have to be independent. In the summers he labored for a big construction company, which was paving Wilshire Boulevard, then still a dirt road. The company was required to provide a huge surety bond, which would reimburse the city if they failed to perform on time. Since Leon was bright, exceptional at math, and articulate in English, his foreign-born employers designated him as their representative to negotiate with the bond company. Leon learned a quick lesson in life when he was paid four times as much in his bond commission as he had earned in construction labor. During that summer he was admitted to the prestigious California Institute of Technology. Unable to pay the tuition, Leon did the next best thing: he formed his own bond company. It was 1928.

The next year the stock market crashed, but somehow Leon, principled, professional, unpretentious, and self-taught, survived with his fledgling company intact. As his company became successful, Leon's clients became leaders in the developing city. When one client, the Van Nuys family (after whom the Los Angeles suburb is named) built a new office building on Wilshire Boulevard they offered him space, where he stayed for the next quarter century. Leon Saliba became a leader in the Lebanese community of Los Angeles and in his Orthodox Christian Church (in Lebanese, *salib* means cross, and *saliba* means follower of the cross). He and his wife had six children and sent them to college and graduate school. In the 1970s a New York Stock Exchange insurance company offered to acquire his company. Independent at age sixty, Leon retired to pursue his passion for golf from his house adjacent to the tenth hole of his country club.

Leon's wife of fifty-five years passed away when he was eighty-three. When she died, Leon had a choice. He could live out his years in an assisted living facility, or he could take care of himself at home. Leon chose independence. As Leon approached 100 he began to have the symptoms and signs of severe aortic stenosis (aortic valve narrowing). Referred to our center, we had to give Leon some further bad news. In addition to severe aortic stenosis, he had severe stenosis in his left anterior descending coronary artery (the one known as "the widow maker"). Although otherwise healthy, Leon had reached the end of the line. He would be lucky to survive another six months. But in the past year or two, my former fellow, Dr. Raj Makkar, had become a world leader in a new research therapy. Raj agreed to replace Leon's aortic valve without surgery, but first he would have to protect the heart with a stent across the stenosis in his LAD. After Leon recovered from the coronary angioplasty, if he was still alive with his aortic stenosis, Raj would replace the valve. Leon recovered from the stent placement without a hitch. The time had come to replace his aortic valve.

Raj would replace Leon's diseased aortic valve using a technique invented by another former fellow, Dr. Alain Cribier, from the days when I was director of our research program. I have long since handed the reins to others, but I take pride in knowing that over four decades, my mentors and I taught so many creative young cardiologists who advanced our specialty. In 1985, now returned to Rouen, Cribier became deeply frustrated by seeing elderly patients with severe aortic stenosis condemned to death because they were deemed inoperable based on age. So he attempted to open the stenosed valve by passing a deflated balloon into the narrowed valve orifice and then inflating it with great force. His initial results were dramatic: the patients were immediately relieved of symptoms. But just as with coronary angioplasty, the aortic valves also restenosed within a year or so.

Cribier had an intuition: what if restenosis in aortic valves was the same process as restenosis in coronary arteries? If so, after it was opened, could aortic valve restenosis also be prevented by a stent? He tested his idea in autopsied hearts with aortic stenosis. He got himself a synthetic aortic valve used by the surgeons, mounted it within a cylindrical stent, and put a balloon catheter inside the synthetic valve. When he inflated the balloon, it forced open the stenosed valve, which was flattened against the aortic wall, leaving his synthetic valve as its replacement. Most important, he also discovered that the stent was stuck there . . . he could not remove it, even with forceful tugging. That was the easy part: how in the world could he transport his valve-in-stent into its position between the ventricle and aorta without opening the chest?

Cribier decided he needed engineering help. He approached medical device companies to design and mount a valve within the stent, and place the entire assembly on a catheter-tipped balloon. His experience with manufacturers recalled Andreas Gruentzig and balloon angioplasty two decades earlier. Cribier could interest absolutely no one. So with a couple of engineers and interventional cardiologist Martin Leon in the United States, they formed their own company.

Cribier initially faced (need I say, the usual) withering criticism from members of the cardiology establishment, who were easily able to identify ridiculous ideas. First they said that such a valve could not be created. But if it was, it would be impossible to deliver the valve into the aorta. And even if a valve could be maneuvered into the aorta, it most assuredly would obstruct the coronary arteries, killing the patient in the process. Cribier, like so many risk-takers in our Golden Era, ignored the experts. He began implanting his new valve in patients who had no surgical option. When he had irrefutably proven his point by treatment of forty patients he finally was able to attract a medical device company. Edwards Laboratories, which four decades earlier had triggered the valve surgery revolution with the Starr-Edwards valve, acquired his little company. With the Edwards Laboratories' expertise in valve manufacturing, clinical trial design and execution, and sponsorship of educational programs, a new era was born. For me personally, the story comes full circle as our fellow from the 1970s Alain Cribier teaches his technique to our fellow of the 1990s Raj Makkar, and Raj in turn teaches the next generation. Cardiology gives meaning to my life when it reminds me, like my own mentors, a teacher never knows where his influence ends; he affects eternity.

I WILL BE your eyes as Raj replaces Leon Saliba's severely diseased aortic valve. Prior to the procedure, Leon has a multislice computerized angiogram of the chest, abdomen, and pelvis (CAT scan), which Raj uses to determine the best size of the replacement valve. In the catheterization laboratory, we see the past merge with the present and the future. Team members insert a balloon catheter (the one I helped develop forty years earlier) in Leon's pulmonary artery for continuous monitoring of cardiac function. A pacemaker wire (recall Paul Zoll's pacemaker) is passed into the right ventricle. Using the wire exchange technique (recall Mason Sones's angiogram), a catheter is placed just above the aortic valve for injecting X-ray dye. Raj makes an incision above the leg artery and passes a catheter with a deflated two-inch long balloon near its tip (recall Andreas Gruentzig's angioplasty). As his assistant injects X-ray dye to visualize Leon's aortic valve, Raj slides the deflated balloon across the stenosed aortic valve. He inflates and deflates the balloon several times, making the valve opening large enough for his next maneuver, which will be to insert his new valve.

Raj now exchanges catheters. The new catheter carries a synthetic aortic valve mounted within a stent (recall Albert Starr's valve). The valve-in-stent over a balloon has been carefully crimped so that the diameter of the whole catheter assembly apparatus is about a quarter of an inch in diameter (recall Ulrich Sigwart's stent crimped on a balloon). That makes it less than a quarter of the original valve diameter. Now its diameter is small enough that Raj can slide it into an artery in Leon's leg. When fully reexpanded the valve will be more than an inch in diameter.

Raj passes the valve-in-stent across Leon's aortic valve. Satisfied that he has properly positioned it, Raj orders the pacemaker to be briefly turned on at a rate of 180 to 200 beats per minute. At a heart rate of 200, the quivering heart delivers very little blood flow across the valve. It's a critical step, because without it, the force of blood flow exiting the ventricle can make the valve flutter like a sheet in a wind tunnel while the balloon is being expanded. Raj stares intently at the pressure monitor, to be sure that Leon's blood pressure falls precipitously, indicating pacing is having the desired effect. After several seconds, Raj inflates the balloon, causing his new valve-in-stent to instantly plaster the diseased valve flat against the aortic wall. He keeps the balloon inflated for a few seconds, then deflates it. Leon has a new aortic valve. The whole miraculous replacement, pacing-inflation-deflation, has occurred in a period of about ten seconds, maybe less. Satisfied with the new valve's position, Raj calls for an echocardiographic recording to document that the new valve is opening and closing properly, performs a final injection of contrast material confirming that Leon's coronary arteries remain open. Raj removes his catheter. An assistant sews up the incision. The entire procedure including anesthesia, "skin-to-skin" in medical slang, has taken about an hour. As Raj pulls off his mask and gloves, Leon awakes. Raj wants the patient to be awake and talking before he leaves the laboratory.

For me, among all the amazing developments that I have seen in my fifty years of medicine, this ranks as the most visually astounding. Raj has replaced Leon's valve without cracking open his chest, without using a heart-lung machine and without stopping and restarting the heart.

The next day Leon is sitting in a chair, and on day three he is ready for discharge. Had Leon been treated by open heart surgery, he would face several months of significant discomfort as his chest wall, separated during surgery, knit itself back together. Instead, his principal aggravation would be a week or two of lesser discomfort from the sites of the catheter insertions.

The first devices were approved in Europe in 2007. By 2009, 4,500 aortic valve procedures were performed. In the next year the number of procedures doubled. By 2011, the annual number had quadrupled over just two years. The first reports of mitral valve replacement are now appearing. Raj has done a few. Replacement of valves without surgery, the latest in a series of unimaginable breakthroughs, will be the next great advance in Cardiology's Golden Era.

Today is Leon's two-year follow-up. He is now 103. He comes with

two of his children. His son Tom proudly tells me that Leon, independent as always, likes to sit on his patio and wave at the golfers as they pass
in their carts. The regulars, of course, all know Leon and beam as they
wave back. Tom says that Leon brightens each person's day. He certainly
brightens mine.

Leon smiles as Raj and I congratulate him on his good health. As I
shake his hand, he thanks me. Embarrassed, I say, "Don't thank me, Leon,
thank Raj. I had nothing to do with this." And Raj puts his arm around
my shoulder and says, "Yes you did, Papa Jim, yes you did."

CONGENITAL HEART DISEASE: TINY HEARTS WITH TINY DEFECTS

HEART SURGERY IN infants with congenital heart defects is made
exceptionally challenging by two factors not encountered in adults: the
heart is tiny, and no two congenital heart abnormalities are identical. If
only, on the day before the operation, a surgeon could hold each child's
heart in his hands, examine its every nook and cranny, and then thoroughly plan the surgical procedure with associates. This year that impossible dream became reality.

At the University of Louisville's engineering school scientists fed
thousands of digital cross X-ray images of little fourteen-month-old Roland C's heart into a 3-D printer. The printer built a precise replica of his
heart by laying down thin layers of a flexible plastic polymer similar in
consistency to heart muscle, about 250 layers per inch.

As Louisville cardiac surgeon Dr. Erle Austin planned surgery on Roland's tiny heart, he asked that Roland's heart model be reconstructed
two times its actual size in three separate sections so that he could touch
every part of its interior, view it from every angle, eliminate uncertainty,
and plan his incisions with great precision.

As Surgeon Austin explained to the Louisville *Courier-Journal*: "Some
people think when you do heart surgery, you go in and can see everything.
Well, to see everything, you have to slice through vital structures. Sometimes the surgeon has to guess at what's the best operation." The model of

little Roland's heart made it clear that Austin could tunnel between the aortic valve and a ventricle, avoiding multiple exploratory incisions. "Once I had a model, I knew exactly what I needed to do and how I could do it. It was a tremendous benefit." Unanticipated anatomic disasters will soon be a distant memory for tomorrow's cardiac surgeons.

In the past year, we witnessed a futuristic application of 3-D printing in living hearts. Collaborators at the University of Illinois at Urbana-Champaign and Washington University in St. Louis programmed a 3-D printer to replicate a high resolution digital image of an individual rabbit heart. From this model, they created a thin elastic "sock" that perfectly encloses the heart. The elasticity of the membrane allows it to move synchronously with each heartbeat, just like the heart's own pericardium, but with a twist. Within this man-made pericardium the engineers place a network of electrodes that monitor both the heart's electrical and mechanical function. When it detects a disordered heart rhythm, the sock can deliver an electric shock to terminate arrhythmias like ventricular fibrillation.

But now let's let our imagination wander even further. What if we could replace the plastic in our 3-D printer with human cells? Reminiscent of the apparent problem of oxygenation faced by creators of the heart-lung machine, many cells are too delicate to survive the current printing process technique. But some tissue is easier than others. Human ears have been bioprinted; human skin for burn victims is in testing. A human liver is on the drawing board. Can hearts be far behind? It only seems a matter of time until bioprinting enters the mainstream of medicine, creating a future that seems almost beyond our imagination.

CORONARY HEART DISEASE: THE NEXT WONDER DRUGS ARE . . . ?

CAD AS YOU now know is due to excess cholesterol trapped in the blood vessel wall, some of which elicits an inflammatory reaction. For years we have been bedeviled by what to do for patients whose blood cholesterol remains high despite potent cholesterol-lowering therapy. Cardiology's

newest potential "wonder drugs," the ones that treat the previously untreatable, have just appeared on the far horizon. Their discovery illuminates another wonderful twist in pursuit of science.

The principal mechanism by which statins lower cholesterol is by de-
creasing its synthesis. But like many drugs, statins have what we call a
negative feedback loop, the yin-yang of pharmacology. Statins also increase
the expression of a substance called PCSK9 that destroys LDL receptors
that pull cholesterol out of the circulating blood. So PCSK9 limits the
effectiveness of statins in lowering blood cholesterol.

One way to stop PCSK9 from destroying the LDL receptor is with
an antibody. Last year in the *Journal of the American College of Cardiology*,
we had a stunning report of a small randomized trial of patients already
treated with the potent drug atorvastatin (Lipitor) who were given the antibody. LDL was further reduced by 40% to 70% in these patients. The
PCSK9 freed up the statin to have its full effect on LDL lowering. So the
drug is additive to the effect of statins. Today I can envision what I never
even imagined: a future in which virtually all our patients can live with a
blood cholesterol level in the desirable range.

PCSK9 inhibition is a classic example of a magical thing simply waiting for our intuition to grow sharper. At this early stage, PCSK9 seems
like the ideal adjunct to statin therapy. As yet there is no prohibitive short-
term toxicity with the drug.

Since there are several potential methods for inhibiting PCSK9, I am
now watching a mad scramble among pharmaceutical research teams to
find the ideal formulation. Yet cardiologists are already imagining the
meaning of the capacity to lower LDL to an ideal level in every one of
their patients. As lipidologist Dr. Robert Vogel speculated in an editorial
accompanying this publication of the early PCSK9 antibody results,
"Brown and Goldstein won a Nobel Prize for their identification of the
LDL receptor in 1985 . . . the therapeutic triumph of statins logically follows their pioneering efforts. So may PCSK9 inhibition."

On the horizon is a potential miracle treatment for people with high
LDL cholesterol (LDL-C). In their animal laboratories, scientists at Harvard and the University of Pennsylvania claim to have reduced LDL-C
permanently with a single injection. Here's how it's done: you permanently
disrupt the function of the PCSK9 gene. Harvard cardiologist Dr. Kiran

Musunuru reports his technique reduces LDL-C by 35 to 40%, an effect comparable to statin drugs: "The kicker is we were able to do that with a single injection, permanently changing the genome [the structure of the individual gene]. Once that changes, it's there forever . . . it's not too much of a leap to think that if it works in mice, it will work as well in humans." The two-step method of reengineering gene structure has promise for many inherited diseases. The first step is to create a break in the DNA sequence of the target gene. The reengineered gene is then attached to a virus that carries the new modified gene to the liver, where it takes up permanent residence. In effect, with one shot, a patient would be transformed into an individual like those who naturally have the good loss-of-function mutation in their PCSK9 gene. Before this approach can be used in humans, however, proof of effectiveness and safety in humans will be required, a process that may require five to ten years.

BUT WHAT ABOUT the other central feature of CAD, the inflammation response that creates vulnerable plaques? Recall that the key features of vulnerable plaques are its feverish temperature, its profusion of inflammatory cells, and its thin cap poised to rupture. Since unstable angina and heart attacks are caused by the rupture of vulnerable plaques, shouldn't we target the inflammatory process as well? We know that by reducing cholesterol accumulation, statins have an anti-inflammatory effect, but what would happen if we supplemented that with an anti-inflammatory drug?

Last year, an intriguing anti-inflammatory candidate emerged from Australia. Colchicine is an old, very familiar drug for the treatment of gout. Investigators Drs. Stephan Nidorff and his boss Peter Thompson noted something very strange: their patients taking colchicine for gout and other inflammatory conditions seemed to have a markedly reduced frequency of heart attacks. So they initiated a clinical trial of low dose colchicine in 532 stable CAD patients already being treated with a statin, memorably christening the trial LoDoCo. Their results, published in the prestigious *Journal of the American College of Cardiology*, astonished the cardiologic world. The fall in unstable angina, heart attack, sudden death, and stroke between the treated and untreated groups was an unprecedented

67%: over three years it fell from 16% to just 5%. In comparison, statin trials find about 30% reduction in events.

LoDoCo is a small trial, but it is already the harbinger of several much larger ongoing anti-inflammatory drug trials. Take a moment to imagine the impact on our society if these results are validated. As I said in my accompanying editorial written with Dr. Robert Vogel, LoDoCo "suggests a new concept: the lipid effects of statins may predominantly inhibit atherogenesis, whereas specific anti-inflammatory agents, such as colchicine, may work synergistically with statins to inhibit plaque rupture. If the results can be confirmed, this study may one day stand as the seminal trial in the use of anti-inflammatory therapy to cool off hot hearts."

Taken together with lifestyle modification, the PCSK9 and new anti-inflammatory drugs are quite simply a potential knockout blow to CAD. When I entered cardiology those many years ago, Bobby Dylan rasped, "the answer my friend, is blowing in the wind." Who could then imagine then that one of the greatest would be an answer to the scourge of the twentieth century? But today I can.

27

"ATTENTION MUST BE PAID"

For masterpieces are not single and solitary births; they are the outcome of many years of thinking in common, of thinking by the body of the people, so that the experience of the mass is behind the single voice.

—Virginia Woolf, English author

LET'S END OUR story where we started—with Willie the Phillie. As Willy Loman's wife laments in *Death of a Salesman*, "Willy Loman never made a lot of money. His name was never in the paper. He's not the finest character that ever lived. But he's a human being . . . So attention must be paid. He's not to be allowed to fall into his grave like an old dog. Attention, attention must finally be paid to such a person."

Our story began when a vulnerable plaque in the wall of Willie's coronary artery ruptures as he sleeps at home. Cholesterol gruel within the inflamed atheroma erupts like molten lava into his flowing bloodstream. A clot begins to form over the torn shards of the blood vessel surface. How big will the clot become? As the clot builds in Willie's artery, blood flow around it slows. A contracting segment of heart muscle, deprived of sufficient oxygen, sends an urgent message to his brain: "I'm choking to death." Willie experiences chest pain. He takes a nitroglycerin to dilate the coronary artery but the drug has no effect, because the cause of the pain is no longer a stable atheroma; it is a blood clot. Over the next half hour, the clotting stabilizes, and Willie's chest pain resolves. The clot was not large enough to completely block the vessel. Willie has just experienced an episode of unstable angina. Although his symptoms have disappeared, the sinister clot remains. Willie has more episodes of chest pain over the next few days.

On the final day, as I begin my examination, the clot finally completely occludes his coronary artery. Unrelenting chest pain, more severe than any of his prior episodes, begins anew. As Willie the Phillie collapses, gasping, pleading for help, I realize that I have no tools to save him. Because a large muscle segment is deprived of oxygen, his heart contracts ineffectively. I see this as I monitor the progressive fall in his blood pressure. Next, an electrical impulse arriving to stimulate the oxygen starved muscle segment is rerouted, causing the ventricle to contract at triple speed. I detect this as I palpate his pulse, feeling the sudden increase in heart rate. The badly injured ventricle cannot sustain this rate for more than a minute or two, and the ventricle fibrillates. Now with no effective cardiac contraction, Willie has no blood flow to his brain. His eyes roll back as he loses consciousness five seconds later. My resuscitation of Willie is a shambles. I am slow to initiate chest compressions after Willie loses consciousness. I politely allow a minute to pass with no chest compression as the anesthesiologist inserts his tube. The defibrillator is not readily available and arrives far too late to save him.

But now, let's raise Willie from his bed, and ask him to stroll with us through the ensuing decades of what might have been, what came to be in the years that followed. In the mid-1960s during my Los Angeles medical residency, hospitals created programs to train doctors and nurses in the ABCs of cardiac resuscitation. Just a year or two after Willie died, I would not have stumbled through the procedure as I did. Willie would have had a modest chance of being resuscitated in his ward bed.

By the time I arrive in Boston in the late 1960s, Willie would have been admitted directly to a coronary care unit from the emergency room. With our bedside monitors we detect disordered cardiac rhythms long before his final episode and place him on preventive therapy. If he breaks through our preventive therapy into ventricular fibrillation, a specially trained nurse delivers a shock less than a minute after its onset. His chances of leaving the hospital would be good.

In those same Boston years when Willie first sees me for chest pain, I am able to perform a coronary angiogram, where I discover a single atheroma in the proximal portion of his left anterior descending artery. I refer Willie for bypass surgery, which completely relieves his angina, and protects him when the atheroma ruptures in his coronary artery.

As the 1970s open I return to Los Angeles to direct the Myocardial Infarction Research Unit. We resuscitate Willie, then monitor his heart function, which allows us to give him a spectrum of new drugs to sustain him through the crisis. His heart is badly damaged, but he survives.

As we enter the 1980s, the sudden onset of the ECG manifestation of a heart attack on the monitor beside Willie's bed triggers an immediate intravenous infusion of the clot busting drug, t-PA. Half an hour after we begin the infusion, the clot in his coronary artery dissolves. Having the good fortune to have his heart attack in a hospital, Willie's heart is only minimally damaged by the brief half hour of complete coronary occlusion.

A few years later, now mentoring younger doctors, instead of clot-dissolving therapy I counsel referrals for immediate coronary angioplasty. Willie is wheeled into the cath lab located adjacent to the CCU, where an interventionalist opens the clot-clogged vessel within a few minutes. Fully opened, the vessel does not reocclude, and Willie leaves the hospital with minimal heart damage.

Skip again to the early 1990s when I stop by to see Willie as chief of cardiology in that long-forgotten outpatient clinic of yesteryear. I suggest we order a blood lipid panel. His LDL cholesterol is 190 mg/dl. I "drape the crepe" with Willie about his risk for heart attack. Willie buys into my plan. I refer him to both a nutritionist and a smoking clinic. Since his bad cholesterol is far outside the normal range, I prescribe a statin. His angina episodes diminish in frequency within a few weeks. By year-end he is angina-free. Willie becomes one of those patients you see every year.

It's the present and today is his annual visit. Willie now follows a prudent diet and he walks a brisk mile almost every day. With thirty less pounds he no longer reminds me of Babe Ruth. In the years I have been seeing him several of the statins have gone off patent. I have put him on the most potent one, which has lowered his LDL cholesterol to 70 mg/dl with no side effects. I turn the conversation to the Phillies finally winning the World Series in 2008, but he cuts the conversation short. "Gotta go, Doc, it's my grandson's high school graduation," he says. We both know that the atheroma is still there, but now it's fast asleep, and together we'll keep it that way. But the final victory lies in an imagined future, when from his youth Willie embraces all the tenets of a healthy lifestyle. Atheromas do not form in his coronary arteries, and so he never appears in my office.

The last step in my own odyssey comes when I step down to return to what is my professional passion, mentoring through teaching clinical research and patient care. Today it seems to work well for both parties: in our clinical case conferences, I pontificate and the cardiology fellows act like I still know what I am talking about. When I leave the conference perhaps someone says of the former little boy listening under his father's mahogany table that the science is gone, and only the compassion remains. That's OK. For me, the journey itself was the reward. My profession and I began in ignorance; we made our share of blunders in the early years, and ultimately succeeded (mine, modestly) with equal doses of persistence and good fortune. If, from time to time, we lost contact with the essential values of our profession during that passage, we found our way back. If we did not find solutions, we discovered how to ask new questions. Our future remains forever beyond our grasp, but our past gives us hope.

As Willie closes the door, I muse about this brief segment of human history. Where does it stand among the greatest contemporary scientific achievements of its era? The Manhattan Project brought together our most brilliant physicists to create a weapon that ended the war with Japan. Its legacy, however, became the painful deaths of many innocent Japanese and seven decades of unresolved world conflict over nuclear weapons. The Moon Landing achieved a dream of mankind for thousands of years. Its legacy remains relatively small, as the U.S. federal government abandons manned space flight. Discovery of the double helical structure of DNA will surely someday be the last century's greatest scientific achievement, but its legacy will be defined in this century. I suggest that cardiology's Golden Age deserves a place on the short list of the last half century's scientific wonders. We successfully operated on a damaged heart, achieved mankind's millennia-old dream of restoring life after sudden death, replaced the function of our heart and lungs with a machine, replaced a failing heart with a new one, discovered dramatically effective treatments for heart attacks, and concluded our symphony with the clash of cymbals by transforming the scourge of the twentieth century into a preventable disease.

As I survey this tapestry of ongoing cardiovascular breakthroughs I see an international village, peopled with patients, iconoclasts, risk-takers, persisters, and entrepreneurs standing shoulder to shoulder, proud of their individual emotional, scientific, and technological achievements that together have no parallel in the history of medicine. We were ordinary people caught up in an extraordinary time, an era of courage, daring, resourcefulness, serendipity, and ingenuity. It's true, friend Willie.

Attention has been paid.

NOTES

Prologue

Intuition and induction in science. In *Pluto's Republic: Incorporating the Art of the Soluble and Induction and Intuition in Scientific Thought.* New York: Oxford University Press, 1992, British physiologist Dr. Peter Medawar distinguishes induction and intuition in the processes of scientific discovery. Induction is reasoning from specific facts to general principles. In research this approach is also called the Scientific Method, wherein a hypothesis forms the basis of data collection. Intuition, on the other hand, is the ability to understand immediately, without the need for conscious reasoning. Medawar links intuition and induction, observing that a flash of intuition often triggers inductive research.

Life expectancy in the United States since 1950. Many population and economic data sets are available at www.data360.org/dataset.aspx?Data_Set_Id =338.

CAD mortality rate. Fox KA, Steg PG, Eagle KA, Goodman SG, Anderson FA Jr, Granger CB, et al. Decline in rates of death and heart failure in acute coronary syndromes, 1999–2006. *JAMA.* 2007;297(17):1892–1900.

Global burden of disease. Lozano R, Naghavi M, Lim SS, et al. Global and regional mortality from 235 causes of death for 20 age groups in 1990 and 2010: A systematic analysis for the Global Burden of Disease Study 2010. *Lancet.* 2012;380:2095–2128.

Risk factors for diseases. Lim SS, Vos T, Flaxman AD, et al. A comparative risk assessment of burden of disease and injury attributable to 67 risk factors and risk factor clusters in 21 regions, 1990–2010: A systematic analysis for the Global Burden of Disease Study 2010. *Lancet.* 2012;380:2224–2260.

Current heart disease and stroke statistics. Go AS, Mozaffarian D, Roger VL, Benjamin EJ, Berry JD, Borden WB, et al., on behalf of the American Heart Association Statistics Committee and Stroke Statistics Subcommittee. Heart Disease and Stroke Statistics—2013 Update: A Report from the American Heart Association. *Circulation.* 2013;27(1):e6-e245.

President William Clinton's coronary disease. The details of Bill Clinton's medical history can all be found in public records. One source is Timeline: History of Former President Bill Clinton's heart problems and procedures at articles .nydailynews.com/2010-02-11/news/27056090_1_quadruple-bypass-surgery -chest-pains-and-shortness-coronary-arteries and another is www.doctorzebra .com/prez/z_x42cardiovascular_risk_g.htm.

1. A Day Like All Days

The mansions of Beverly Hills. The colossal mansions and grounds were first made famous by Douglas Fairbanks and Mary Pickford when they built Pickfair in 1919. The Roaring Twenties brought movie legends Gloria Swanson, Will Rogers, Charlie Chaplin, Tom Mix, John Barrymore, Buster Keaton, Harold Lloyd, Jack Warner, Clara Bow, Marion Davies, and Rudolph Valentino, each with their own extravagant mansions. Later the deaths of mobster Bugsy Siegel, Marilyn Monroe, and Jayne Mansfield brought unwelcome notoriety.

Cedars-Sinai Medical Center. The medical complex includes a multi-specialty 958-bed teaching hospital with approximately 2,000 physician staff members, 2,000 volunteers, and 10,000 employees. The teaching program encompasses over 230 principal investigators and 350 trainees in 60 post-graduate medical education programs and 800 research projects. The research program includes centers in cardiology, gastroenterology, neuroscience, immunology, surgery, organ transplantation, biomedical imaging, cancer, genetics, gene therapy, and stem cells. The cardiology program has been ranked in the nation's top 15 centers since the inception of *U.S. News & World Report* rankings. Cedars Sinai cardiac transplant program has the world's largest annual number of surgeries. See en.wikipedia .org/wiki/Cedars-Sinai_Medical_Center.

The probability of coronary disease. In the late 1970s one of my brilliant multifaceted fellows, Dr. Howard Staniloff, MD, showed me a pathology book about "false-positive" laboratory chemistries (tests which indicate disease when none is present). We had a mutual epiphany because we were bedeviled by the same problem, false positive and false negative results, in stress testing. My colleague Dr. George Diamond and I created a system for determining the probability of CAD in every patient before and after testing. Around the world, cardiologists adopted the new method. It is still in worldwide use today, known as the Diamond-Forrester classification. I will not give details, but if you are interested, google Diamond-Forrester and you'll find more than you want to know. The manuscript is: Diamond GA, Forrester JS. Analysis of probability as an aid in the clinical diagnosis of coronary-artery disease. *N Engl J Med*. June 14, 1979;300(24):1350–1358.

2. "What Man Meant for Evil, God Meant for Good"

Pericardial tamponade throughout history. A less fortunate victim of a penetrating chest wound in 1898 was the empress of Austria and queen of Hungary, nicknamed Empress Sissi. She was stabbed while boarding a boat, and over several hours developed cardiac tamponade. Her story, along with the history of cardiac tamponade, is told in: Meyer P, Keller P-F, Spodick DH. Empress Sissi and cardiac tamponade: An historical perspective. *Am J Cardiol*. 2008;102(9):1278–1280.

Treatment of pericardial tamponade. The mortality rate for tamponade has changed little in the last century, due largely to the rising proportion of more lethal injuries caused by gunshot wounds. Kang N, Hsee L, Rizoli S, Alison P. Penetrating cardiac injury: Overcoming the limits set by Nature. *Injury*. 2009; 40:919–927.

Ludwig Rehn publishes his experience. Rehn L: On penetrating cardiac injuries and cardiac suturing. *Arch Klin Chir*. 1897;55:315. On the Internet you will find many sites stating Chicago surgeon Daniel Hale Williams performed the first successful open heart surgery. Williams's surgical procedure, performed in 1893, however, like Rehn's, involved closure of a wound on the heart's surface, and was not open heart surgery. Williams did not publish his experience. Nonetheless, Williams's experience was a first in the United States, and is remarkable because he was an African American operating in the Jim Crow era of the late 1800s.

The early years of cardiac surgery. Several books recount the events of the early years of cardiac surgery as described in the notes to chapter 14. An excellent shorter version is: Stephenson LW. History of Cardiac Surgery. In: Cohn LH, Edmunds LH Jr, eds. *Cardiac Surgery in the Adult*. New York: McGraw-Hill; 2003:3–29.

War, doctors, and medical advances. The birth of cardiac surgery was not the German war machine's first inadvertent contribution to medicine. In World War

I, their use of mustard gas against British soldiers near Ypres, Belgium, led to the discovery of one of the first-ever effective anti-cancer drugs, nitrogen mustard. The dislocating experience for physicians in wartime is documented in: Fishbein M. *Doctors at War.* New York: E. P. Dutton; 1945.

Publication of the new surgical technique. Harken DE. Foreign bodies in, and in relation to, the thoracic blood vessels and heart; techniques for approaching and removing foreign bodies from the chambers of the heart. *Surg Gynecol Obstet.* July 1946;83:117–125.

Paget's and Billroth's comments about cardiac surgery. Stephenson LW, Ruggiero R, eds. *Heart Surgery Classics.* Boston: Adams Publishing Group, 1994. Includes a section entitled, "The Very Beginnings," with Harken's allusion to English surgeon Steven Paget's comment that surgery of the heart had reached its natural limits, taken from: Paget S. *Surgery of the Chest.* London: John Wright; 1896. Theodor Billroth's comments are the subject of Schober KL: The quotation about the heart: Comments on Theodor Billroth's attitude towards cardiac surgery. *J Thorac Cardiovasc Surg.* 1981;29:131.

Harken's mentor fails at mitral valve surgery. Cutler EC, Levine SA. Cardiotomy and valvulotomy for mitral stenosis. *Boston Med Surg J.* 1923;188:1023.

Harken's safety pin. Harken was a raconteur. Knowing him, a story told at dinner could have been apocryphal, but it was not. Late in his life he reiterated it in a living history that now appears on the Internet in an interview by Dr. W. Gerald Rainer: www.ctsnet.org/sections/residents/pioneerinterviews /article-1.html.

Pathologists' food obsession. A charming discussion of pathologists' broader use of kitchen terms in noncardiac organs is found in Patel F. Culinary delights in kitchen pathology. *J Hosp Med.* March 2002;63(3):180–181.

3. A River of Blood

The career of Charles Bailey. His distinguished surgical career is recalled in a series called *Profiles in Cardiology*, edited by Drs. J. Willis Hurst and W. Bruce Fye. The profile of Bailey is: Weisse AB. Charles Bailey. *Clin Cardiol.* 2005;28:208–209.

Bailey's recollection of his experience in Philadelphia. Bailey's comments are extracted from transcribed interviews of sixteen prominent cardiologists of this era, compiled in a superb historical book: Weisse AB, *Heart to Heart: The Twen-*

tieth Century Battle against Cardiac Disease: An Oral History. New Jersey and London: Rutgers University Press; 2002.

How the mitral valve functions. For a simple ninety-second video of how the valve works, see www.youtube.com/watch?v=rguztY8aqpk.

4. The Pain of the Pioneer

"although man meant it for evil, God meant it for good." The translation of the Bible varies with the version. The full quote from the 2012 International Standard version is: "As far as you're concerned, you were planning evil against me, but God intended it for good, planning to bring about the present result so that many people would be preserved alive," King James Bible (Cambridge Ed.) Genesis 50:20.

Mitral valve surgery before Bailey, Harken, and Brock. At least two surgeons preceded Harken and Bailey, as told in: Treasure T, Hollman A. The surgery of mitral stenosis 1898–1948: Why did it take 50 years to establish mitral valvotomy? *Ann R Coll Surg Engl.* March 1995;77(2):145–151, and in Gonzalez-Lavin L, Bailey, CP, Harken, DE. The dawn of the modern era of mitral valve surgery. *Ann Thorac Surg.*1992;53:916–919. The English surgeon Dr. Henry Souttar performed successful mitral valve surgery on one fifteen-year-old patient in 1925 but never repeated the procedure, and Harken's mentor Dr. Elliot Cutler had one patient survive for four years after cutting out part of the mitral valve.

Harken's recollection of his early experience in the army and in Boston. Harken DE. The emergence of cardiac surgery. I. Personal recollections of the 1940s and 1950s. *J Thorac Cardiovasc Surg.* 1989;98(5 Pt 2):805–813.

5. A Hill of Bones

William Mustard's surgical career. In 1976, William Mustard was awarded the title of Officer of the Order of Canada "in recognition of his many achievements in the field of medicine, particularly as a cardiac surgeon of international repute" and in 1995, he was posthumously inducted into the Canadian Medical Hall of Fame.

Bigelow develops hypothermia for cardiac surgery, but does not bring it to clinical application. Bigelow WG, Callaghan JC, Hopps JA. General hypothermia for experimental intracardiac surgery. *Am J Surg.* 1950;132:531–37. Bigelow did not have a surgical practice in which hypothermia was relevant, and so no patients were referred to him.

Lewis reports his success with hypothermia in ASD, but does not successfully pursue alternative methods of open heart surgery. Lewis FJ, Taufic M. Closure of atrial septal defects with the aid of hypothermia: Experimental accomplishments and the report of one successful case. *Surgery.* 1953;33:52.

Lillehei's surgeries. Detailed descriptions of all of Lillehei's surgeries (without patient pseudonyms) and wonderful personal stories are found in: Miller GW. *King of Hearts: The True Story of the Maverick Who Pioneered Open Heart Surgery.* New York: Times Books; 2000. Miller's book, which involved eight years of research, served as a major source of the information about Lillehei and his patients. Lillehei's note and the Gittens' poignant response is taken from this book.

Lillehei reports his success with cross-circulation. Lillehei CW, Cohen M, Warden HE, et al. The results of direct vision closure of ventricular septal defects in eight patients by means of controlled cross-circulation. *Surg Gynecol Obstet.* 1955;101:446.

University politics. Thoroughly researched information on Lillehei and his environment is found in: Goor DA. *The Genius of C. Walton Lillehei and the True History of Open Heart Surgery.* New York: Vantage Press; 2007.

Differences in perception. In *The Portable Atheist,* Philadelphia, PA: Da Capo; 2007, Christopher Hitchens examines the issue of perception: "Owners of dogs will have noticed that, if you provide them with food and water and shelter and affection, they will think you are God. Whereas owners of cats are compelled to realize that, if you provide them with food and water and affection, they draw the conclusion that they are God."

Lillehei's perception of historic events. Rosenberg JC, Lillehei CW. The emergence of cardiac surgery. *Lancet.* 1960;80:201–214, and Lillehei CW. The birth of open-heart surgery: Then the golden years. *Cardiovasc Surg.* 1994;2(3):308–17.

The fate of cross-circulation. Lillehei ignored the contradictory mix of adulation and ethical contempt, performing another forty-five cross-circulation procedures in 1954–1955. His in-hospital mortality rate was 38%. On the other hand among those who survived 49% were alive thirty years later. History has judged these results, in the context of that era, to represent success.

6. An Impossible Dream

Sam Bachner and Dr. Alfredo Trento. Unlike the other patients and their doctors in this book, these names are not pseudonyms, and none of their identifying personal details are altered.

Surgery for disadvantaged children in other countries. This was before the time of the Larry King Foundation and other charities that now handle such expenses for a limited number of deserving children each year.

Gibbon's initial success in animals before World War II. Gibbon JH. Artificial maintenance of circulation during experimental occlusion of pulmonary artery. *Arch Surg.* 1937;34:1105–1131.

John Gibbon's years at Harvard, service in World War II, and life in Philadelphia. A wealth of details concerning Gibbon's life and his first successful surgery (including the patient's real name) can be found in: Schumaker, Jr, Harris B, *A Dream of the Heart: The Life of John H. Gibbon, Jr., Father of the Heart-Lung Machine.* Santa Barbara, CA: Fithian Press; 1999. And in: Romaine-Davis A. *John Gibbon and His Heart-Lung Machine.* Philadelphia, PA: University of Pennsylvania Press; 1991.

Dennis passes Gibbon in development of the human heart-lung machine. Dennis C, Spreng DS, Nelson GE, et al. Development of a pump oxygenator to replace the heart and lungs: An apparatus applicable to human patients, and application to one case. *Ann Surg.* 1951;134:709. This report of use of a heart-lung machine in a patient preceded Gibbon's surgery by two years. Without survivors. Dennis temporarily gave up the attempt to use the device in patients.

Oxygenation before Gibbon and Björk. Adding oxygen to blood had never garnered scientific interest since its discovery by the famed French chemist Antoine Lavoisier. Among those whose academic careers were abruptly cut short, Lavoisier must stand alone. During the French Revolution Robespierre falsely accused Lavoisier of adulterating tobacco, leading to his arrest and beheading on the same day.

The many efforts at developing a heart-lung machine, as recalled by a surgeon who participated in the era. Stoney WS. Evolution of cardiopulmonary bypass. *Circulation.* June 2, 2009;119(21):2844–2853.

Houston surgeon Michael DeBakey reminiscences. DeBakey M. John Gibbon and the heart-lung machine: A personal encounter and his import for cardiovascular surgery. *Ann Thorac Surg.* December 2003;76(6):S2188–94.

Gibbon's modest report of his success. Gibbon JH Jr. Application of a mechanical heart and lung apparatus to cardiac surgery. *Minn Med.* March 1954; 37(3):171–185.

Gibbon's view of the history of the heart-lung machine. Gibbon JH Jr. The development of the heart-lung apparatus. *Am J Surg.* 1978;135:608–619 and Gibbon JH Jr. The gestation and birth of an idea. *Phila Med.* 1963;59:913.

Harken's view of Gibbon's withdrawal. Cooper DKC. *Open Heart: The Radical Surgeons Who Revolutionized Medicine.* New York: Kaplan Publishing; 2010. Harken never hesitated to express his opinion.

The Iceman recalls the emergence of open heart surgery. Kirklin JW: The middle 1950s and C. Walton Lillehei. *J Thorac Cardiovasc Surg.* 1989;98:822.

7. Electrifying Discoveries

Historical account of Claude Beck's experience in defibrillation. Sternbach GL, Varon J, Fromm RE. The resuscitation greats: Claude Beck and ventricular defibrillation. *Resuscitation.* 2000;44:3–5.

Beck's manuscript describing resuscitation by defibrillation. Beck CS, Pritchard WH, Feil HS. Ventricular fibrillation of long duration abolished by electric shock. *JAMA.* December 13, 1947;135(15):985.

Mirowski reports success with the implanted automatic defibrillator. Mirowski M, Reid PR, Mower MM, et al. Termination of malignant ventricular arrhythmias with an implanted automatic defibrillator in human beings. *N Engl J Med.* 1980;303:322.

The history of development of the implantable defibrillator. Kastor JA. Michel Mirowski and the automatic implantable defibrillator. *Am J Cardiol.* 1989;63:977–982. The implantable defibrillator was the ultimate advance in delivering a defibrillation shock to a fibrillating heart. Implanted in a patient's chest wall, the defibrillator analyzes each ECG complex, and when ventricular fibrillation is detected fires a shock. This was the device that fired in Dick Cheney's driveway, saving his life.

The history of electrophysiology. Horowitz LN. Clinical cardiac electrophysiology: history, rationale, and future. *Cardiol Clin.* August 1986;4(3):353–364.

Fabrice Muamba post-hospital video. www.youtube.com/watch?v=kyySdtYsh6E.

8. The Heart That Skipped a Beat

Wounded soldier with heart block. Dr. Eckart's medical account of this story appears in *Pacing Clin Electrophysiol* 2008;31:635–638.

Dr. Paul Zoll recounts the history of his first successful human pacemaker.
Dr. Zoll's quoted comments are extracted from transcribed interview in: Weisse
AB. *Heart to Heart.*

"Lies the rub." This phrase appears in Shakespeare's *Hamlet.* The derivation of
"rub" is from a term for the spin put on a ball to make it curve. Events also often
come at us with spin, rather than straightforwardly.

Dr. Paul Zoll announces the development of his pacemaker. Zoll PM. Resuscitation of the heart in ventricular standstill by external electric stimulation.
N Engl J Med. 1952;247:768–771.

The relationship of heart rate to longevity. Levine HJ. Rest heart rate and life
expectancy. *J Am Coll Cardiol.* October 1977;30(4):1104–1106.

Slowing heart rate in mice prolongs life. Several hundred mice were fed normal feed or feed containing digoxin, a drug that slowed their heart rate. The
treated mice lived longer than control mice (50% survival 850 vs. 700 days) and
had slower heart rates (266 vs. 563 beats/min.). A confounding factor was that
the treated mice had a lower body weight and starvation can extend rodent longevity. Coburn AF, Grey RM, Rivera SM. Observations on the relation of heart
rate, life span, weight and mineralization in the digoxin-treated A/J mouse. *Johns
Hopkins Med J.* 1971;128:169–193.

Who designed the first pacemaker? In 1950 Canadian engineer John Hopps
and cardiac surgeon Dr. Wilfred Bigelow (he of the freezing groundhogs) built
an external pacemaker using a vacuum tube and power from an AC wall socket,
which carried a hazard of inducing ventricular fibrillation. In the late 1960s
Dr. Bernard Lown introduced direct current (DC) defibrillation in his Boston
CCU, during the years of my training at Peter Bent Brigham Hospital.

9. Singed Wings

The career of Earl Bakken. After his retirement from Medtronic, Bakken built a
home in Hawaii, where he now lives. He has given back to society in many ways,
one of which is the funding and creation of the modern new North Hawaii Community Hospital for the residents of the big island of Hawaii.

The Lillehei tax evasion debacle. The story is well told in both of the Lillehei
biographies: Miller GW. *King of Hearts,* and Goor DA. *The Genius of C. Walton
Lillehei and the True History of Open Heart Surgery.*

Lillehei is ostracized in Minneapolis society. Lillehei's biographer reports his personal experience in: Goor DA. *The Genius of C. Walton Lillehei and the True History of Open Heart Surgery.*

10. How to Win a Nobel Prize

Forssmann reports his results and departs cardiology for urology. Forssmann W. Catheterization of the right heart. *Klin Wochenschr.* 1929;8:2085. His publication was ignored by most, and belittled by others.

Werner Forssmann recalls his breakthrough heart catheterization with Nurse Ditzen. Forssmann provides an entertaining description of his experience in Forssmann W. *Experiments on Myself:Memoirs of a Surgeon in Germany.* Trans. H Davies (New York: St. Martin's Press; 1974): pp. xiv, 352.

The award citation for the 1956 Nobel Prize in Medicine. The Nobel chronicles. 1956: Werner Forssmann (1904–1979); André Frédéric Cournand (1895–1988); and Dickinson Woodruff Richards Jr (1895–1973). *Lancet.* May 29, 1999;353(9167):1891.

11. One Man's Disaster Is Another Man's Breakthrough

Sones and Shirey describe the new technique of coronary angiography. Sones FM, Shirey EK. Cine coronary arteriography. *Mod Concepts Card Dis.* 1962;31:735. Sones was not drawn to writing manuscripts when there were catheterizations to be performed, so there was a substantial gap between his first coronary angiogram and his first description in the scientific literature.

Historical accounts of coronary angiography and coronary angioplasty. An extensive body of historical information, photos, and videos about angiography and angioplasty is available at www.ptca.org/archive/bios/sones.htm.

The life and times of Mason Sones. A thoroughly colorful description of Sones and his lab is given by his biographers David D. Monagan and David O. Williams in *Journey into the Heart: A Tale of Pioneering Doctors and Their Race to Transform Cardiovascular Medicine* (New York: Gotham; 2007). This superb, eminently readable book served a significant resource for the personal stories and quotes about Sones. The quotes from Sones and Proudfit are taken from this book.

The role of serendipity in medical breakthroughs. Meyers MA. *Happy Accidents: Serendipity in Modern Medical Breakthrough.* New York: Arcade Publishing; 2007. Sones's discovery of coronary angiography has a prominent place in Meyers's entertaining stories of serendipity in medical research.

12. When the Pampas Came to Cleveland

Beck and Vineberg try to revascularize the heart. Beck CS. The development of a new blood supply to the heart by operation. *Ann Surg.* 1935;102:805, and Vineberg AM. Development of an anastomosis between the coronary vessels and a transplanted internal mammary artery. *Can Med Assoc J.* 1946;55:117. Neither man's approach stood the test of time.

René Favaloro recalls his childhood. Weisse AB. *Heart to Heart.* Cooper DKC. *Open Heart.*

Favaloro stuns the world with his successful bypass surgery. Favaloro RG. Saphenous vein autograft replacement of severe segmental coronary artery occlusion. *Ann Thorac Surg.* 1968;5:334. At the same time, George Green and others were pursuing bypass surgery using the internal mammary artery. Green GE, Stertzer SH, Reppert EH. Coronary arterial bypass grafts. *Ann Thorac Surg.* 1968;5:443.

Favaloro's idealism in his own words. Several of René Favaloro's quoted comments in this chapter are extracted from his transcribed interview in: Weisse AB. *Heart to Heart.*

The postoperative management of coronary bypass surgery. In the mid-1990s with National Institutes of Health (NIH) support, I was one of the principal investigators on the largest-ever angiographic trial on the long-term effects of lowering cholesterol levels in patients after CABG. We compared aggressive lowering of LDL cholesterol (LDL-C) levels (to <100 mg/dl) to the current standard (130 mg/dl). Aggressive statin therapy resulted in a 30% reduction in revascularization procedures and 24% reduction in clinical events during 7.5 years of follow-up. Consequently, long-term cholesterol lowering therapy is now considered mandatory following bypass surgery.

René Favaloro's legacy as viewed by fellow Argentines. Hannah Vinter. Shot Through the Heart: The Life and Death of René Favaloro. *Argentina Independent.* July 29, 2010.

Richard Cheney's medical history. Although I am privy to details of Mr. Cheney's management through the practice of cardiology, because I have used a patient's name, I have strictly confined my accounting to published sources of information, including his autobiography.

13. Expanding Horizons

Albert Starr recalls his laboratory. Weisse AB. *Heart to Heart.*

Albert Starr recalls a moment of intuition. Starr A. A cherry blossom moment in the history of heart valve replacement. *J Thorac Cardiovasc Surg.* 2010;140(6):1226–1229.

Starr and my mentor Jeremy Swan. Both men became consultants for Edwards Laboratories, and through their many meetings, became good personal friends. Both were also skiers. Starr made a diagnosis of CAD on himself when he developed angina pectoris on the ski slopes.

Starr describes his success with replacement of diseased mitral valves. Starr A, Edwards ML. Mitral replacement: Clinical experience with a ball-valve prosthesis. *Ann Surg.* 1961;154:726. For many years the Starr-Edwards ball-in-cage prosthesis dominated valve surgery. After years of being slammed against the cage struts, some of the balls became misshapen.

14. "The Ship Has Weather'd Every Rack, the Prize We Sought Is Won"

Cardiac transplantation before Shumway. Stephenson LW. History of Cardiac Surgery. In: Cohn LH, Edmunds LH Jr, eds. *Cardiac Surgery in the Adult.*

Shumway and Lower report their early success with heart transplantation in animals. Lower RR, Shumway NE. Studies on orthotopic homotransplantation of the canine heart. *Heart Surg Forum.* 1960;11:18.

Christiaan Barnard reports his success. Barnard CN. A human cardiac transplant: An interim report of a successful operation performed at Groote Schuur Hospital, Cape Town. *S Afr Med J.* 1967;41:1271.

Barnard was actually scooped by three years. Hardy JD, Chavez CM, Hurrus FD, et al. Heart transplantation in man and report of a case. *JAMA.* 1964;188:1132.

Shumway's recollection of his years with Lillehei. Cooper, DKC. *Open Heart.* David K.C. Cooper is himself an eminent transplant surgeon who helped bring it to the United Kingdom. His book is a fascinating account of the many surgeons who practiced in the golden era of cardiac surgery. He was a friend of both Norman Shumway and Christiaan Barnard. His work was an invaluable resource, and many of the quotes from Shumway, Barnard, Lower, and Hardy can be found in this book.

Shumway's obituary recalls his accomplishments, his unique surgical persona, and his self-effacing sense of humor. Oransky I. Norman Shumway. *Lancet.* 2006;367:896–897.

"I am God." The words were uttered by actor Alec Baldwin in the movie *Malice.*

The differing account of Barnard's first transplant. McRae D. *Every Second Counts: The Race to Transplant the First Human Heart.* New York: G.P. Putnam's Sons; 2006.

The attitude toward organ transplantation between races. Malan M. *Heart Transplant: The Story of Barnard and the "Ultimate in Cardiac Surgery."* Johannesburg: Voortrekkers; 1968.

Christiaan Barnard counters his critics and telling view of himself and his career. Barnard C, Curtis BP. *Christiaan Barnard: One Life.* New York: Macmillan; 1969.

Transplant recipients with unusual achievements. All the names in this paragraph are real and have received extensive public acclaim.

15. Merging Streams

The history of electrophysiology. Several authors have traced developments before and after Beck, Zoll, Bakken, and Lillehei. Among them is: Lüderitz B. Historical perspectives of cardiac electrophysiology. *Hellenic J Cardiol.* 2009 January-February 2009;50(1):3–16.

Dr. Paul Zoll publishes a description of external defibrillation, along with an advertisement. Zoll PM, Linenthal AJ, Gibson W, Paul MH, Norman LR. Termination of ventricular fibrillation in man by externally applied electric countershock. *N Engl J Med.* 1956;254:727–732.

Successful CPR is announced by investigators at Johns Hopkins. Kouwenhoven WB, Jude JR, Knickerbocker GG. Closed-chest cardiac massage. *JAMA.* 1960;173:1064–1067.

Cedars-Sinai physicians publish the first description of a coronary care unit but are forgotten by history. My colleague Dr. Morris Wilburne was a cardiologist at the old Cedars of Lebanon Hospital (now Cedars-Sinai Medical Center) in the early 1960s. Although he and his collaborator Dr. Joshua Fields clearly had the concept, they did not succeed in bringing the unit to a functioning reality. Consequently histories of CCUs had accorded them absolutely no recognition until 2011 when contemporary cardiology's historian Dr. Bruce Fye unearthed an abstract written by Wilburne establishing his priority as the first to describe a CCU (Wilburne M. The coronary care unit: A new approach to treatment of acute coronary occlusion [Abstract]. *Circulation.* October 1961;24:1071). Nonetheless, Hughes Day remains secure as the first to bring the CCU to realization. Science is consistent, if not entirely fair. Once again, implementation trumped idea. History remembers the person who makes an idea work, not the one who first has the idea. The story is recounted in: Fye WB. Resuscitating a *Circulation* abstract to celebrate the 50th anniversary of the coronary care unit concept. *Circulation.* 2011;124:1886–1893.

The first CCU is established in the United States. Day HW. Preliminary studies of an acute coronary care area. *Lancet.* 1963;83:53–55. Day established his CCU in 1962, and published in the following year. Desmond Julian succeeded in establishing his CCU very soon after Day, so I am inclined to give joint credit. Science historian Thomas Kuhn, who wrote about paradigm shifts, has this comment about simultaneous innovation: "To the historian discovery is seldom a unit event attributable to some particular man, time, and place." As Julian notes in his history of the CCU (see below), in 1809 Dr. Allan Burns in his book *Observations on Some of the Most Frequent and Important Diseases of the Heart* (reprint New York: Hafner Pub. Co.; 1964), in his chapter entitled "On disease of the coronary arteries and on syncope anginosa," writes "where, however, the cessation of vital action is very complete, and continues long, we ought to inflate the lungs, and pass electric shocks through the chest."

Dr. Desmond Julian recalls the rocky history faced by advocates of the CCU. In: Julian DG. The history of coronary care units. *Br Heart J.* June 1987;57(6):497–502.

Dr. Bernard Lown expands the concept of CCUs to early identification of risk. Lown B, Fakhro AM, Hood WB Jr, Thorn GW. The coronary care unit: New perspectives and directions. *JAMA.* 1967;199:188–198.

Coronary care units become a breakthrough in treatment of heart attack. Killip T, Kimball JT. Treatment of myocardial infarction in a coronary care unit: A two year experience with 250 patients. *Am J Cardiol.* 1967;20:457–464.

For every great scientific advance there are naysayers. Bloom BS, Peterson OL. End results, cost and productivity of coronary-care units. *N Engl J Med.* 1973;288:72–78.

The invention of the balloon-tipped catheter. Who thought of the balloon? Chonette recalls the idea emerged from the meeting but does not recall the participants. Ganz thought the idea might have been his, but maybe not. Marcus heard later from someone, maybe Swan, that a young Edwards engineer standing at the back of the room volunteered the idea. Unfortunately, Swan did not record his recollection of the event. Marcus likens the dilemma to the 1950s movie classic *Rashomon*, which shows divergent versions of "the truth" from the point of view of four participants. Director Kurosawa leaves the question unanswered, and so must we.

The first bedside measurement of cardiac function in critically ill patients. Forrester JS, Diamond G, Chatterjee K, Swan HJ. Medical therapy of acute myocardial infarction by application of hemodynamic subsets (first of two parts). *N Engl J Med.* 1976;295:1356–1362. My memory of my early years of managing many critically ill patients is now a montage of images. The description of some critically ill patients (e.g., Alexi Kroon) is a composite of these images.

The falling rate of in-hospital mortality with heart attack. Hanssen M et al. French Registry on acute ST-elevation and non ST-elevation myocardial infarction 2010. FAST-MI 2010. *Heart.* May 2012;98(9):699–705.

The history of management of heart attack. Braunwald E. Evolution of the management of acute myocardial infarction: A 20th century saga. *Lancet.* 1998;352:1771–1774.

16. The Clot Busters

Pathologists do not find clots in coronary arteries at autopsy. Maroo A, Topol EJ. The early history and development of thrombolysis in acute myocardial infarction. *Thromb Haemost* 2004;2:1867–1870. Topol went on to become a thought leader in his generation of cardiologists. He has recently written a nonfiction bestseller: Topol E. *The Creative Destruction of Medicine: How the Digital Revolution Will Create Better Health Care.* New York: Basic Books; 2012.

Sol Sherry recalls the early years of thrombolytic therapy. Sherry S. The origin of thrombolytic therapy. *J Am Coll Cardiol.* October 1989;14(4):1085–1092.

A Russian pioneers the modern era of thrombolytic therapy of acute myocardial infarction. Russian cardiologist Dr. Evgeny Chazov had performed the procedure in Moscow some years earlier, but his publication had escaped notice because we read only the Western scientific literature, demolishing my idea that I had dictated an account of the first intracoronary infusion of a thrombolytic in acute myocardial infarction. When you think you are first, I learned, you usually are not. Chazov EI, Matveeva LS, Mazaev AV, Sargin KE, Sadovskaia GV, Ruda MI. Intracoronary administration of fibrinolysin in acute myocardial infarct. *Ter Arkh.* 1976;48:8–19.

17. The Birth of Biotechnology

The creation of Genentech. In celebration of seventy-five great entrepreneurs, *Bloomberg Businessweek* magazine posted Robert Swanson and Herbert Boyer's "Giving Birth to Biotech" on October 17, 2004. The article is available at www .businessweek.com/stories/2004-10-17/robert-swanson-and-herbert-boyer -giving-birth-to-biotech.

The transatlantic battle over the most cost-effective thrombolytic agent in acute myocardial infarction. The sometimes hilarious confrontation is described in: O'Donnell M. Battle of the clotbusters. BMJ. 1991;302:1259–1261.

How America emerged as a leader in biotechnology. In *Genentech: The Beginning of Biotech.* Chicago: University of Chicago Press; 2011, Sally Smith Hughes, the author, with twenty years of experience in the field of science writing, weaves together interviews with corporate leaders, capitalists, and scientists in biotechnology to describe the creation of Genentech.

What happened to Genentech? The tumultuous merger with Roche. Details of the issues in the $46.8 billion acquisition in March 2009 are nicely presented in "Anatomy of a Merger: 'Hostile Deals Become Friendly in the End, Right?'": Knowledge@Wharton (knowledge.wharton.upenn.edu/article.cfm?articleid=2579).

18. A Balloon in Zürich

The life and times of Charles Dotter, the pioneer of interventional radiology. Payne MM. Charles Theodore Dotter: The father of intervention. *Tex Heart Inst J.* 2001;28(1):28–38.

Andreas Gruentzig recalls the development of his original coronary angioplasty device. Gruentzig's notes were published by his friend and professional colleague Spencer King. In the years after Gruentzig's recruitment to Atlanta, King became a world leader in interventional cardiology. King SB. Angioplasty from bench to bedside to bench. *Circulation.* 1996;93:1621–1629.

Andreas Gruentzig's breakthrough human coronary angioplasty procedure in Zürich. Adolph Bachmann's name is recognized by every interventional cardiologist in the world. So I have not given him a pseudonym nor altered any details of his history.

Origin of "grabbing the brass ring." Years ago there were thousands of merry-go-rounds in the United States; only hundreds remain. A few of these are "brass ring" carousels. Riders can reach up once a rotation to grab a ring above them. The rider who grasps a brass ring gets a free ride.

The drama of the first successful angioplasty recalled by its participants. Doctor Bernhard Meier, who assisted Gruentzig, and the patient Adolph Bachmann discuss the event in a two-minute video clip at www.ptca.org/videos .html.

A view of Gruentzig written by his boss. Hurst JW. Andreas Roland Gruentzig, M.D.: The teaching genius. *Clin Cardiol.* January 1986;9(1):35–37. Hurst, author of the era's principal textbook in cardiology, was chief of cardiology at Emory University.

A view of Gruentzig by his biographers David Monagan and David Williams. Monagan D, Williams DO. *Journey into the Heart: A Tale of Pioneering Doctors and Their Race to Transform Cardiovascular Medicine.* New York: Gotham Books; 2007. Williams is an internationally acclaimed interventional cardiologist now practicing at Harvard's Brigham and Women's Hospital after many years on the staff of Brown University.

19. Conquering Atlanta

"Goyishe kopf." In my years at Cedars Medical Center, I have learned a lot of Yiddish words. *Goyishe kopf,* is a humorous term for "dumb non-Jew," of which I am one.

Aaron Stein's doctor. I chose not to use Aaron's doctor's real name because of the circumstances preceding my referral of Aaron to his care.

Gruentzig considers leaving Atlanta. In *Journey into the Heart,* Gruentzig's biographers David D. Monagan and David O. Williams suggest that he considered leaving Atlanta to move to California. I can confirm this speculation, based on conversation with those who discussed the option with him.

The crash of the Beechcraft Bonanza. The most comprehensive description of the last minutes of Gruentzig's flight that I have seen appears in the book by Monagan and Williams referenced in the previous note. Although the cause of the crash was not definitively established, a reasonable speculation is that Gruentzig became confused about his true direction. Confronted with a disparity between his own instincts and information from his instruments in an atmosphere in which he could see neither the ground nor the horizon, he incorrectly believed he had an instrument malfunction.

Gruentzig discusses his approach to patient care. An interview of Gruentzig made a month before his death appears at www.ptca.org/archive/bios/gruentzig .html.

20. Pricking Andreas's Balloon

ST segment elevation prior to an exercise stress test. After our Myocardial Infarction Research Unit segued into the NIH-sponsored Specialized Centers of Research (SCOR), for many years my clinical job was to direct the cardiac stress laboratory. Having conducted many hundreds of stress lab tests, I never allow a test to begin without prior evaluation, and am present throughout the test. None of my patients had a heart attack or cardiac arrest.

The changing mortality rate from CAD in the modern era. Dudas K, Lappas G, Stewart S, Rosengren A. Trends in out-of-hospital deaths due to coronary heart disease in Sweden (1991 to 2006). *Circulation.* January 4, 2011;123(1):46–52.

Geoffrey Hartzler's colorful life within and outside cardiology. Hartzler's career is engagingly portrayed in Kahn JK. Profiles in cardiology: Geoffrey O. Hartzler. *Clin Cardiol.* 2004;27:58–59. A section edited by Drs. J. Willis Hurst and W. Bruce Fye.

Time to treatment is crucial in acute myocardial infarction. Rathore SS, Curtis JP, Chen J, Wang Y, Nallamothu BK, Epstein AJ, Krumholz HM; National Cardiovascular Data Registry. Association of door-to-balloon time and mortality in patients admitted to hospital with ST elevation myocardial infarction: National cohort study. *BMJ.* May 19, 2009;338:b1807.

Why restenosis occurs following angioplasty. Forrester JS, Fishbein M, Helfant R, Fagin J. A paradigm for restenosis based on cell biology: Clues for the development of new preventive therapies. *J Am Coll Cardiol.* 1991;17:758–769.

The origin of stents. Roguin, A. Stent: The man and word behind the coronary metal prosthesis. *Circ Cardiovasc Interv.* 2011;4:206–209.

21: Why Do Atheromas Form in Blood Vessels?

The limitations of bypass surgery. Preston TA. Marketing an operation: Coronary artery bypass surgery. *J Holistic Med.* 1985;7(1):8–15.

When bypass surgery clearly saves lives. To be cardiologically correct, revascularization by PCI or CABG clearly reduces mortality in acute coronary syndromes (unstable angina and acute myocardial infarction) and probably does so in two specific coronary anatomic conditions, left main coronary artery stenosis and selected patients with disease in all three coronary arteries.

The familial component of risk for CAD. Ranthe MF. *J Am Coll Cardiol.* 2012;60(9):814–821.

Separating diet from genetics in CAD risk. Yano K, Reed DM, McGee DL. 1984. Ten-year incidence of coronary heart disease in the Honolulu Heart Program: Relationship to biologic and lifestyle characteristics. *Am J Epidemiol.* 1984;119(5):653–666.

The half-century confrontation over the role of cholesterol. San Diego lipidologist Dr. Daniel Steinberg, one of the leading combatants, recounts the fascinating battle in his book: Steinberg D. *The Cholesterol Wars: The Cholesterol Skeptics vs the Preponderance of Evidence.* New York: Academic Press/Elsevier, Inc.; 2007.

22. Plaque Rupture, Heart Attack, and Sudden Death

The life and influence of Russell Ross. An affectionate portrait of Ross is provided by his biographer and fellow dentist Dr. Henry Slavkin in: Slavkin HC. Atherosclerosis, Russell Ross and the passion of science. *J Am Dent Assoc.* August 1999; 130(8):1219–1222. An excellent account of the impact of his iconoclastic thinking in cardiology is given by a leader in atherosclerosis research in the next generation, Dr. Peter Libby of Harvard in: Libby P. Russell Ross, PhD. Visionary basic scientist in cardiovascular medicine. *Nature Medicine.* 1999;5:475.

Ross sends atherosclerosis research in a new direction. Ross R, Glomset JA. Atherosclerosis and the arterial smooth muscle cell: Proliferation of smooth muscle is a key event in the genesis of the lesions of atherosclerosis. *Science.* 1973;180(4093): 1332–1339.

The discovery of ruptured plaque in unstable angina. In the mid-1980s my team developed a new technique, which used flexible fiberoptics to provide images of the surface of coronary arteries in the catheterization laboratory. We discovered that patients with unstable angina "always" had a damaged blood vessel surface with a small nonocclusive clot. The report appeared in: Forrester JS, Litvack F, Grundfest W, Hickey A. A perspective of coronary disease seen through the arteries of living man. *Circulation.* March 1987;75(3):505–513.

The modern understanding of plaque rupture. One of cardiology's hottest topics in the 1990s was the mechanisms responsible for plaque rupture. Forrester JS. Role of plaque rupture in acute coronary syndromes. *Am J Cardiol.* October 19, 2000;86(8B):15J–23J. Falk E, Shah PK, Fuster V. Coronary plaque disruption. *Circulation.* August 1, 1995;92(3):657–671.

23. A Moldy Gift

The scientific and corporate issues in the evolution of statins. Jie JL. *Triumph of the Heart: The Story of Statins.* New York: Oxford University Press; 2009.

Akira Endo's recollection of his discovery of statins. Endo A. The origin of the statins. *Atheroscler Suppl.* October 2004;5(3):125–130.

The cost effectiveness of widespread use of statins in prevention of CAD. Grabowski DC, Lakdawalla DN, Goldman DP, Eber M, Liu LZ, Abdelgawad T, Kuznik A, Chernew ME, Philipson T. The large social value resulting from use of statins warrants steps to improve adherence and broaden treatment. *Health Aff.* October 2012;31(10):2276–2285.

An objective analysis of the components of diet in promoting or inhibiting the development of CAD. Hu FB, Willett WC. Optimal diets for prevention of coronary heart disease. *JAMA.* November 27, 2002;288(20):2569–2578.

The Mediterranean diet vs. the low fat diet. The trial, called the PREDIMED trial, has an appendix with 14 points by which you can rate your own diet. It seems to me to be extremely difficult to score 14, but it may be possible to raise your score by several points. Estruch R, Ros E, Salas-Salvadó J, et al. Primary prevention of cardiovascular disease with a Mediterranean diet. *N Engl J Med.* 2013; at www.nejm.org.

24. Yosemite

The chest thump. Tragically, there is also a tiny millisecond "vulnerable window" in the cardiac cycle during which a thump on the chest can induce an electric shock that induces ventricular fibrillation. The condition is called commotio cordis, the cause of the rare sudden death in young athletes struck by a baseball, or a chest blow in martial arts (for a tragic video example see www.youtube.com /watch?v=LLtzT2bXVGI).

Electrical energy delivered over time. Although some of us understand volts and amps, few of us recognize joules. A joule is a measure of electrical energy over time: 1 volt×1 amp for 1 second=1 joule.

The duration of successful and failed CPR. Goldberger ZD, Chan PS, Berg RA, et al. American Heart Association Get With The Guidelines-Resuscitation (formerly the National Registry of Cardiopulmonary Resuscitation) Investigators. Duration of resuscitation efforts and survival after in-hospital cardiac arrest: An observational study. *Lancet.* October 27, 2012;380(9852):1473–1481. In children, CPR longer than twenty minutes is not necessarily futile: Matos RI, Watson RS, Nadkarni VM, et al. Duration of CPR and illness category impact survival and neurologic outcomes for in-hospital pediatric cardiac arrests. *Circulation.* 2013;127(4):442–451.

Factors influencing when to terminate resuscitation. The issues in termination of CPR are discussed in: Nolan JP, Soar J. Duration of in-hospital resuscitation: When to call time? *Lancet.* 2012; 380(9852):1451–1453.

Probability of successful CPR when it occurs in the hospital. An analysis of 64,000 in-hospital cardiac arrests in 435 U.S. hospitals between 2000 to 2008 found that in about half (31,000) of the patients CPR resulted in return of the patient's spontaneous circulation. Only 10,000, however, survived to discharge. For the patients whose independent circulation was restored, the average duration of the CPR was twelve minutes, whereas for nonsurvivors, the average CPR lasted twenty minutes.

Revival after prolonged CPR. The Internet has a story that closely parallels Greta's experience. The video can be found at www.youtube.com/watch?v =yapZZTGRp94.

Organized medicine's perspective on the Schiavo case. The history of her illness, and the ethical issues from a physician perspective are found, with an audio interview at: Quill TE. Terri Schiavo—A tragedy compounded. *N Engl J Med.* 2005;352:1630–1633. Dr. Quill is a professor of medicine, psychiatry, and medical humanities and the director of the Center for Palliative Care and Clinical Ethics at the University of Rochester Medical Center, Rochester, New York.

Terri Schiavo's right to live. The case evoked passion, sometimes from unexpected sources. Judicial and medical authority is condemned in: Hentoff N. Terri

Schiavo: Judicial murder. *Village Voice.* March 22, 2005. Amazon.com lists ten books dedicated to the Schiavo debate.

Greta's recovery and return to good health. As mentioned in my introductory author's note, Greta is two patients' stories combined. The two young women had very similar histories, and both had good outcomes. The first Greta was my patient. I use her story to introduce one of the primary themes that reappears throughout my book: a central conundrum in the practice of medicine is the uncertainty inherent in diagnosis, in treatment, and in research. I merged her story with our second Greta, because her story, which runs from her entry into the cath lab to Yosemite, represents the single most dramatic outcome that I have ever encountered in my forty-some years in cardiology. And of course, her dramatic recovery encapsulates so many of our breakthroughs in the life of a single person. I interviewed both Jon Jackson and our second Greta and her husband with my friend Jon in March 2013.

The public verdict on removal of Schiavo's feeding tube. In March 2005, the Gallup poll asked, "As you may know, on Friday the feeding tube keeping Terri Schiavo alive was removed. Based on what you have heard or read about the case, do you think that the feeding tube should or should not have been removed?" The results: 56% of Americans agreed that it was the right thing to do, while 31% disagreed.

25. Conquering CAD in Our Lifetime

Analysis of national health data trends for high blood pressure and LDL cholesterol over the past twenty-five years. Egan BM, Li J, Qanungo S, Wolfman TE. Blood pressure and cholesterol control in hypertensive hypercholesterolemic patients. *Circulation.* 2013; DOI: 10.1161/circulationaha.112.000500. Available at circ.ahajournals.org.

The impact of healthy diet upon patients already on drug therapy. Dehghan M, Mente A, Teo KK, Gao P, Sleight P, Dagenais G, et al. Ongoing Telmisartan Alone and in Combination With Ramipril Global End Point Trial (ONTARGET)/Telmisartan Randomized Assessment Study in ACEI Intolerant Subjects With Cardiovascular Disease (TRANSCEND) Trial Investigators. Relationship between healthy diet and risk of CVD among patients on drug therapies for secondary prevention. A prospective cohort study of 31,536 high-risk individuals from 40 countries. *Circulation.* 2012; 112.103234.

The importance of diet in the clinical practice of cardiology. See www.theheart .org/article/1481799.

The impact of exercise on disease prevention. Lee IM. Effect of physical inactivity on major non-communicable diseases worldwide: An analysis of burden of disease and life expectancy. *Lancet.* 2012;12:61031–61039.

The NCAA compiles a comprehensive database on sudden death in athletes. Harmon KG, Asif IM, Klossner D, Drezner JA. Incidence of sudden cardiac death in national collegiate athletic association athletes. *Circulation.* 2011;123: 1594–1600.

The number of athletes in the United States is huge and increasing. According to the American College of Cardiology's Section of Sports and Exercise Cardiology, among athletes younger than thirty-five years of age, 44 million now participate in organized sports. We have 7.7 million high school athletes and 463,000 college athletes. Athletes older than thirty-five years of age are particularly engaged in endurance sports. Marathoners have increased from 353,000 in 2000 to over 500,000 in 2011. U.S. triathlon memberships increased from 21,300 to more than 146,000 in the same time frame.

The most recent published survey of sudden death in NCAA athletes identified an event rate of four to six deaths per year. Suicide and drug deaths in this group greatly exceed cardiovascular death, and by comparison annual automobile fatalities in the same age group are about 2,500-fold more common. Nonetheless the cardiovascular SD rate in college athletes is higher than that reported in high school athletes, possibly due to the longer exposure to rigorous training over longer periods of time. Sudden death was more common in Division I athletes, and African American college athletes were at substantially greater risk for cardiac sudden death than white athletes, as were male compared to female athletes. Maron BJ, Haas TS, Murphy CJ, Ahluwalia A, Rutten-Ramos S. Incidence and causes of sudden death in U.S. college athletes. *J Am Coll Cardiol.* 2014;63(16):1636–1643.

Is your athletic kid at risk? Corrado D, Basso C, Rizzoli G, Schiavon M, Thiene G. Does sports activity enhance the risk of sudden death in adolescents and young adults? *J Am Coll Cardiol.* 2003;42:1959–1963; and Meyer L et al. A 30-year review incidence, causes, and survival trends from cardiovascular-related sudden cardiac arrest in children and young adults 0 to 35 years of age. *Circulation.* 2012;126:1363–1372.

Risk during athletic competition in France. Marijon E, Tafflet M, Celermajer DS, Dumas F, Perier MC, Mustafic H, et al. Sports-related sudden death in the general population. *Circulation.* 2011;124:672–681.

Modern statistics on sudden death in marathons. Kim JH, Malhotra R, Chiampas G et al. Cardiac arrest during long-distance running races. *N Engl J Med.* 2012;366:130–140.

The cost and effectiveness of screening athletes. Halkin A, Steinvil A, Rosso R, et al. Preventing sudden death of athletes with electrographic screening. *J Am Coll Cardiol.* 2012;60:2271–2276.

The 2012 London Olympics. Preventing sudden cardiac death on the world's biggest athletic stage. July 23, 2012. Lisa Nainggolan and Michael O'Riordan. cardiacscreeningcenter.com/wp-content/uploads/2012/07/CARDIAC_ARREST _IN_OLYMPIC_ATHLETES.pdf.

The issue of childhood obesity and diabetes. Hamman RF, Pettitt DJ, Dabelea D, et al. Estimates of the burden of diabetes in United States Youth in 2009. American Diabetes Association 2012 Scientific Sessions. June 9, 2012; Philadelphia, PA. Abstract 1369-P.

The obesity epidemic. The Global Health Estimates, which provides a comprehensive and comparable assessment of mortality and loss of health due to diseases and injuries for all regions of the world, is arguably our most reliable and comprehensive source for such information. It is compiled by the World Health Organization.

The new American College of Cardiology/American Heart Association guidelines for the treatment of cholesterol would increase the number of individuals eligible for statin therapy by 12.8 million people, 81% of whom are individuals without known cardiovascular disease. According to investigators from the Duke Clinical Research Institute published in *The New England Journal of Medicine,* among the 115 million U.S. adults now aged forty to seventy-five years old, 49% would be eligible to receive a statin, and among those aged sixty to seventy-five years old, 87% of men would now be eligible, based on their ten-year risk of cardiovascular disease. My view, and that of many cardiology thought leaders, is the guidelines swing too far toward initiating statin treatment late in life.

The 2014 American Heart Association Statistical Update provides eight bullet points:

- 21% of men, 16% of women, and 18% of students in grades 9 to 12 use cigarettes.
- Secondhand smoke exposure declined from 53% to 40% between 2000 and 2008.
- In grades 9 through 12, 18% of girls and 10% of boys do not engage in ≥60 minutes of exercise at least once a week despite recommendations that children do so 7 days per week.
- 30% of adults engage in no aerobic leisure-time physical activity.

- Less than 1% of Americans meet at least 4 of 5 healthy dietary goals. Among adults, the percentage reaching goals were: fruits and vegetables 12%; fish, 18%; sugary drinks, 52%; and whole grains, 7%. Only 29% of children aged 12 to 19 met goals for low sugary drinks.
- 154.7 million U.S. adults (68%) are overweight or obese, and 35% are obese.
- 24 million children (32%) aged 2 to 19 years are overweight or obese. From 1974 to 2010, the prevalence of obesity in children 6 to 11 years of age increased from 4% to 19%.
- Obesity is associated with marked excess mortality, diabetes mellitus, CAD, stroke, and heart failure, and other health conditions, including asthma, cancer, end-stage, renal disease, and degenerative joint disease.

The falling prevalence of CAD in U.S. soldiers. Webber BJ, Seguin PG, Burnett DG, Clark LL, Otto JL. Prevalence of and risk factors for autopsy-determined atherosclerosis among US service members, 2001–2011. *JAMA.* 2012;308(24):2577–2583.

Projected CAD mortality rate in 2020. Huffman MD, Lloyd-Jones DM, Ning H, Labarthe DR, Guzman Castillo M, O'Flaherty M, et al. Quantifying options for reducing coronary heart disease mortality by 2020. *Circulation.* June 25, 2013;127(25):2477–2484.

26. The Present Creates the Future

A critical assessment of the benefits and limitations of cardiac stem cell therapy. Forrester JS, Makkar RR, Marbán E. Long-term outcome of stem cell therapy for acute myocardial infarction: Right results, wrong reasons. *J Am Coll Cardiol.* June 16, 2009;53(24):2270–2272.

Our experience with cardiac stem cell infusion in patients. Makkar RR, Smith RR, Cheng K, Malliaras K, Thomson LE, Berman D, Czer LS, Marbán L, Mendizabal A, Johnston PV, Russell SD, Schuleri KH, Lardo AC, Gerstenblith G, Marbán E. Intracoronary cardiosphere-derived cells for heart regeneration after myocardial infarction (CADUCEUS): A prospective, randomised phase 1 trial. *Lancet.* March 10, 2012;379(9819):895–904.

Edward Sukyas. He tells his experiences in Kowacky K. Walking to his own beat. *Discoveries*, www.cedars-sinai.edu/Patients/Programs-and-Services/Heart-Institute/Walking-to-His-Own-Beat.aspx All the names in this story are real.

Reducing the cost of hospitalization for heart failure. Several devices hold promise. One, invented by my mentee Dr. Neal Eigler, measures the pressure that causes congestion in the lungs. Comparing the year before and after its use in thirty-five patients, the number of hospitalizations fell from fifty-one to twelve, and days of hospitalization fell threefold.

The most recent perspective on the wireless defibrillator. The wireless pacemaker and defibrillator era begins. The complexity and politics of FDA decisions for approval of new technology has led most device manufacturers to initiate clinical trials in Europe. Introduction of effective new devices is often several years longer in the United States than in Europe. The situation represents the conflict inherent in innovation vs. regulation. See Tiny, wireless pacemaker due to be launched in Europe at www.bbc.com/news/technology-24535624, and Aziz S, Leon AR, El-Chami MF. The subcutaneous defibrillator: A review of the literature. *J Am Coll Cardiol.* April 22, 2014;63(15):1473–1479. doi: 10.1016/j.jacc.2014.01.018. Epub 2014 Feb 12.

Our experience with aortic valve replacement without surgery. Chakravarty T, Jilaihawi H, Doctor N, Fontana G, Forrester JS, Cheng W, Makkar R. Complications after transfemoral transcatheter aortic valve replacement with a balloon-expandable prosthesis: The importance of preventative measures and contingency planning. *Catheter Cardiovasc Interv.* February 21, 2013. doi: 10.1002/ccd.24888.

The FDA approval of the mitral valve clip. I am particularly proud that one of my mentees, Dr. Saibal Kar, has the nation's largest experience with this device, and has traveled the world teaching its use to others. The FDA's description of the device appears at: www.fda.gov/MedicalDevices/Productsand MedicalProcedures/DeviceApprovalsandClearances/Recently-ApprovedDe vices/ucm375149.htm.

The story of the infant with heart defect is told by the engineers and doctors. See www.courier-journal.com/article/20140221/NEWS01/302210103/Child -s-heart-fixed-Kosair-Children-s-Hospital-help-3-D-printing.

Organ printing. For videos of this remarkable process, see www.singularityweblog .com/3d-printing-is-bio-printing-the-future-of-organ-replacement/.

PCSK-9 inhibitors for lowering blood cholesterol. The preliminary results with PCSK9 inhibitors indicate it is additive to statin drugs, and may be particularly useful in patients who cannot tolerate statins. Roth EM, McKenney JM, Hanotin C, Asset G, Stein EA. Atorvastatin with or without an antibody to PCSK9 in primary hypercholesterolemia. *N Engl J Med.* 2012;367:1891–1900.

One of the nation's leading lipidologists reviews the information about this new drug class. Stein EA. Low-density lipoprotein cholesterol reduction by inhibition of PCSK9. *Curr Opin Lipidol.* December 2013;24(6):510–517.

The fascinating background story of how a treatment for gout may lead to a breakthrough in preventing heart attack. Vogel RA, Forrester JS. Cooling off hot hearts: A specific therapy for vulnerable plaque? *J Am Coll Cardiol.* January 29, 2013;61(4):411–412.

GLOSSARY

anastomosis: a connection created at surgery. For example, during coronary bypass surgery, the surgeon creates an anastomosis between the internal mammary artery and one of the coronary arteries. At bariatric surgery, creating anastomoses between parts of the gastrointestinal tract promotes weight loss.

angina (or angina pectoris): chest pain, most commonly exercise induced, and due to coronary artery disease.

angiogram: an X-ray image of a blood vessel.

angioplasty: repair of a blood vessel, as with a balloon-tipped catheter.

aorta: the artery which connects the heart to the rest of the body, separated from the left ventricle by the aortic valve.

arrhythmia: a disorder of the heart's electrical system resulting in very rapid or very slow heart rate, which may be accompanied by dizziness, fainting, or even sudden death.

arteriosclerosis: a word used interchangeably with *atherosclerosis*.

artery: a blood vessel that carries blood to organs and tissue, as opposed to a vein which carries blood away from organs.

atheroma: a mass of fatty and cellular material that forms in the wall of a blood vessel. Also called a plaque.

atherosclerosis: disease of the blood vessels characterized by multiple atheromas.

atrial septal defect: a congenital heart abnormality in which the muscular wall between the right and left atrium has a hole in it.

atrium: a collecting chamber. In the heart, the right and left atria collect blood before delivering it to the right and left ventricles.

bariatric: having to do with obesity.

capillary: the microscopic blood vessels between the termination of arteries and the beginning of veins. Tissue nutrients and waste products are exchanged by the blood through the walls of the capillaries.

cardiac output: the volume of blood the heart pumps in a minute.

cardiogenic shock: a life-threatening condition in which the heart's pumping function is so compromised that it can no longer maintain an adequate blood pressure or delivery of blood to vital organs.

cardiovascular: having to do with the heart and blood vessels.

catheter: a hollow tube. In cardiology we insert catheters into blood vessels.

complete heart block: failure of transmission of the normal electrical impulse from the atrium to the ventricle, resulting in very slow heart rate, fainting, and even sudden death.

defibrillate: to eliminate fibrillation. In the heart, either the atrium or the ventricle can fibrillate.

defibrillator: a device that delivers an electric shock to either the atrium or the ventricle, with the goal of returning the electrical system to a normal rhythm. Defibrillators are used in treatment of both atrial and ventricular fibrillation.

diastole: the period of the heart's relaxation.

electrode: a specialized structure, often at the end of a wire, designed to transmit an electrical pulse. For instance, electrical impulses from a pacemaker or defibrillator are transmitted to an electrode that is in contact with the heart muscle or the skin.

esophagus: the muscular tube that connects the mouth to the stomach.

fibrillation: uncontrolled wormlike quivering of muscle fibers. Atrial fibrillation results in diminished "priming" of the ventricular pump, and is not life threatening. Ventricular fibrillation results in absence of blood flow, and results in brain death within four minutes or less.

heart failure: the condition in which the pumping function of the heart is inadequate. When heart failure is mild to moderate, blood backs up into the lungs, causing pulmonary congestion. When heart failure is even more severe, cardiogenic shock develops.

hemostat: a surgical clamp that looks somewhat like a pair of scissors.

infarction: death of living tissue.

hypertension: high blood pressure.

hypertrophy: excessive growth of tissue. In cardiology, the term is most commonly used with the ventricles, e.g., left ventricular hypertrophy is a common complication of hypertension.

lipid: fat.

lipoprotein: a particle consisting of fat and protein. In the blood, lipoproteins are insoluble fats made soluble by binding to protein, allowing fats to be transported throughout the body

lumen: the canal within a tube, e.g., the coronary artery lumen.

mitral valve: the one-way valve that separates the left atrium from the left ventricle.

myocardial: having to do with the muscle (*myo*) of the heart (*cardia*).

myocardial infarction: a heart attack

orifice: the mouth of a tube. For instance, at coronary angiography we insert a catheter into the orifice of a coronary artery.

oxygenated: possessing oxygen. Blood is oxygenated in the lungs, returned to the left atrium, then pumped by the left ventricle into the aorta for distribution throughout the body.

pacemaker: a specialized tissue or device that governs a rhythmic biologic activity. The heart possesses a natural pacemaker that can be replaced by an electronic device.

percutaneous: through the skin, e.g., replacement of a heart valve using a prosthesis mounted on a catheter is a percutaneous procedure.

pericardial tamponade: compression of the heart by fluid trapped between the sac that surrounds the heart (pericardium) and the heart itself.

pericardium: a tough, inelastic sac that surrounds the heart.

prosthesis: an artificial replacement for a normal structure, e.g., a prosthetic heart valve.

pulmonary: having to do with the lungs.

pulmonary artery: the vessel that carries deoxygenated blood from the right ventricle to the lungs.

pulmonary capillary pressure: the distending force within the small vessels in the lungs. This pressure increases when pumping of the left ventricle is inadequate. Increased pulmonary capillary pressure causes the symptoms of congestive heart failure.

statin: a class of drugs that lowers blood cholesterol by both inhibiting its synthesis and by increasing its uptake by the liver.

stem cell: a cell that, when it divides, replaces itself, and also differentiates to other more-specialized cell types.

stenosis: narrowing. In the heart, both valves and arteries develop stenosis that restricts blood flow. Typical examples are mitral valve stenosis, aortic valve stenosis, and coronary artery stenosis.

stent: a device used to keep a hollow tube open. In CAD, stents are frequently used following balloon angioplasty.

suture: the fibrous thread used in stitching or the stitch itself.

systole: the portion of the heart's cycle during which it is contracting. The numerator in blood pressure is recorded during systole.

tetralogy of Fallot: a congenital heart abnormality consisting of four abnormalities: pulmonary valve stenosis, right ventricular hypertrophy, ventricular septal defect, and displaced aorta.

thrombolysis: dissolving a clot.

thrombus: the medical term for a blood clot.

tricuspid valve: the one-way valve that separates the right atrium from the right ventricle.

unstable angina: chest pain that threatens to go on to become a full-blown heart attack.

valve insufficiency: the condition when a one-way valve allows backflow. Valve insufficiency is also called regurgitation.

venous: having to do with veins.

ventricle: a chamber. In the heart, the right ventricle pumps deoxygenated, venous blood to the lungs; the left ventricle pumps oxygenated blood to the body.

ventricular septal defect: a hole in the wall between the right and left ventricle.

INDEX